W0043425

VIROLOGY MONOGRAPHS

DIE VIRUSFORSCHUNG IN EINZELDARSTELLUNGEN

CONTINUING / FORTFÜHRUNG VON

HANDBOOK OF VIRUS RESEARCH

HANDBUCH DER VIRUSFORSCHUNG

FOUNDED BY / BEGRÜNDET VON

R. DOERR

EDITED BY / HERAUSGEGEBEN VON

S. GARD · C. HALLAUER · K. F. MEYER

10

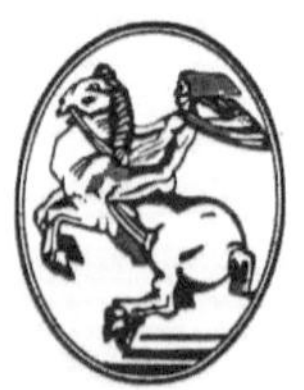

1971

SPRINGER-VERLAG

WIEN NEW YORK

LYMPHOCYTIC CHORIOMENINGITIS VIRUS

BY

F. LEHMANN-GRUBE

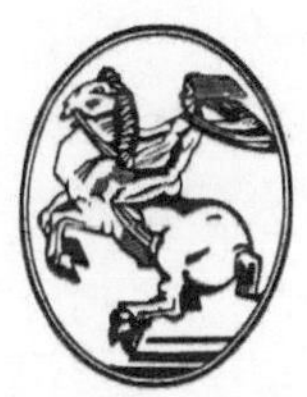

1971

SPRINGER-VERLAG

WIEN NEW YORK

Softcover reprint of the hardcover 1st edition 1971
Library of Congress Catalog Card Number 70-167276
Printer: R. Spies & Co., A-1050 Wien

ISBN-13:978-3-7091-8278-9 e-ISBN-13:978-3-7091-8276-5
DOI: 10.1007/978-3-7091-8276-5

The writing of this review was made possible
by the patience and encouragement
of my wife Käthe

Lymphocytic Choriomeningitis Virus

By

F. Lehmann-Grube[1]

Hygiene-Institut der Philipps-Universität, Marburg/Lahn

With 16 Figures

Table of Contents

[1] Author's address: Heinrich-Pette-Institut für experimentelle Virologie und Immunologie an der Universität Hamburg, Martinistraße 52, D-2 Hamburg 20, Germany.

I. Introduction

Of the ever increasing number of viruses known to affect man and higher animals, the virus of lymphocytic choriomeningitis (LCM) was one of the first to be discovered. Indeed, this virus has been known and maintained in the laboratory by passages in a relatively simple host, the mouse, for 35 years. Yet our knowledge of its properties is still scanty when compared with the wealth of information available for other viruses, some of which have come to our attention much more recently. There are at least four reasons which may help to explain this seeming paradox. (1) The early belief that the LCM virus was the frequent cause of human diseases had soon to be abandoned; infections of man with this virus are rare. (2) By way of contrast, laboratory infections are not uncommon and they frequently run severe and even fatal courses. (3) Until recently, the only means of titrating the virus was by mouse inoculation, a method in which accuracy and economy are poorly correlated. (4) The virus is of unusual lability, being quickly inactivated under conditions which leave other viruses intact. Thus, when balancing medical and theoretical importance against personal hazard and technical difficulties, the result was quite unfavorable, and lack of interest was really not surprising.

In the last few years, however, the situation has gradually changed and an increasing number of workers have turned their attention to this virus. In the book "The Production of Antibodies", F. M. Burnet and F. Fenner (1949) drew attention to the basic biological significance of the peculiar relationship between the LCM virus and its natural host, the mouse. Together with Owen's erythrocyte chimerism in cattle twins (Owen, 1945), the lifelong carrier state in mice, so painstakingly investigated by E. Traub, formed the basis of what was to become in the following years one of the central and most fruitful themes of immunologic research; the concept of self-recognition and immunological tolerance. It was also Burnet who pointed out that the continuous coexistence of virus and host could only be perpetuated if the virus had "virtually no power to damage the embryonic tissues in which it multiplies" (Burnet, 1955) which led J. Hotchin (1958; Hotchin and Cinits, 1958) to postulate that an immunologic conflict between virus and host was the cause of disease and death of the adult mouse infected with the LCM virus.

Thus, the relationship between LCM virus and the mouse has become a matter of great interest in immunology, and work on this virus begins to function as a link uniting virologists with immunologists in their search for answers to at least some of the riddles of immunology which are still unsolved in spite of the efforts of so many.

In this review, an account as complete as possible[1] is given of the present state of knowledge of this virus. Emphasis is placed on host-virus interactions, but all other aspects, be they virological or medical, are not neglected.

---

1) The survey of the literature on which this study is based was terminated on December 31, 1969.

A. Definitions

In order to provide for unambiguous reading, definitions are given as follows. Lymphocytic choriomeningitis refers to any illness caused by the LCM virus. Closer characterization, especially in respect of human diseases, is done by referring to syndromes, *e.g.* LCM meningitis, LCM encephalomyelitis. According to this definition, lymphocytic choriomeningitis is not a clinical entity and will not be used as such, not even in connection with the experimental illness in monkeys and mice for which this name was originally coined.

A sharp distinction is made between infection and disease, the former denoting invasion of the macroorganism or the cell by the agent followed by its multiplication, and the latter referring to all pathological consequences thereof. Latent infection is the persistent and nonpathogenic multiplication of the virus in contrast to subclinical infection which runs a limited course like most infections but remains clinically inapparent (ANDREWES, 1958). The obvious disadvantage of this definition is the difficulty — if not impossibility — of proving in the individual case the complete absence of pathological alterations. Thus, latency is always relative in the sense that the sensitivity of our tools determines whether a chronic infection may be classified as such (LEHMANN-GRUBE, 1967b).

A carrier state is the lifelong coexistence of the virus with the mouse, regardless of whether signs develop or not. It is used synonymously with persistent infection. "Vital" = "viral, immunologically tolerated, acquired latent infection" (HOTCHIN and CINITS, 1958; HOTCHIN, 1958) or "persistent tolerated infection" (HOTCHIN and WEIGAND, 1961a; HOTCHIN, 1962a) are to be avoided because these terms imply mechanisms which may or may not be applicable.

Pathogenicity is used descriptively as an absolute term referring to signs of disease or death upon infection. In contrast, virulence is used in a relative sense, meaning pathogenicity per number of infectious units inoculated. Both are functions of the interaction between a particular host and a particular strain of virus and will not be used to characterize the property of a virus strain *per se*.

The immunologic terms in this presentation are defined as follows (see Fig. 1). Immunity is one state of an organism after its first interaction with an antigen (immunogen). Upon new contact with the antigen, immune reactions occur which may lead to immune phenomena, *e.g.* protection. Thus immunity, as used here, denotes an antigen-specific alteration, and immunologically specific protection towards a pathogen is but one of the possible consequences. A special case of immunity is allergy which is defined as the specific alteration of an organism after interaction with an antigen (allergen) in the sense that a new contact with the allergen leads to pathologic immune phenomena. It should be stressed that this definition of allergy — though conforming with today's usage — is different from the one given originally by VON PIRQUET (1906). The term allergic reaction is used synonymously with immunologic conflict.

Another state of an organism is immunological tolerance (= immunological paralysis) which is the specific hypo- or nonresponsiveness induced by an antigen (tolerogen). This phenomenon will be more fully defined in connection with the LCM disease in adult mice.

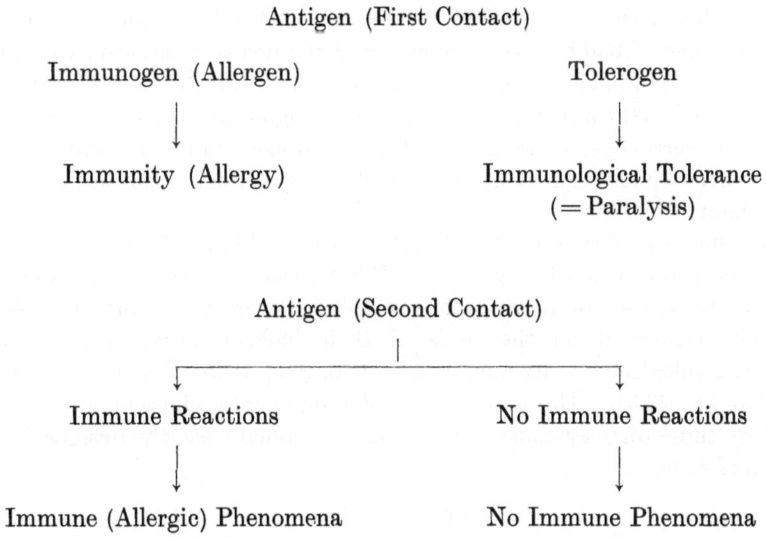

Antigen (First Contact)

Immunogen (Allergen) → Immunity (Allergy)

Tolerogen → Immunological Tolerance (= Paralysis)

Antigen (Second Contact)

Immune Reactions → Immune (Allergic) Phenomena

No Immune Reactions → No Immune Phenomena

Fig. 1. Immunological terms as used in this review

B. History

The LCM virus was discovered by ARMSTRONG and LILLIE (1934) when they passaged intracerebrally in monkeys material from patient "C. G." who had died in 1933 in St. Louis, U.S.A., from what had appeared to be St. Louis encephalitis. The disease in these animals resembled simian experimental St. Louis encephalitis until the sixth transfer when a monkey was employed which had withstood inoculations with the St. Louis virus twice previously. Unexpectedly, this monkey also fell ill with signs of a disease which differed from those observed in previous passages. A virus was isolated which was not that of St. Louis encephalitis. From the pathological picture it produced in the central nervous system of monkeys and mice after intracerebral inoculation, it was designated as the "virus of experimental lymphocytic choriomeningitis". Its true source was never established. It might have come from the patient having been carried along with the St. Louis agent which would mean that C. G. had been infected with two viruses concurrently. Alternatively, it might have originated in one of the monkeys despite the fact that none of the other monkeys used at that time was found to have had the infection.

Already in this first report Armstrong and Lillie noted the similarity between the experimental monkey disease and Wallgren's acute aseptic meningitis of man. The evidence for the suspected causal relationship was soon provided by RIVERS and SCOTT (1935; 1936b; SCOTT and RIVERS, 1936) who isolated viruses from five patients with acute abacterial meningitis followed by increase of neutralizing antibody in three, and by ARMSTRONG and DICKENS (1935) who detected neutralizing antibody in four patients, four years, three-and-one-half years, one year, and two months, respectively, after having experienced this syndrome, with serological conversion from negative to positive in one of them. Armstrong and

Dickens concluded that the etiologic agent responsible for Wallgren's "méningite aseptique aiguë" had been discovered and that a new disease entity which they named "benign lymphocytic choriomeningitis" had thus been established. It cannot be denied that this generalized conclusion might have been justified at that time. It has, nevertheless, caused a great deal of confusion in the medical literature for many years which even today is not completely straightened out, as will be discussed later.

In the same year, TRAUB (1935a; 1935b) reported that a colony of albino mice at Princeton in the state of New Jersey, U.S.A., was infected with a virus. The identity of the viruses of Armstrong and Lillie, Rivers and Scott, and Traub, respectively, suspected on the basis of their biologic properties, was soon established serologically (ARMSTRONG and DICKENS, 1935; RIVERS and SCOTT, 1936a; TRAUB, 1935b). The name, virus of lymphocytic choriomeningitis, was accepted by those directly concerned and has remained since the designation for this group of viruses.

C. Classification

Until recently, no serious efforts were made towards the classification of the LCM virus, and the occasional attempt to give it a home with one of the already existing major groups, *e.g.* myxo- or arboviruses, did not find the approval of other investigators.

A few years ago, WEBB (1965) noted that there were biological similarities between Machupo, a member of the Tacaribe group of viruses (PINHEIRO *et al.*, 1966), and LCM virus, but she failed to detect a serologic relationship by cross complement fixation tests. More recently, MURPHY *et al.* (1969) made a detailed comparison by thin section electron microscopy and found both viruses to be strikingly similar morphologically. Identical structures were seen in culture cells infected with the Tacaribe virus. Murphy and his colleagues proposed that LCM, Machupo, Tacaribe, and related viruses be placed in a new taxonomic group but that the details of this classification should not be worked out before more had become known in particular of the immunologic relationships between these viruses.

This knowledge was procured by W. P. ROWE, W. E. PUGH, P. A. WEBB, and C. J. PETERS (personal communication). They found that antisera against a variety of Tacaribe group viruses stained LCM virus-infected Vero cells by indirect immunofluorescence. The reciprocal relationship was not as clear-cut. LCM-specific antibody could be shown by the same method to be bound to Amapari virus-infected cells, but in an irregular fashion or not at all to cells infected with other members of the Tacaribe group. None of the Tacaribe group antisera fixed complement in the presence of four to eight units of LCM virus antigen. However, with 32 to 64 units of antigen low titers of complement-fixing activities were detected in Machupo and Pichinde virus antisera. LCM virus antisera were negative in complement fixation tests with Tacaribe and Amapari virus antigens.

On the basis of these morphologic and serologic findings, it seemed justified to collect LCM and the Tacaribe complex viruses in a new taxonomic group. Interested investigators from various countries (W. P. ROWE, F. A. MURPHY, G. H.

BERGOLD, J. CASALS, J. HOTCHIN, K. M. JOHNSON, F. LEHMANN-GRUBE, C. A. MIMS, E. TRAUB, P. A. WEBB, J. Virol., in press) proposed the name arenoviruses (from *Arenosus L. sandy*) which was chosen to reflect the characteristic fine granules in the virus particles as seen by electron microscopy.

Definition of the arenoviruses is as follows. They are lipid solvent sensitive, contain RNA, and share a group-specific antigen which is demonstrable by immunofluorescence and, in some cases, by complement fixation tests. Virus particles are pleomorphic ranging in diameter from 50 to 300 nm, with a mean of 110 to 130 nm. They consist of a dense, well-defined unit-membrane envelope with closely spaced projections and an unstructured interior containing a variable number of electron-dense granules which have diameters of 20 to 30 nm. The presence of these granules is the most characteristic feature of these viruses. Virus particles are released from infected cells by budding. At the present time, recognized members of the arenovirus group are LCM, Lassa and the Tacaribe viruses with Tacaribe, Junin, Machupo, Amapari, Tamiami, Pichinde, Parana, and Latino. The LCM virus is considered the prototype of the group.

II. Properties of the Virus

By way of introduction it has to be stressed that we are not dealing with the LCM virus but with numerous strains which, although reacting uniformly when tested serologically, possess quite different properties. This fact will have even more consequences when discussing the biological phenomena. Here as well as there we have to be content giving, so to speak, average information, pointing out differences where they are of importance.

A. Effects of Physical and Chemical Treatments

The great lability of the LCM virus was noted in the first reports (LÉPINE *et al.*, 1937c). Some stabilization was achieved by use of buffered glycerin (LÉPINE *et al.*, 1937c; YAMADA, 1940a; 1940b). It was also observed (SMADEL *et al.*, 1939a; 1939b) and has repeatedly been confirmed since (LEHMANN-GRUBE, 1960; PFAU and CAMYRE, 1967) that the infectivity of the LCM virus is well protected by even low concentrations of serum or purified proteins. The data of LACORTE *et al.* (1968) show that a suspension of infected mouse brain had retained some of its infectivity after storage at 4° C for as long as 120 days. Ackermann's observation that $\log_{10}$ four infectious units were lost after 24 hours at 37° C in the presence of ten per cent horse serum (ACKERMANN, 1961b) is not in agreement with most observations on this point.

In an essentially protein free medium the WE strain was rapidly inactivated by traces of detergent, freezing and thawing, storage at —60° C, and ultrasonication. When suspended in phosphate-buffered saline, the half life at 37° C of this strain was found to be as short as 16 to 20 minutes which contrasts markedly with 28 hours for poliovirus type 1, determined under identical conditions (LEHMANN-GRUBE, 1968). Whether other strains are significantly less prone to inactivation would have to be determined. CAMYRE and PFAU (1968) observed differences of stability at 4° C between the WCP, CA 1371, and Traub strains,

As long as the assay of the virus has to be based upon infectivity, the preservation of this property is essential for its purification and characterization. The incorporation into the buffer of Ficoll, Macrodex (Knoll AG, Germany; dextran with an average molecular weight of 60,000), polyvinylpyrrolidone, starch, sucrose, sorbitol, or dimethylsulfoxide had no significant effects on thermal stability. The infectivity was well protected by calf serum, albumins (egg, bovine serum), and Haemaccel (Behring-Werke, Germany). Of these, Haemaccel appeared to be most useful; nonantigenic and of relatively small molecular weight (35,000), this substance may be expected to interfere least with experimental manipulations. Surprisingly, Eagle's amino acids increased heat stability. A diluent consisting of 0.1 per cent Haemaccel and amino acids in phosphate-buffered saline was more extensively tested and was found to protect the virus against thermal as well as mechanical (repeated freezing and thawing, ultrasonication) inactivation. However, as may be seen in Table 1, even under these conditions maintenance of

Table 1. *Rate of Inactivation of LCM Virus, Strain WE, in Phosphate-Buffered Saline Plus 0.1 per cent Haemaccel and Eagle's Amino Acids; Influence of pH*
[From F. Lehmann-Grube: Arch. ges. Virusforsch. **23**, 202 (1968)]

Time of incubation at 37° (minutes)	pH 6.0	pH 7.0	pH 8.0
0	6.75[1]	6.50	6.63
15	n.t.[2]	6.36	n.t.
30	6.67	6.17	6.36
60	6.31	6.13	6.14
90	6.17	6.36	6.42
120	6.13	n.t.	5.94
180	5.94	6.28	5.83
Regression coefficient[3]	−0.004,705	−0.000,523	−0.004,114
Half life (minutes)	64	574	73

[1] $\log_{10}$ ID_{50}/ml.
[2] Not tested.
[3] Titer upon time.

a neutral pH was found to be essential (Lehmann-Grube, 1968). It is my experience that maintenance of a neutral pH is not that critical if the virus is suspended in a diluent containing serum.

Pfau and Camyre (1967) reported increased stability of the virus if tris-(hydroxylmethyl)amino methane was incorporated into the menstruum. However, the stabilizing property of this substance manifested itself only in the presence of protein. In screening experiments no protection was obtained with sodium glutamate, dimethylsulfoxide, and the sulfates of sodium, magnesium, potassium, and calcium. Thermal inactivation of LCM virus was increased by the incorporation of $MgCl_2$ or $CaCl_2$ at one M concentrations into the suspending medium (Pfau, 1965a). Thus, LCM virus belongs to the class of viruses which are more rapidly inactivated in the presence of high concentrations of divalent cations (Wallis and Melnick, 1962).

For those working with this virus it is important to know that its infectivity may be lost at low temperatures even if the diluent contains protective substances such as proteins (VOLKERT and HANNOVER LARSEN, 1965c). At —20° C the titer of an infectious mouse brain suspension was found to drop 1000-fold within four weeks (SKINNER and KNIGHT, 1969). LEHMANN-GRUBE (1968) observed that some preparations gradually lost infectivity at —60° C while others — prepared under apparently identical conditions — were perfectly stable. According to ACKERMANN (1961a), virus is best stored frozen at pH 7.5 to 8.0; at lower pH values it quickly loses its infectivity.

It has already been pointed out that lability as used here only refers to infectivity. Whether its loss is due to a breakdown of the particle or results from minor alterations on the virus surface is not known. It has been proposed that loss of infectivity is apparent rather than real and is a consequence of reversible clumping of the virus (PFAU, 1965b). While this hypothesis may have its merits, the available evidence does not seem to be in support of it (LEHMANN-GRUBE, 1968).

In common with most other viruses, that of LCM is rapidly inactivated by irradiation with ultraviolet light (HAVENS *et al.*, 1943). MILZER and LEVINSON (1949) reported that a four per cent homogenate of guinea-pig brain, infected with the highly virulent J. P. strain, was completely inactivated when exposed to ultraviolet light at continuous flow for 0.3 sec. LACORTE *et al.* (1968) did not observe inactivation of the virus by irradiation with radium. None of these reports is suitable for quantitative evaluation.

ROGERS (1951) demonstrated that LCM virus — together with Colorado tick fever and encephalomyocarditis, but not eastern, western, St. Louis, and Japanese encephalomyelitis viruses — was inactivated by merthiolate diluted 1:10,000 or more, but HEYL *et al.* (1948) had not seen such an effect.

In spite of its great lability, LCM virus retains infectivity upon lyophilization. This was first shown by RIVERS and SCOTT (1936a) who freeze-dried an emulsion of infected mouse brain and, later, by WOOLEY (1939) who employed pieces of infected tissue.

B. Attempts at Purification

From the foregoing it is not surprising that efforts to concentrate and purify the virus have met with difficulties. PFAU (1965a) had some success by differential precipitation with protamine sulfate or methanol; ammonium sulfate was less useful. Concentrating the virus by dialysis with the help of polyethylene glycol (carbowax) resulted in poor recovery, although carbowax itself had no effect on the virus. Almost 80 per cent of the infectivity was recovered at the interface between infectious cell culture fluid and a rubidium chloride cushion after ultracentrifugation.

The usefulness of the methanol precipitation was confirmed and the method standardized by PEDERSEN (1966). He achieved a 50-fold reduction of volume with an accompanying loss of infectivity of approximately 50 per cent. As based on OD_{278} measurements, the specific infectivity, defined as infectious units per mass of protein, was estimated to have risen about seven-fold. Essentially the same results were obtained by SLENCZKA and LEHMANN-GRUBE (unpublished) with methanol and also with acetone, the latter at a final concentration of 25 per cent. Again, purification was accompanied by a loss of infectivity of up to 50 per cent, which could not be avoided by varying the buffers used for resuspending the precipitates. Acetone at a final concentration of 50 per cent inactivated most of the infectivity.

Pfau (1965b) investigated the possibility of purifying the virus by fluorocarbon treatment. Freon 113 (trichlorotrifluoroethane) was not quite satisfactory but with Freon 114 (dichlorotetrafluoroethane) up to six extractions could be made without a significant loss of infectivity. By combining differential centrifugation and Freon 114 treatment, the specific infectivity had risen by a factor of 252. More recently, Pfau (1969) reported to have purified the virus 3000-fold by combining methanol precipitation with adsorption to and elution from calcium carbonate followed by ultracentrifugation. Since his starting material was serum free fluid from infected cell cultures, this degree of purification must be regarded as an important accomplishment.

The behavior of the virus in density gradients was studied by Pfau (1965a). Using the Traub strain, great losses were experienced with rubidium chloride, cesium chloride, potassium tartrate, and sucrose although in each case it could be shown that the compounds themselves in comparable concentrations either had no effect on the infectivity or even stabilized it. In the case of cesium chloride, results were not improved by adding 0.02 per cent albumin to the gradient or varying its pH.

Later, Camyre and Pfau (1968) observed significant differences between virus strains. In a potassium tartrate gradient, the previously used Traub strain rapidly lost its infectivity. In contrast, the WCP and CA 1371 strains were fully recovered. The results were unsatisfactory with Ficoll or sucrose gradients.

C. Size and Morphology

From filtration experiments with graded collodion membranes, the diameter of the infectious unit of the WE strain was estimated by Rivers and Scott (1936a) to be not greater than 100 to 150 nm but, as Rivers (1939) pointed out, the data would have permitted a considerably smaller estimate. This work was extended by Scott and Elford (1939) who arrived at a size of 40 to 60 nm by collodion membrane filtration and of 37 to 55 nm by ultracentrifugation experiments. Casals-Ariet and Webster (1940) determined by filtration the size of the infectious unit of their strain "II. S.F." and found it to be 33 to 50 nm in diameter.

These experiments were done and interpreted on the assumption that all infectious units are of equal size. This may turn out to be wrong. Electron micrographs have revealed great variation in particle size, with a range from 50 to 300 nm (Dalton *et al.*, 1968). Of course we do not know yet whether these are all infectious, and, hence, the question of the size of the infectious unit cannot be considered as having been answered satisfactorily.

Pfau (1965b) determined the sedimentation rate of the virus. When infectious cell culture fluid was employed, infectivity was pelleted with a rate of 178 S or more. After purification of the virus by fluorocarbon treatment and centrifugation, infectivity sedimented with particles corresponding to S rates of 76 or more. This difference was real and not dependent on viscosity of the suspending medium. An explanation is lacking.

As just mentioned, DALTON *et al.* (1968) were successful in visualizing the virus. They have presented electron micrographs of sectioned primary African green monkey kidney and established mouse cells infected with the Fo-2 and CA 1371 strains of LCM virus. These pictures indicate that the individual particles not only vary considerably in size but, furthermore, exhibit great pleomorphism. Some have spiked surfaces. They seem to be released from the cell surface by a budding process. Cores in the usual sense cannot be made out but up to eight dense granules with diameters of 20 to 30 nm are seen in the centers of the particles. They disappeared upon treatment with RNase but not with DNase or pronase and were regarded as representing the — possibly multiple — genome(s) of the virus.

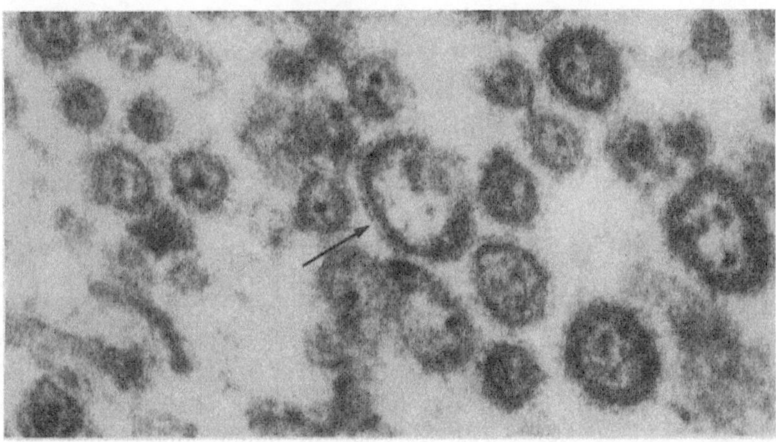

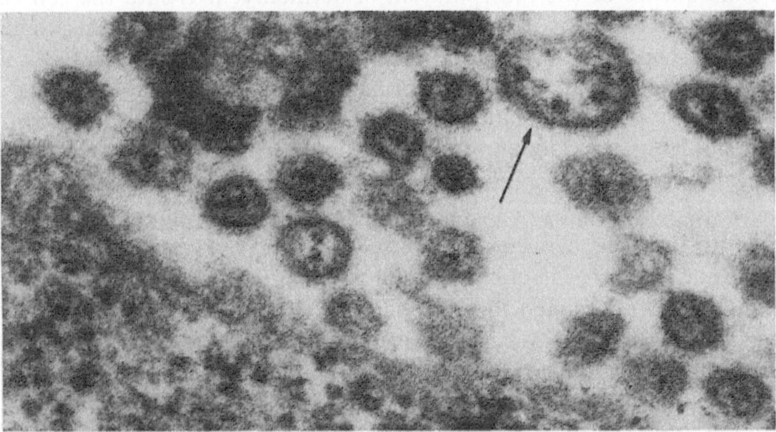

Fig. 2. Electron micrographs of BHK-21 cells two days after infection with LCM virus, strain WE. Groups of virus particles containing single or multiple "cores" may be seen. At least six such structures are present in the largest particle in the lower half of the figure (arrow). Projections on the outer surface of the virus are particularly distinct on the particle indicated by an arrow in the upper half of the figure. Magnification *ca* 130,000 ×. (Kindly supplied by Dr. R. W. Compans.)

The morphologic characteristics of the LCM virus have been confirmed by R. W. Compans (personal communication). He infected BHK-21 cells in suspension with the WE strain. Two days later the pelleted cells were fixed with glutaraldehyde and osmium tetroxide and then embedded in epoxy resin. Thin sections were stained with lead citrate, followed by uranyl acetate. Representative micrographs are presented in Figure 2. (I am grateful to Dr. Compans for his permission to make use of these pictures prior to their publication.) Variation of size, pleomorphism, spiked surfaces, and multiple "cores" are clearly recognizable. The viral identity of the structures seen with the electron microscope in LCM virus-infected cells was confirmed by Abelson *et al.* (1969) with the aid of labeled LCM-specific antibody (see Section III. B. 3).

Recently, Pfau (1969) reported to have succeeded in visualizing the virus by means of the negative staining technique. He concentrated the infectivity released into the medium of infected L cell cultures and saw viral structures with icosahedral symmetry, 36 to 40 nm in diameter. It is hoped that photographs will soon become available to aid in the further analysis of the structural details of the virus.

D. Chemical Composition and Buoyant Density

Although only circumstantial evidence is available, there can be little doubt that the virus of LCM belongs to the RNA viruses. Pfau *et al.* (1965) found no significant inhibition of its multiplication in L cells in the presence of 5-fluoro- and 5-bromo-2'-deoxyuridines at concentrations which affected vaccinia but not vesicular stomatitis viruses. Barlow and his colleagues (Barlow *et al.*, 1965; Barlow and Keller, 1965b; Barlow *et al.*, 1966) obtained similar results with 5-fluoro-, 5-iodo-, 5-bromo-2'-deoxyuridines; concentrations which reduced herpesvirus multiplication in BHK-21 cells by a factor of $\log_{10}$ four or five had insignificant effects on LCM virus. LCM-specific immunofluorescence, likewise, was not inhibited by these compounds.

The consequence of the incorporation of actinomycin D into the cell culture medium is not as clear-cut. Pfau *et al.* (1965) saw no effect at all, but Slenczka and Lehmann-Grube (1967) obtained erratic results. While occasionally no inhibition became apparent, in most experiments the multiplication of LCM virus, WE strain, in L cells was significantly reduced (Fig. 3). Similar equivocal effects had been observed by Cooper (1966) with poliovirus in human cell lines. He traced the differences of response to properties of the calf sera in growth and maintenance media. Apparently lack of insulin made the virus multiplication more susceptible to the drug. We therefore varied the conditions under which the cells were maintained prior to infection with and without actinomycin; none were found which consistently eliminated the variability of the results. However, even when there was depression of LCM virus multiplication, it was always much less than that of vaccinia virus under otherwise identical conditions. It may be added that we observed some inhibition of Mengo virus — although to a lesser degree than that of LCM virus — with similar variability from experiment to experiment (Slenczka and Lehmann-Grube, unpublished). Thus, as other RNA viruses, that of LCM is inhibited to some extent by actinomycin which may or may not be due to blocking of DNA transcription. Recently, Buck and Pfau (1969), using the Traub strain of virus, saw no inhibition of its multiplication in L cells up to a concentration of actinomycin D of 0.4 μg per ml. At 0.5 and 0.8 μg per ml the virus multiplication was 90 per cent inhibited which points to an unusual dose-response relationship. Surprisingly, actinomycin at a concentration as low as 0.1 μg per ml markedly depressed the later part of the growth curve where virus multiplication had practically come to a standstill, although the drug by itself could be shown not to influence the infectivity. In other cells, LCM virus multiplication was found to be reduced to ten per cent with concentrations of actinomycin D as low as 0.1 μg per ml.

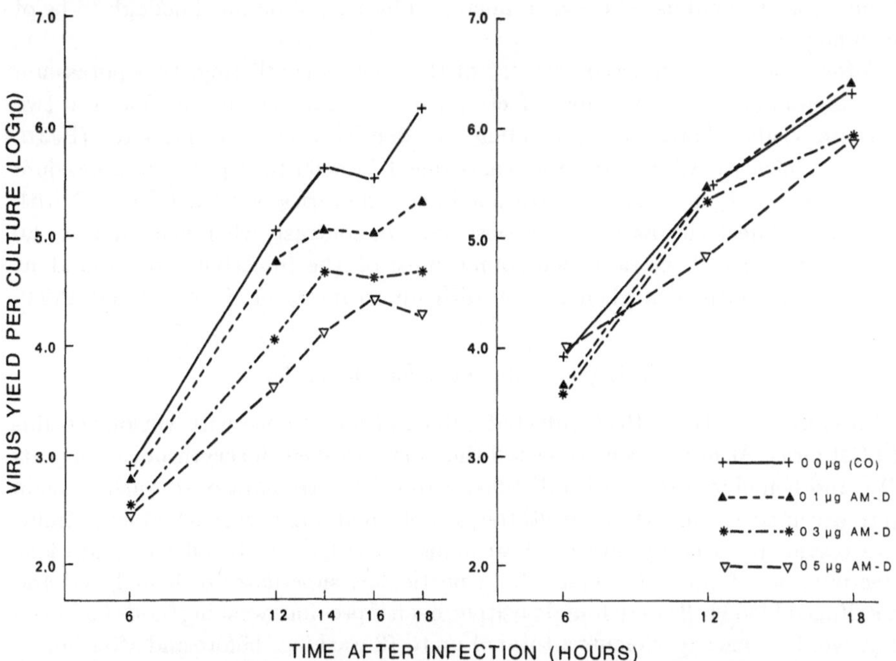

Fig. 3. Influence of actinomycin D on replication of infectious LCM virus, strain WE, in L cells. Virus was added to Petri cultures at a multiplicity of $10^{-2.3}$ in 0.5 ml of maintenance medium. After adsorption at *ca* 22° C cultures were rinsed three times, and maintenance medium, prewarmed to 37° C and containing the indicated concentrations of the drug, was added (time O). Cell-associated virus was released by ultrasonication, and total infectivity (medium plus cells) was determined in L cell tube cultures. Results from two of several essentially identical experiments are shown. [W. SLENCZKA and F. LEHMANN-GRUBE: Zbl. Bakt., I. Abt., Ref. **206**, 526 (1967).]

Further evidence that the LCM virus contains RNA may be adduced from the electron microscopy study already mentioned (DALTON *et al.*, 1968), from the characteristics of acridine orange staining of infected cells (BARLOW *et al.*, 1965; 1966), from the inhibition of virus multiplication in L cells by 6-azauridine (BUCK and PFAU, 1969), and in KB cells by 1,3-bis(chloroethyl)-1-nitrosourea (SIDWELL *et al.*, 1966), and from the observation that antigen could be demonstrated by immunofluorescence in infected cells treated with arabinosyl cytosine (CAMPBELL *et al.*, 1968).

If we know little of the nucleic acid core of the virus, we know even less of its outer components. Infectivity is rapidly destroyed by ether treatment (STOCK and FRANCIS, 1943; ANDREWES and HORSTMANN, 1949; PFAU, 1965b; SLENCZKA and LEHMANN-GRUBE, unpublished) indicating that the virion contains lipids. It is furthermore susceptible to soaps, detergents, and — probably — bile salts. Very early, ARMSTRONG *et al.* (1936) had found that of all the tested body fluids from experimentally infected monkeys, only the bile was free of infectivity. Later STOCK and FRANCIS (1943) tested a variety of fatty acids and detergents for their virus-inactivating capacities and found chaulmoogric, linoleic, linolenic, myristic, oleic, and ricinoleic acids as well as "Zephiran", "Duponol LS", and "Aerosol OT" to be effective. No loss of infectivity was observed by VOLKERT *et al.* (1964) and PFAU (1965a) by treatment of the virus with DNase, RNase, trypsin, and pronase. Certainly, these data are not sufficient to permit speculation as to the structure of the virus. The published electron micrographs are not detailed enough to be of much help here.

Information concerning the density of the virus is conflicting. In a potassium tartrate gradient, the remaining infectivity of the Traub strain was found in two of three visible bands corresponding to densities of 1.24 and 1.15 (PFAU, 1965a). When the WCP virus was centrifuged in a 60 to 2 per cent potassium tartrate gradient, three bands corresponding to densities of 1.24, 1.20, 1.17 with most of the infectivity at 1.24 were observed. In contrast, when using a 45 to 20 per cent gradient of the same compound, most of the infectivity was found at density 1.17 which is a phenomenon difficult to interpret (CAMYRE and PFAU, 1968).

E. Interaction with Erythrocytes

SHWARTZMAN (1943; 1944) infected guinea-pigs and mice with various strains of LCM virus. At intervals he collected the blood, washed the erythrocytes repeatedly, and hemolyzed them with distilled water. The stromata were washed again up to seven times, and serum, erythrocytes, stromata, and various washing fluids were tested for virus by intracerebral mouse inoculations. In all test materials, infectivity was frequently detected. In particular, supernates of hemolyzed and centrifuged blood cells were found positive, even if previous washing fluids had been negative. In some experiments a total of up to 13 washings before and after hemolysis failed to remove completely the virus from the cells. These findings were interpreted to indicate that "the virus is firmly associated with the stromatic material of erythrocytes". From the results obtained with different strains, it was further concluded that consistent infectivity of erythrocytes was produced by strains with a high virulence for the species.

Both these conclusions are difficult to accept. Complete separation of virus from any kind of cells is notoriously hard to achieve and since all the virus assays were done qualitatively, with disregard of the initial virus concentrations, little may be said of the significance of residual virus. What makes the interpretations even less convincing is the fact that signs of the disease developed in mice three to four days after inoculation of strains FA and T and three days after WWS which had been passaged in mice. It may be accepted as a rule that the manifestation of an LCM virus infection in a mouse never becomes apparent before the fifth day (see Section V.A. 1) and that a deviation from this rule raises suspicion as to the true identity of the agent. In similar though less extensive experiments, LÉPINE *et al.* (1937c) had infected monkeys and mice with the French strain and had found whole blood and the plasma derived from it to be equally infectious;

washed erythrocytes had been free from infectivity. Erratic results were obtained by Traub (1938b) who worked with viremic blood from carrier mice. The question of adsorption to red cells should be taken up anew, but rather than to test for infectivity associated with the cells, loss of virus from the supernatant fluid after contact with the cells and centrifugation should be used as the criterion for attachment.

Hamacher (1956) tested the ability of virus, strains WE and 0, to agglutinate red blood cells from hen, newborn chick, mouse, rat, hamster, guinea-pig, rabbit, sheep, horse, rhesus monkey, and man. Conditions were varied as to cell concentration (0.25, 0.5, 1.0 per cent), buffer composition, and temperature (4°, 22°, 37° C). Neither allantoic fluid nor homogenized chorioallantoic membranes from infected eggs nor homogenized lungs from infected guinea-pigs and homogenized infected guinea-pig brain "extracted" with various solvents brought about visible hemagglutination.

F. Soluble Antigen

It was demonstrated first by Howitt (1936/37; 1937) and, independently, by Lépine *et al.* (1938a; 1938b) that tissue homogenates from LCM virus-infected mice and guinea-pigs fix complement in the presence of appropriate immune sera. We now know that multiplication of LCM virus *in vivo* and *in vitro* is always associated with the formation of complement-fixing antigen. In guinea-pigs, its concentration was found by Smadel *et al.* (1939b; Smadel and Wall, 1941) to be correlated with the virulence of the virus strain.

Smadel and his coworkers (Smadel *et al.*, 1939a; 1939b; Smadel and Rivers, 1939) proved this antigen to be soluble (s) in the sense that it did not sediment with the virions during ultracentrifugation. The slight activity of the washed virus itself was referred to the presence of adsorbed s-antigen. Smadel *et al.* (1939a; 1940) characterized the s-antigen as follows. In solution the activity was not affected by storage for months at 3° C, although initially spontaneous irreversible flocculation occurred, or by pH changes over the range 4.5 to 9.0. The activity was slightly affected at 50° or 56° C and more so by temperatures above 56° C and by a pH of 3.0. The antigen could be concentrated and partially purified by freeze-drying or ethanol precipitation. Ammonium sulfate fully precipitated the activity but recovery was incomplete, with albumin and globulins having about equal shares of the specific activity. In the latter the antigen was predominantly associated with the water soluble pseudoglobulin rather than with the insoluble euglobulins. Purified and concentrated antigen was precipitated by hyperimmune guinea-pig sera. Conversely, complement-fixing and precipitating antibodies could be absorbed beyond detectability from such sera by s-antigen; it is significant that the neutralizing titers were not affected. Smadel and Wall (1940) inoculated non-infectious s-antigen repeatedly into guinea-pigs but could not induce either complement-fixing or neutralizing activities or immunity. However, pre-existing complement-fixing antibody was boosted with s-antigen to high titers (see Section II. C. 2).

Further studies on the LCM virus antigen from infected mouse and guinea-pig tissues were presented in a brief note by Barlow and Mustico (1965; 1966). They found it to be unaffected by heating at 60° C for one hour or by changes of pH from three to nine. On an Ouchterlony plate three distinct bands, named A_1, A_2, A_3, were seen. By differential centrifugation and gel filtration, the major antigen, A_1, could be separated. Resolution of A_2 and A_3 was not accomplished. Treatment of the antigens with trypsin and pepsin destroyed most of their complement-fixing activities and also abolished their precipitability. Absorption of an antiserum with A_1 resulted in 80 per cent loss of complement-fixing activity; it also decreased the neutralizing titer, which did not occur after absorption with A_2—A_3.

A comparison of the studies by Smadel and his associates and Barlow and Mustico shows up significant differences of both physical properties and specificities. In particular, while Smadel's data did not suggest sharing of components by virions and s-antigen, Barlow's findings indicate that the A_1 antigen consists of fragments of the virus particles. No doubt, further work has to be done before final conclusions may be drawn.

Hannover Larsen (personal communication) prepared complement-fixing antigen from infected mouse organs by means of the acetone extraction method of Grešícová and Casals (1963). When inoculated repeatedly together with Freund's adjuvant, mature mice responded with low levels of complement-fixing antibody for a short period. When inoculated repeatedly into newborn mice, no tolerance or later protection to challenge was induced.

III. Interaction of Virus with Cells in Culture

The number of different cells in culture which may be infected by the LCM virus is practically unlimited; indeed, no mammalian cell culture system seems to be known which does not support multiplication of one or the other virus strain. In spite of high virus yields which are often obtained, cytopathic alterations are usually absent.

A. Range of Host Cells

As far back as 1940 the virus of LCM was reported to multiply in cells maintained *in vitro*. MacCallum and Findlay (1940) passaged the original English strain of Findlay *et al.* (1936) 270 times in Maitland type cultures of minced chick embryos at intervals of three to four days. Around the 66th passage the disease in mice inoculated with the culture fluid changed markedly, a phenomenon which will be dealt with further below (see Section IX). Two other virus strains were sub-cultivated in the same fashion 35 and 38 times, respectively, without apparent changes.

Propagation of the WE strain in monolayer cultures of chick embryo fibroblasts was noted by Benson and Hotchin (1960). Ackermann (1961a), working with the WE strain, found that it multiplied in primary cell cultures from different sources, including monkey, mouse, pig, and embryonic bovine kidney and mouse embryo, as well as in established H.Ep. 2, KB, and Detroit 98 cell lines. Highest titers were reached in cultures of FL, permanent human amnion, cells. Benda and Činátl (1962) reported on the propagation of LCM virus strains in a great variety of primary cells and established cell lines. The WE strain multiplied in all of them, reaching highest titers in primary monkey kidney and human embryo and in established cynomolgus monkey heart, L, and H.Ep. 2 cells. In this laboratory, chick embryo fibroblasts and primary kidney cultures from monkey, rabbit, guinea-pig, calf as well as established KB, BHK-21, L, and Vero cells are routinely employed for the propagation of the WE strain.

ŘEHÁČEK (1965) investigated the ability of cell cultures prepared from *Hyalomma dromedarii* ticks to propagate 22 different viruses. All members of the arbovirus group readily multiplied in the cells. Of the other tested viruses, which included LCM, encephalomyocarditis, Newcastle disease, polio 1, vaccinia, vesicular stomatitis, and pseudorabies viruses, only LCM virus multiplied in the tick cell cultures to a comparable extent.

B. Characteristics of Virus Multiplication

1. Adsorption

In a preliminary fashion, BENDA and ČINÁTL (1962) reported on the adsorption of WE and K strains of LCM virus to primary monkey kidney cells in tube cultures at 36° C. Half the infectious virus had disappeared after 30 to 45 minutes from two ml of culture fluid. This, however, held only with small virus doses. The kinetics of adsorption of Traub virus to L cells in suspension was studied by PEDERSEN and VOLKERT (1966). Using as an index the proportion of cells with immunofluorescence after 20 hours of incubation following the adsorption period, they found a maximum of 85 per cent of the cells showing immunofluorescence after 80 minutes. The significance of this figure is difficult to assess. In the same paper an experiment is described which clearly shows that spread of virus still occurred after adsorption had been terminated by washing of the cells. In experiments performed by ACKERMANN (1961a) adsorption was not separated from multiplication, thus making an analysis impossible.

In concluding this section, it has to be stated that little is known of the adsorption kinetics of LCM virus to cells *in vitro*.

2. Propagation of Infectious Virus

The kinetics of multiplication of the WE strain in tertiary mouse embryo cells was determined in some detail by ACKERMANN (1961a). After infection with low multiplicities, maximal titers of 10^8 mouse LD_{50} per ml were reached between 24 and 36 hours. With a multiplicity of 832 mouse LD_{50} per cell, the highest concentration of infectivity was reached 12 hours earlier. Ackermann found more infectious virus to be cell-associated than free in the medium. According to OLDSTONE *et al.* (1969), embryo cells in culture from SWR/J mice produce more infectious LCM virus than cells from C3H embryos. DEIBEL *et al.* (1965) followed the multiplication in chick embryo cells of an adapted WE strain. After infection with a low multiplicity, new infectious virus appeared cell-associated at 16 hours and was released into the medium between 4 and 12 hours later. A maximum of virus yield was attained after approximately 72 hours. It was calculated that each cell had produced at least 16 infectious units, of which most remained cell-associated. BARLOW and KELLER (1966) investigated the multiplication of the UBC (= WE) strain in BHK-21 cells. New virus appeared between 6 and 12 hours after infection and peak titers were reached on the second day. BROWN and KIRK

(1969) infected BHK-21 clone S13 cells with the same strain of virus at a multiplicity of 0.1 LD_{50} (mouse) and followed the development of infectivity in medium and cells (disrupted by freezing and thawing). Maxima of $10^{8.0}$ and $10^{8.3}$ LD_{50} per ml, respectively, were attained on the third day. Multiplication of the CA 1371 strain in primary monkey kidney cells was followed by Oldstone and Dixon (1968c) after infection with high and low multiplicities.

A detailed study of the behavior of the Traub strain of LCM virus in L cell suspension cultures after infection with two different multiplicities was reported by Pedersen and Volkert (1966). With a multiplicity of three LD_{50} (mouse) per cell the latent period was said to be less than three hours. It was followed by a steep increase of the infectious virus in the medium reaching a maximum of more than 10^8 LD_{50} per ml at 26 hours. When the multiplicity was lowered to 0.03 LD_{50} per cell, the latent period was lengthened to seven hours and the maximum titer in the medium ($10^{7.5}$ LD_{50} per ml) was reached after 47 hours. There was always significantly less virus associated with the cells broken up by freezing and thawing than in the medium. It should be mentioned that these multiplicities may only be used in a relative sense. Infectious titers of the Traub virus are three times lower when

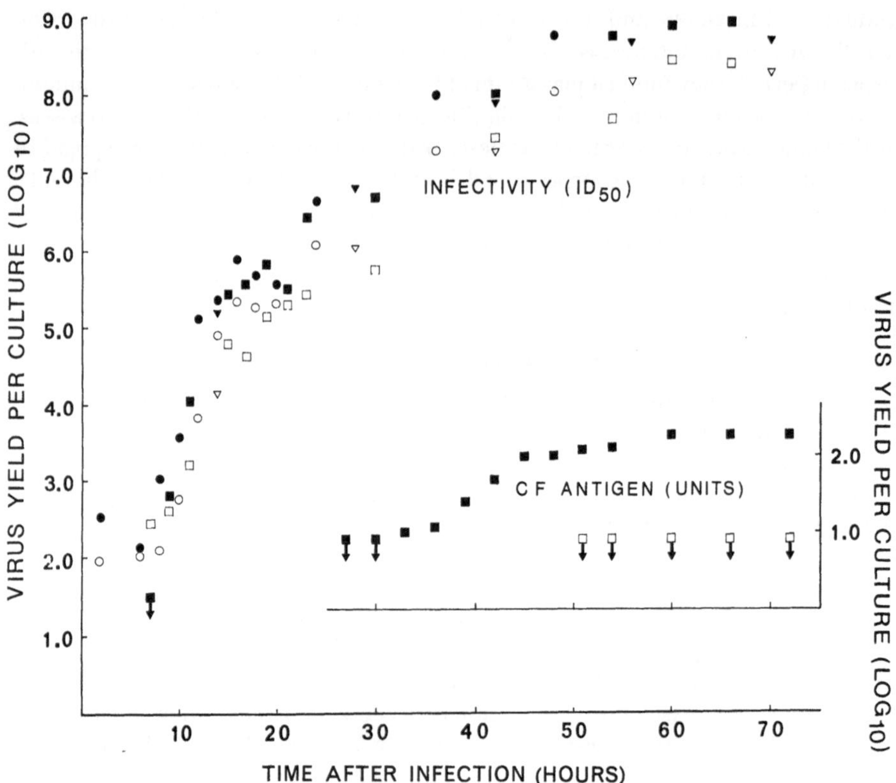

Fig. 4. Multiplication of WE strain LCM virus in L cells as determined by infectivity assay in L tube cultures and complement fixation test.
Closed and open symbols denote virus associated with cells and virus released into the medium, respectively. Differently shaped symbols represent different experiments. [F. Lehmann-Grube and W. Slenczka: Zbl. Bakt., I. Abt., Ref. 206, 525 (1967).]

titrated in L cells (ID_{50}) as compared with the mouse (LD_{50}) (LEHMANN GRUBE, unpublished). Hence, the actual multiplicities were one and 0.01, respectively.

The eclipse with a more than 1000-fold drop of infectivity after infection with the low but not with the high multiplicity of infection is surprising. Its significance becomes doubtful when it is recognized from the graphs that the initial titer after the infection with a multiplicity of 0.03 was approximately 10^3 times higher than the initial titer after infection with 100 times more virus.

Results which were different in several respects from the above have been obtained by LEHMANN-GRUBE and SLENCZKA (1967), who followed the multiplication of the WE strain in L cell monolayer cultures. After the infection with a multiplicity of 10^{-3} L cell ID_{50} per cell, the first cell-associated virus appeared after approximately eight hours. Infectivity then increased at a fast rate, reached a plateau around the 16th hour, and rose again less steeply six hours later to a peak at around the 48th hour. Throughout, there was more virus associated with the cells broken up by ultrasonication than there was in the medium (Fig. 4).

Table 2. *Kinetics of Production of Virus and s-Antigen (Cell-Associated) in L Cells Infected with LCM Virus, Strain WE, at a Multiplicity of One L Cell ID_{50} per Cell*

Time of incubation at 37°C (hours)	Yield per five cultures (ca 2×10^7 cells)				
	Virus ($\log_{10} ID_{50}$)		s-Antigen ($\log_{10}$ units)		
	Exp. 1	Exp. 2	Exp. 1	Exp. 2	Exp. 3
0	—[1]	—	—	—	<1.0
0.08 (5 min)	—	5.95	—	<1.0	—
0.5	—	6.13	—	<1.0	<1.0
1.0	5.70	—	<1.0	—	—
1.5	—	4.89	—	<1.0	<1.0
2.0	5.41	—	<1.0	—	—
2.5	—	5.06	—	<1.0	<1.0
3.0	5.50	—	<1.0	—	—
3.5	—	5.31	—	<1.0	<1.0
4.0	5.58	—	<1.0	—	—
4.5	—	5.13	—	<1.0	<1.0
5.0	5.20	—	<1.0	—	—
5.5	—	4.91	—	<1.0	<1.0
6.0	5.20	—	<1.0	—	—
6.5	—	5.01	—	<1.0	<1.0
7.0	5.34	—	<1.0	—	—
7.5	—	5.06	—	<1.0	1.45
8.0	5.70	—	1.12	—	—
8.5	—	6.33	—	~1.0	1.69
9.0	7.09	—	1.69	—	—
9.5	—	7.56	—	1.18	1.99
10.0	7.95	—	1.69	—	—

[1] Not tested.

The eclipse and latent period were studied in more detail (Table 2). After the infection of the cells with a multiplicity of one L cell ID_{50}, a moderate drop occurred in the first few hours, not exceeding one $\log_{10}$. New production of infectious virus became apparent eight hours after infection, which signified a latent period not different from the one following a 1000-fold lower infectious dose per cell (see Fig. 4).

Attempts were made by Slenczka and Lehmann-Grube (unpublished) to find explanations for some of the discrepancies obtained with suspension and monolayer cultures, respectively (see above). Strain WE virus was allowed to adsorb at 22° C onto L cells in suspension at multiplicities of 0.3 L cell ID_{50} (corresponding to approximately one mouse LD_{50}). At the end of two hours the cells were washed twice and were then resuspended in Eagle's minimal essential medium supplemented with five per cent calf serum to be further incubated in suspension at 37° C. Aliquots were taken at time intervals. The cells were separated from the medium, washed once, and treated with an ultrasonic drill at 0° C for 45 seconds. Titrations of released and cell-associated virus were performed in L cell tube cultures.

The principal results were as follows. With two different lines of L cells, new infectious virus appeared after 6 to 9 and 9 to 12 hours, respectively, reaching maxima between 24 and 30 hours. There was always significantly less virus in the medium than cell-associated. This latter point was further investigated. Infected cells were disrupted by either freezing and thawing or by ultrasonication and the amounts of infectious virus released by either method were determined. After one freeze-thaw cycle, most infectivity remained associated with the debris but could be released by ultrasonication of the sediment obtained by centrifugation. After the cells had been frozen and thawed three times, again only five per cent of the infectivity was found to have been released as compared with sonication. As before, ultrasonic treatment showed that the missing infectivity was with the sedimented cellular debris, although this time not all of it could be recovered, presumably due to some inactivation.

Further studies of the multiplication of LCM virus, strain WE, in L cell monolayers have been conducted in collaboration with Heide Menzel (unpublished). In repeated experiments, multiplication of virus was followed after infection with multiplicities of 1.0 or 0.001. With higher doses peak virus titers were reached faster, but they were slightly lower than those obtained with the more dilute inocula. A search for L cell clones which would produce larger amounts of infectious virus has failed. Of 18 progeny populations from single cells, not one synthesized more virus than the parent L cells; with most, significantly lower yields were obtained.

In all these virus-host cell systems virus multiplication is self-limited in the sense that once a maximum titer is reached no further increase is attained with continued incubation even where cytopathology is absent. We meet here for the first time a self-regulatory mechanism which is typical for LCM virus-infected cells.

When compared with the WE strain, the Armstrong strain (E-350) multiplied much slower in L cells and reached considerably lower peak titers (Lehmann-Grube, unpublished). Benda and Činátl (1962) and Camyre and Pfau (1968) likewise observed differences in multiplication rates and maximum titers between strains. In a few instances there was no multiplication at all. Remezov and Topleninova (1961) found no evidence of virus multiplication in embryonal human fibroblasts, and Benda and Činátl (1962) reported that the K strain of LCM virus failed to grow in cell lines of human origin. Wilsnack and Rowe (1964) observed neither immunofluorescence nor release of infectious material in CA 1371-inoculated primary hamster kidney cells. Such negative results were probably due to peculiarities of the virus strains. Occasionally, however, the host cells may be the cause. For example, HeLa S3 cells failed to support the multiplication of the WE virus (ACKERMANN, 1961a), which is known to reach high concentrations in most cells cultivated *in vitro*. In HeLa cells maintained in this laboratory the same virus multiplied to low titers. PFAU and CAMYRE (1968) experienced multiplication in one line of HeLa cells but not in three others.

3. Propagation of Antigen(s) as Revealed by Immunofluorescence and Complement Fixation Tests

REMEZOV and TOPLENINOVA (1961) were the first to report on the detection of antigen in LCM virus-infected human lung cells by means of indirect immunofluorescence. As the paper was not accompanied by photographs and the virus strain was not specified, the results are difficult to interpret. Using the direct method WILSNACK and ROWE (1964) found cytoplasmic immunofluorescence in a maximum of 70 per cent of primary monkey kidney cells after infection with the CA 1371 strain of LCM virus. Few cells fluoresced in infected WI 26, primary mouse embryo, and primary rabbit kidney cultures and none in primary hamster kidney cultures. OLDSTONE and DIXON (1968c), using primary monkey kidney cells infected with the same virus, saw immunofluorescence appear prior to new infectivity. Again, spread of infection was limited in the sense that with higher virus dilutions only a proportion of the cells contained fluorescing antigen. Apparently, this is a characteristic of the CA 1371 virus strain. WIKTOR *et al.* (1966) infected WI 38 diploid cells and detected at 12 hours immunofluorescence, which became most intense at 48 hours and faded thereafter, although infectious virus was still present in high titers. MIMS and SUBRAHMANYAN (1966) followed the antigen content of macrophages and embryo fibroblasts *in vitro* from LCM virus carrier mice and from normal mice infected *in vitro* and observed a drop of the proportion of positive cells with time after seeding and infection, respectively. BENDA *et al.* (1965) searched for immunofluorescence in L cells infected with the WE strain. At a multiplicity of approximately 0.5 mouse LD_{50} per cell, intracytoplasmic antigen was first detected nine hours after infection. With a multiplicity approximately 300-fold lower, antigen appeared in the cells after 24 hours. In both cases fluorescing antigen preceded the infectivity in the medium. Irrespective of multiplicity, virtually all cells eventually fluoresced. In a later study these workers detected fluorescing antigen in primary monkey kidney cell cultures as early as six hours after infection with the WE strain of virus at a high multiplicity (HRONOVSKÝ *et al.*, 1969). PEDERSEN and VOLKERT (1966) counted the proportion of immunofluorescence positive L cells infected in suspension with the Traub strain in parallel with the determination of infectious virus in medium and cells (see Section III. A. 2). In contrast to BENDA *et al.* (1965) they first saw cytoplasmic immunofluorescence appear several hours after the infectious progeny in the medium. With two different multiplicities again all cells eventually had become positive. SLENCZKA and LEHMANN-GRUBE (unpublished) infected L cells in suspension with the WE strain virus at a multiplicity of 0.3 L cell ID_{50}. In two experiments performed with L cells from different lines, immunofluorescence became detectable six and eight hours, respectively, after infection, which was slightly earlier than increases of cell-associated infectivities. The proportion of cells exhibiting immunofluorescence rose *pari passu* with the infectivity but never reached 100 per cent; a small proportion of approximately five per cent always remained free of viral antigen. While in most cells the antigen was located in the cytoplasm (Fig. 5), it occasionally was also noticed in the nucleus. This observation contrasts with the majority of other reports, although MIMS (1966) found antigen in some nuclei of cells in carrier mice.

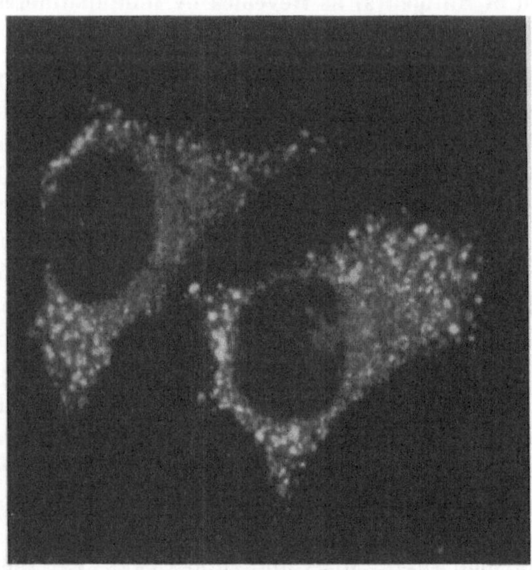

Fig. 5. Virus-specific antigen in L cells, stained with fluorescent antibody, 38 hours after infection with LCM virus, strain WE. (Kindly supplied by Dr. W. Slenczka.)

More recently localization of antigen in infected cells was refined by ABELSON *et al.* (1969) who identified LCM virus antigen with an ingenious new method developed by NAKANE and PIERCE (1966). Antibody, conjugated with horseradish peroxidase, was brought into contact with the infected cells and then made visible cytochemically by its ability to convert diaminobenzidine to a phenazine polymer which is brown in color and strongly osmiophilic. The electron microscope revealed intense staining of the extracellular virions by the labeled antibody. In addition, large cytoplasmic ribosomal aggregates associated with virus-specific antigen were observed in the LCM virus-infected cells. Their localization corresponded to the intracellular antigen as revealed by immunofluorescence.

LCM virus-infected culture cells produce antigen(s) detectable by complement fixation tests. In L cells infected with the WE virus at a multiplicity of one L cell ID_{50}, cell-associated soluble complement-fixing antigen became detectable together with new infectious virus (Table 2). It is worth noting that, even after extensive sonication of the infected cells, less than 50 per cent of the complement-fixing activity was soluble in the sense that it stayed in the supernatant fluid upon ultracentrifugation. The antigen increased significantly in the next few hours, whereby a considerable proportion was released into the medium (LEHMANN-GRUBE, unpublished). The time between infection and detectability of complement-fixing antigen was prolonged when the infectious dose was lowered (see Fig. 4). In contrast, the appearance of new infectious virus was not significantly affected by the multiplicity (see Fig. 4 and Table 2). Undoubtedly this difference reflects the greater sensitivity of the infectivity assay as compared with the complement fixation test. ACKERMANN (1961a) detected considerable amounts of complement-fixing antigen within WE virus-infected mouse embryo cells but little or no release. PEDERSEN and VOLKERT (1966) discovered traces in L cells infected with the Traub strain and no release. Using BHK-21 S13 cells and the WE strain of LCM virus, BROWN and KIRK (1969) found complement-fixing antigen in the medium although more was cell-associated. Whether these differences are real or rather reflect differing sensitivities of the employed assay procedures cannot be decided at present.

It has been pointed out before (see Section II. F) and is also evident from the above data that no final statement may be made as to the relationship between virion and complement-fixing antigen. On the other hand, a complete lack of correlation between infectivity and immunofluorescence was found by LEHMANN-GRUBE *et al.* (1969). Also, some circumstantial evidence points to a connection between complement-fixing and immunofluorescing antigens (BENDA *et al.*, 1965). It may be tentatively concluded that immunofluorescence localizes complement-fixing antigen(s) rather than infectious virus. Of course, it is impossible to exclude the presence of virions in an immunofluorescence positive cell. Conversely, an immunofluorescence negative cell is not necessarily free of virions.

4. Cytopathogenicity

One of the basic characteristics of LCM virus infection is to leave cells in which the virus multiplies intact. However, a few exceptions have become known. Among these are chick embryo fibroblasts, which were found by BENSON and HOTCHIN (1960) to disintegrate following infection with the WE strain virus. DEIBEL *et al.* (1965) confirmed this but found adaptation to be necessary for full cytopathic effects to develop. In other laboratories no such cell destruction was observed with the same virus strain. HOTCHIN and CINITS (1958; HOTCHIN, 1958) failed to induce cytopathology in chick embryo cells with either the WE virus or a strain which had been transferred 36 times through the chorioallantoic membrane and 43 times through the yolk sac of the fertile egg. They noticed, however, that the infected cells were metabolically less active. Apparently, the experimental conditions are rather critical. The occurrence of cytopathology in KB cells infected with an unspecified strain (EAGLE *et al.*, 1956) was confirmed by HOTCHIN and CINITS (1958; HOTCHIN, 1958). It did not attain extensive degrees and was only seen when the infectious dose was large. Cytopathology in WE-infected BHK-21 cells (BARLOW and KELLER, 1965a) was also seen by WIKTOR *et al.* (1966). These latter authors had employed an isolate from a contaminated cell culture. In this laboratory, cell destruction was never observed to occur in the Marburg line of L cells infected as complete monolayers with either WE or E-350 strains. In contrast, actively dividing cells were visibly affected. L cells, obtained from Microbiological Associates, Bethesda, exhibited cytopathology even when infected in the stationary phase (LEHMANN-GRUBE *et al.*, 1969). Cytopathic effects in L cells were also seen by BENSON *et al.* (1961; BENSON, 1962). According to ROWE (personal communication), some LCM virus strains cause cytopathological alterations in Vero cells. I have confirmed this finding with two prototype strains, WE and E-350. Whether the destruction of Vero cells by LCM virus is extensive enough to form the basis for simple assay procedures (see Section XI. A) will have to be determined.

The report by Stulberg *et al.* (1956) on cell destruction in cultures of eight established lines (Detroit) infected with LCM virus is too cursory to allow critical evaluation; no confirmation seems to have been published. Using the J. P. strain of Leichenger *et al.* (1940), Parikh (1961) noted cytopathology after five passages in primary human amnion cells. The reported deaths of mice already on the fourth day after intracerebral inoculation of infectious cell culture fluid makes the identity of the agent rather doubtful. The cytopathogenic variant of Jungeblut and Kodza (1963b) is probably not a strain of LCM virus (see Section IX). The alterations seen by Ackermann (1961b) in mouse embryo cells turned out to have been caused by a contaminating mold (Ackermann, 1961a). The strains of Chastel (1965), reported to destroy chick embryo fibroblasts, cannot be considered to belong to our virus (see Section XII). In conclusion, cytopathology is not a feature of multiplication of the LCM virus although there can be no doubt that, under certain circumstances, cell destruction may occur.

C. Persistent Infections (Carrier Cultures)

Studies of persistent infections with the LCM virus of cells *in vitro* are of great importance for our understanding of the carrier state in mice (see Section V. A. 3). Traub (1962b) and Traub and Kesting (1963) followed the multiplication of strain W over a period of several months in lymph node cultures derived from normal, leukemic, and persistently infected mice. Initially, various elements including lymphocytes were present in these cultures. Later "fibroblast-like" cells resembling "reticulocytes" predominated. A remarkable feature of the continuous production of infectious virus was the pronounced cyclic fluctuation in cultures infected *in vitro*, which subsided after prolonged maintenance; it was less marked in cultures from carrier mice. Apparently, these increases and decreases of virus yields did not occur in the later stages of chronic infections, irrespective of whether they had been initiated *in vivo* or *in vitro*. Cytopathic effects were not observed.

The multiplication of LCM virus in mouse embryo fibroblasts either infected *in vitro* or derived from persistently infected animals was followed for weeks by Benson *et al.* (1961), Traub (1962b), and Traub and Kesting (1963). In spite of continuous virus multiplication no cytopathology became ever apparent.

Benson *et al.* (1961) reported that infection of L cells with the UBC (=WE) strain resulted in cytopathic cell destruction which eventually affected 90 per cent of the cell sheet. The surviving cells continued to grow and, after one month, looked morphologically normal in spite of continuous virus multiplication. Wagner and Snyder (1962) followed the infection of L cells with the WE strain for 27 passages over a period of 154 days. "No consistent cytopathic changes" were noted, although virus was produced all the time. No interferon, but moderate resistance to vesicular stomatitis virus was found (see Section VII. B. 2).

The same system was more fully explored by Lehmann-Grube (1967a). L cell monolayer cultures were infected with the WE strain of LCM virus and cellular and viral multiplications were followed for 39 passages extending over a total cultivation time of 162 days. Neither cytopathology nor reduction of cell counts were ever observed after primary infection (zero passage), but both were regular aspects during the first subcultivation. Retardation of the multiplication of the infected cells was evident in the following two passages, but thereafter these cells were indistinguishable in respect to morphology, as well as growth rate, from the noninfected counterparts, although they continued to produce large amounts of infectious virus. The media of these chronically infected cultures contained no interferon and no interference was detected with vesicular stomatitis virus. The most conspicuous feature was the cyclic fluctuation of the virus yields which was even more marked than the one seen by Traub (see above). It extended over the whole observation period, being most pronounced during the first 15 passages where titers varied between $>10^{7.8}$ and $<10^{1.3}$ LD_{50} per ml of culture fluid.

This characterization of a carrier state of LCM WE virus in L cells was confirmed and extended by LEHMANN-GRUBE *et al.* (1969; LEHMANN-GRUBE, 1969a) with the E-350 strain of Armstrong. Serial cultivation of infected L cells was easily accomplished. Initially, retardation of cellular multiplication and some cytopathic changes were observed. Later, the cells multiplied normally while continuously producing and releasing LCM virus (Fig. 6).

Although approximately 95 per cent of these persistently infected "L (Arm)" cells were infected as shown by immunofluorescence and cloning procedures, patho-

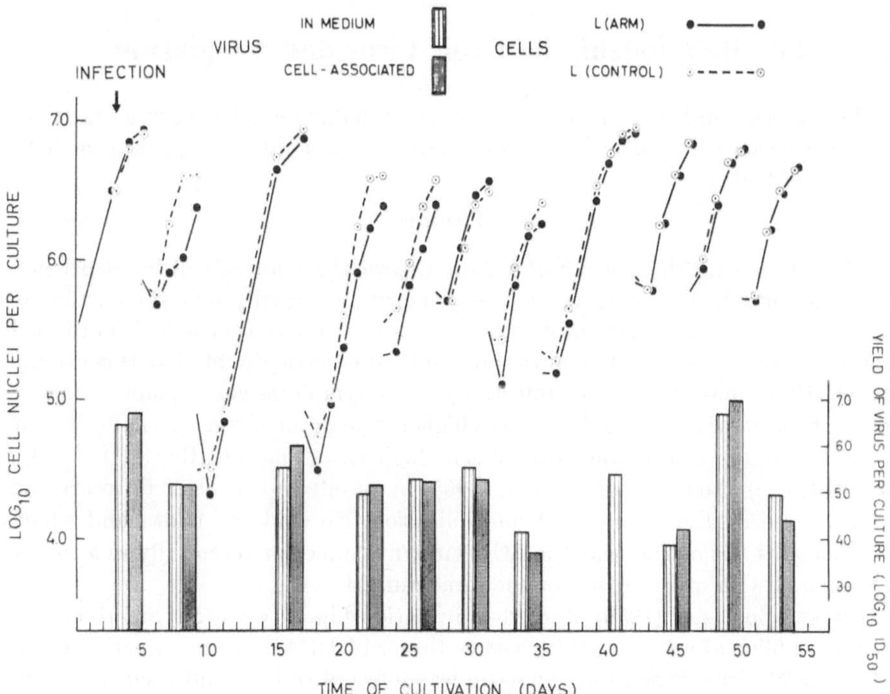

Fig. 6. Initiation of LCM virus-L cell carrier cultures. Multiplication of virus (strain E-350) and cells during the first ten passages after infection. From F. LEHMANN-GRUBE, W. SLENCZKA, and R. TEES: J. gen. Virol. 5, 63 (1969). (With permission of Cambridge University Press, London.)

logical alterations either morphologically (light and electron microscopy) or functionally (multiplication rate and efficiency of plating) were absent. This classifies L (Arm) cells as being latently infected in accordance with the definition given by ANDREWES (1958).

In an attempt to characterize more fully the virus-host cell relationship, the following experimental facts were established. No antigens alien for L cells were found on the surfaces of L (Arm) cells, either by immunofluorescence or by cytotoxicity tests. Most clones from single cells carried LCM-specific antigen in every cell. A few clones were free of the virus. Some cultures derived from single cells consisted of both infected and antigen free cells. This unexpected phenomenon was interpreted as indicating segregation of virus and cells by some unknown mechanism. Homologous interference was complete. Heterologous interference could not be demonstrated (see Sections VII. A. 2 and VII. B. 2).

Treatment of L (Arm) cultures with LCM virus-neutralizing antibody slowly decreased the proportion of antigen-containing cells. This cure was real and, furthermore, not caused by the inhibition of multiplication of L (Arm) cells reacting with antibody. In a preliminary note BENSON (1961a) reported on the elimination of the virus from infected Maitland type mouse tissue cultures by guinea-pig immune serum. These observations indicate that the persistent infection of L cells with the LCM virus was not only perpetuated by a vertical transfer of virus from parent to daughter cells but that horizontal spread played a role.

IV. Relationship between Virus and Neoplasms

The relationship between the LCM virus and malignancy has been a matter of interest ever since Traub's claim that persistent virus infection of mice may be the cause of leukemia.

A. Tumors

When discussing the sources of isolation, several instances will be mentioned where the virus had been discovered in primary and serially maintained tumors (see Section X. A. 4). Isolation of the virus does not prove that it had multiplied within the tumor tissue. Some data, however, leave little doubt that this occurs. TRAUB (1941) determined the infectivity in a lymphosarcoma from a carrier mouse; it was approximately 1000 times higher than in the blood but not different from other organs of the same animal. The high virus concentration ($>10^7$ LD_{50} per g of tissue) found by LEWIS *et al.* (1965) in an infected hamster fibrosarcoma probably also resulted from local multiplication. No evidence is at hand which would support the notion that the LCM virus multiplies preferentially in a tumor as compared with other tissues of the same animal.

POTTER and HAAS (1959) studied the relationship between an amethopterin resistant subline of a lymphocytic ascites tumor of DBA/2 origin, amethopterin, and the LCM virus. When the neoplasm was infected *in vitro* and then carried in nonimmune amethopterin-treated or untreated (BALB/c $\times$ DBA/2) F_1 hybrids, all tested mice were found to be viremic. Apparently, the infected ascites cells released a large amount of virus. When the mice had been immunized with LCM virus prior to transplantation, no virus became detectable in the recipients, and after five such passages the tumor was found to be free of virus; it did not regain its infectious capacity after 12 passages in nonimmune mice. In contrast, when the infected tumor cells were passed to LCM-immune mice which were treated with amethopterin, the virus was not eliminated and viremia became detectable in most animals. Somehow the drug interfered with the specific immune activity of the LCM virus-sensitized host; this is surprising, because amethopterin is thought to suppress the development of immunity rather than established immune responses.

This phenomenon is even more difficult to comprehend when reading the follow-up report by HAAS (1960). Viremia developed during 38 passages of the infected P 288 cells in non-immune mice and the tumor cells were quickly cured in immune mice after one, two, and three passages, respectively, in three transfer series, essentially confirming the previous results. The surprising observation is that after 14 passages of the persistently infected tumor cells in amethopterin-treated immune mice, the drug could be withheld without affecting the development of viremia, provided that the transfer of the tumor was done into the peritoneal cavity of the immune recipient. We are bound to conclude that the immune-mediated cure of the infected tumor cells had become more difficult because of some change in the virus-cell relationship brought about by the prolonged presence of LCM-immune cells and/or antibody together with amethopterin.

BENSON and HOTCHIN (1962) studied the oncogenicity of LCM virus-infected L cells in normal adult, normal newborn, and persistently infected carrier mice and concluded that the virus infection had transformed the L cells into a more oncogenic state. This important claim should certainly be studied in more detail.

B. Leukemias

TRAUB (1941) reported the observation that leukemia occurred more often in a carrier colony than in a noninfected subcolony which had originated from six virus free mice of the same original stock. Whereas the data seem to indicate that a real difference existed, they fail to prove that the higher incidence was caused directly by the virus and not by some other factor, *e.g.* selection, which might or might not have been associated with the persistent viral infection. Later, TRAUB (1962c) reported on the incidence of various forms of lymphatic leukemias in mice free of LCM virus as compared with carriers, and found initially no significant differences. Upon brother-sister mating changes occurred, not only in the LCM virus-infected but also in the control breeding lines, and the conclusion that the chronic virus infection had been responsible for a relatively high incidence of early lymphomatoses in one of the lines was hardly justified. STEWART *et al.* (1957) found no evidence that LCM virus had been responsible for leukemia and parotid gland tumors of mice.

POLLARD *et al.* (1968a) found in four of eight gnotobiotically raised one-year-old carrier mice that the thymuses, lymph nodes, and spleens were "so large as to suggest that they were leukemic". The histological appearance differed from that of lymphatic leukemia and rather resembled reticulum cell sarcoma or plasmacytoma. In a follow-up study POLLARD and SHARON (1969) detected "lymphoma-like" changes in 28 of 54 germ free carrier mice older than eight months. Because of the extensive immuno-proliferation with numerous plasma cells in the organs and the increased levels of globulin in the sera of these mice, the lesions were again classified as plasmacytomas. The control mice were free of such alterations. The relationship between these tumors and LCM virus is difficult to evaluate. The infected mice came from a carrier colony which had been maintained for over 25 years, while the controls were from an entirely different mouse stock, thus making a direct comparison between the two kinds of mice impossible.

Several reports on the beneficial influence of LCM virus on the courses of transmissible leukemias in guinea-pigs and mice will be discussed together with interference phenomena, although we do not know whether the observed sparing effects may be ascribed to genuine viral interference. The same is true of other examples of inhibition of virus-induced tumor development (see Section VII. B. 1).

V. Virus and Macroorganism

In discussing the interaction of this virus with animals and man, a clear distinction between infection and disease has to be maintained (see Section I. A). The number of different species which may be infected with LCM virus is large; response with signs of illness, however, is seen in a few hosts only.

A. Mouse *(Mus Musculus)*

1. Signs of the Disease in Adult Mice

The intracerebral infection of the adult mouse with the LCM virus is followed by a characteristic illness. This has been described by many writers, and rather than add a new version I shall quote Rivers and Scott (1936a) whose description is pre-eminent in conciseness and clarity. "During the first 5 days after inoculation the mice appear well. Occasionally on the 5th, but more commonly on the 6th day, symptoms appear, at which time some of the mice may be found dead although none of them were obviously sick on the preceding day, while others with dirty, ruffled fur, half-closed eyes, and hunched backs remain motionless. When disturbed they occasionally leap up and down in the jar and fall over backwards; but the characteristic reaction, especially when the animals are suspended by the tail, is for them to exhibit coarse tremors of the head and extremities frequently going on to a series of clonic convulsions terminating in a tonic extension of the hind legs. In male mice an erection sometimes occurs during the convulsions. The convulsions, often the cause of death, may also occur spontaneously either in sick mice or even in those that appear to be normal. As a rule, the animals either die within 1 to 3 days after the onset of symptoms or quickly recover in 5 or 6 days. Paralyses have never been observed." The fate of the mouse after peripheral infection depends on the virus strain. With the Armstrong strain (E-350) hardly any signs ensue. After infection with the WE strain of Rivers, a few mice die with indefinite signs of illness. Another strain isolated by the late Dr. C. Armstrong and used by Rowe (1954) was found to be markedly pathogenic with pleural and/or peritoneal effusions after intraperitoneal inoculation; these were so severe as to cause death by respiratory embarrassment in 30 to 70 per cent of the animals when high doses were inoculated. After subcutaneous inoculation most strains are not markedly pathogenic. Disease signs in such mice can be demonstrated by weight measurements which reveal a retardation of growth between the 5th and 12th day or even loss of weight (HOTCHIN and BENSON, 1962; 1963).

TRAUB and KESTING (1963) noted seven to eight days after subcutaneous inoculation of the W strain virus a "more or less extensive s.c. edema in the injected area". Since this observation contrasts with the negative results of most investigators, its significance is difficult to assess. In particular, its relationship with the foot pad reaction (see Section V. A. 2) is unknown.

MAHY *et al.* (1964) assayed the plasma levels of lactate dehydrogenase, aspartate transaminase, alanine transaminase, phosphoglucose isomerase, aldolase, and alkaline phenylphosphatase in intracerebrally LCM virus-infected adult mice and found none of the enzyme activities to be altered on days two, four, or seven, although all animals were dead by day ten.

Working with four isolates from mouse neoplasms of uncertain identity, but also with a laboratory strain, STEWART and HAAS (1956) made the usual observation that subcutaneous inoculation into mature mice led to an inapparent, immunizing infection. However, if the virus was mixed with freshly minced fetal mouse tissue, the subcutaneous inoculation was followed by a fatal disease. To my knowledge, this peculiar phenomenon was never investigated further. Likewise unexplained is the modifying effect of Evans blue dye on LCM virus infection. In mice that received virus into the foot pad and concurrently or up to two days later 0.25 ml of a 0.5 per cent solution of Evans blue intravenously no local foot pad response developed; instead, these mice became sick and died. Evans blue given on the third day or later had no such an effect; nor did it cause illness by itself. A similar consequence of dye inoculation was seen in mice infected subcutaneously but not in those infected intracerebrally or intraperitoneally (CUTIE and SIKORA, 1965).

2. Foot Pad Response

The existence of a local virus-mediated reaction was described by ROGER and HOTCHIN (1962; HOTCHIN, 1962b; ROGER, 1963b). The foot pads of mice respond to the inoculation of the LCM virus with swelling and gross edema, the beginning and duration of which are dose dependent. Otherwise many mice remain free of signs of a disease but become immune. A proportion develops a severe illness (see below).

Various virus strains passaged in mice, guinea-pigs, or eggs as well as triple plaque-purified material were effective. No response was seen with heated viral or uninfected control materials. By quantal titration, the foot pad was found to be somewhat less susceptible to the virus than the brain after intracerebral inoculation.

A more extensive analysis was conducted by ROGER and ROGER (1963a; 1963b; 1964a; 1964c). At limiting dilutions some mice did not react locally even though they had been infected as evinced by later immunity to intracerebral challenge. Thus the titer based on infection may be higher than the one based on the local response, which is reminiscent of the difference between ID_{50} and LD_{50} after intracerebral inoculation (see Section XI. A. 1) and may best be explained along similar lines, *i.e.* spilling of virus into the blood stream. As regards the general disease, three courses were distinguished: (1) the mice died with cerebral signs less than 15 days after infection; (2) they succumbed to a runt disease between days 15 and 21; (3) they survived.

The proportion of mice dying acutely varied significantly between colonies, ranging from 8.7 to 35.7 per cent. The survival times in these animals were not different. Since the mice from different colonies that had survived the first peak of mortality were indistinguishable, the authors concluded that every colony is made up of two subpopulations called "S" and "R", signifying susceptibility or resistance to the acute disease, respectively. "S" and "R" were thought to be controlled by genetic factors unrelated to sex. From the finding that the mean survival time after intracerebral inoculation was shorter than the mean survival time after foot pad inoculation (of those mice which died acutely) but that in both cases the individual observations were normally distributed with equal standard deviations, it was hypothesized that two types of infection occur after foot pad inoculation; a local one where the virus is confined to the site of injection and a systemic one which follows the occasional dissemination of the virus after a breakdown of the lymphatic barriers; in this latter case the ensuing disease was thought to be identical to the one following the intracerebral inoculation with a delay caused by the initial local retention.

The latter part of this hypothesis can hardly satisfy. It does not account for the fact that subcutaneous inoculations almost never and intraperitoneal inoculations rarely cause the cerebral disease, although mice may be very sick after peripheral infection and even die. Nor does it explain why some mice may be infected by the foot pad route, yet show no local response (ROGER and ROGER, 1964c). As may be expected, the general disease following the foot pad inoculation is associated with spread of the infection. ROGER and ROGER (1966) found virus in the brains of 40 mice which had died acutely or with some delay after infection *via* the foot pad; no dissemination of the virus could be demonstrated in ten mice which had reacted locally only.

HOTCHIN and BENSON (1963) determined the lethality in two mouse colonies after foot pad inoculation of two UBC (=WE) substrains. Few of either "Swiss" or "Albany" mice died when M/B_7 was inoculated. However, when M/B_7 L_{11} was employed — which differed from the former by having been passaged 11 times in mouse livers — the pattern of lethality was markedly different. Only 3.3 per cent "Swiss" mice succumbed as against 40 per cent "Albany" mice. These data indicate that death after the foot pad inoculation is not only a function of the mouse strain but is determined by an interaction of both virus and host.

3. Carrier State

In December 1934, Traub, then working at Princeton, N.J., discovered a virus in the institute's mouse stock which presumably had not been there the previous year. Upon intracerebral inoculation of sterile broth into apparently healthy animals a small proportion developed signs of disease. From their brains an infectious agent was isolated which caused death in the majority of previously uninfected mice after intracerebral inoculation and also killed most guinea-pigs (TRAUB, 1935a; 1935b; 1936a). In his first reports, Traub noted the similarity of alterations caused by his virus with those described by ARMSTRONG and LILLIE (1934) and within a short time the serological identity of the two viruses as well as their identity with the agents isolated from man by RIVERS and SCOTT (1935) was established. The origin of the new isolate remained obscure. No viremia was found in 102 house mice trapped on the premises. However, after intracerebral inoculation of another group of 45 such mice, five did not respond. Pooled (?) blood from four of these drawn one month later was viremic. In yet another series, three wild mice had been infected intraperitoneally without signs and challenged intracerebrally 38 days later. Pooled serum taken 78 days after the intracerebral test contained virus (TRAUB, 1936c). Although the possibility cannot be excluded that the infectivity in the blood stemmed from the experimental infection, these observations are compatible with the most likely explanation that the virus had been introduced into the colony by infected house mice.

The analysis of the numerous experiments performed by TRAUB and reported between 1936 and 1939 (1936a; 1936b; 1936c; 1938b; 1939a; 1939b) is made difficult by the fact that a distinction between protection due to immunity and apparent protection due to persistent infection was initially not always made. When first recognized approximately half the animals were involved in the epidemic. Of these, roughly two thirds were carriers with virus in blood and organs and the remainder were actively immune. Dams transmitted the virus to their offspring; carriers of both sexes caused horizontal spread within and even between cages. As a rule, neonatally or congenitally infected mice remained carriers for the rest of their life. Those infected at a higher age underwent clinical or subclinical infection but often recovered to be subsequently protected. As TRAUB (1938b) pointed out, "the more immature the mouse tissues are at the time of infection, the more regularly the virus persists in them". Carriers shed the virus with nasal secretions and urine. The very efficient horizontal and vertical transmission is illustrated by the observation that in subcolonies where close contact between animals was provided soon all were resistant to challenge; by 1937 all mice of the infected colony had become carriers, intrauterine infection being then the only mode of transmission.

Initially up to 100 per cent of the mice born to carrier mothers exhibited pathological signs. These consisted of what today would be called runting and were first in evidence around the seventh day after birth; they lasted for approximately one month. Lethality in these mice was rather high. It should be mentioned that overt disease in congenitally infected carriers must be considered to be exceptional. Most workers observed few or no signs of disease in mice born to infected mothers. In 1937 the virus-host relationship had changed markedly, mice born to carriers now being practically healthy (TRAUB, 1938b). TRAUB (1939b) concluded that both mice and virus had changed towards a mutual adaptation which he called a "perfect parasitism".

In the following years, Traub's observations were confirmed and extended. As a rule, carrier dams transmit the virus to their offspring with an efficiency close to 100 per cent (HAAS, 1954; TRAUB, 1960a; LEHMANN-GRUBE, 1964b), although a few exceptions have been reported. TRAUB (1939b) mated neonatally infected female carrier mice with noninfected males and found four of nine litters free of virus, although all mothers had been shown to be viremic before and after parturition. SEAMER (1965a) reported that among 42 infants from first litters born to mothers which had been made carriers by infection after birth and which had been shown to be viremic before and after delivery, 11 were free of virus. Of these, two were resistant to intracerebral challenge, two succumbed with accelerated responses, and seven died of typical LCM. Later, the same mothers gave birth to viremic progeny only. Mice of the second to the fourth generation were always carriers. Such differences between first and later litters seem to be exceptional.

Transmission of the virus from female carrier mice to their offspring occurs *in utero* (TRAUB, 1936c; 1939b). From his extensive experimentation, TRAUB (1960a) drew the conclusion that the ova were infected, possibly before implantation into the mucosa of the uterus. Mims' demonstration by means of immunofluorescence that in persistently LCM virus-infected mice reproductive cells are found infected (MIMS, 1966) lends support to this hypothesis. Thus, carrier mice may be infected from day one of their existence. Of course, we do not know whether such ova may be fertilized and develop normally.

The state of mice born to normal females infected during pregnancy varies. In Traub's initial studies (TRAUB, 1936c), three of four litters were free of virus when mothers were inoculated intracerebrally or intravenously before parturition. HAAS (1941) found 10 of 14 litters to have the virus when the mothers had been infected 1 to 11 days before delivery. LEHMANN-GRUBE (unpublished) did not succeed in inducing the carrier state *via* the pregnant female. As shown by TRAUB (1960a) only a rather narrow time span during pregnancy permits the transfer of virus from the mother to the fetuses.

Recently, MIMS (1969) reported studies concerning the effects on mice eight to nine days pregnant and their fetuses after intravenous and foot pad inoculations of the WE strain of LCM virus. The intravenous route proved to be significantly more virulent for pregnant than for normal mice. After the intravenous inoculation of 10^3 LD_{50}, infectivity in the placenta appeared on the first day and rose to high concentrations. Histopathology was observed by day five. In the fetuses, virus did not appear before the fifth day; one day later they were dead. When 10^7 LD_{50} were inoculated, the virus concentration in the placenta was 10^8 LD_{50} per g after 30 hours and had risen to $10^{9.6}$ on the third day. At these times, the fetuses contained less than $10^{3.8}$ and $10^{5.4}$ LD_{50} per g, respectively. The mothers were well on the fifth day, but the fetuses died between days two and four. As judged from distribution of immunofluorescing antigen, infection probably spread from foci in the placenta to yolk sac and amnion and thence to the fetus. No evidence was obtained that the virus was carried to the fetuses with maternal blood.

When mice seven to eight days pregnant were infected with the Armstrong virus, the offspring was uninfected and normal.

TRAUB (1960a) determined the role the father may play in transmitting the virus. One half the litters born to normal mothers mated with persistently infected fathers had virus. Litters following infected ones were always free of virus. Pertinent data were also presented by SKINNER and KNIGHT (1969). When persistently infected male mice were mated with specific pathogen free females, the babies had no virus when examined within two to three days of birth, but many were resistant when challenged later. At the age of three or more weeks a few mice had infectious tissues or excreted virus with urine indicating that they were persistently infected. Apparently transmission of virus to the progeny occurred either after birth directly from the father or through the acutely infected mother but not *via* the male sperm.

TRAUB (1960b) assayed the virus contents of blood, spleens, and reproductive organs of adult carriers and found the concentrations to be higher than in mice infected when five weeks old and killed six to seven days later. In inbred carrier mice, established by neonatal infection, marked differences between strains with respect to virus concentrations in blood and organs were noted by OLDSTONE and DIXON (1968a; 1968b) with lowest titers in C3H, higher ones in $B_{10}D_2$ Old Line, and highest in SWR mice. VOLKERT and HANNOVER LARSEN (1965c) found slightly lower titers in C3H as compared with AKR mice, but the differences were not nearly so great as the ones seen by Oldstone and Dixon.

TRAUB (1961b) measured the complement fixation activities in many different organs of carrier mice. Highest concentrations were found in spleens and lymph nodes. No organ was consistently free. WILSNACK and ROWE (1964) studied the distribution of antigen by means of the immunofluorescence method in young adult carrier mice from a colony established approximately 40 generations previously by HAAS (1941). Infected cells in liver, kidney, spleen, lungs, intestines, heart, and uterus were found with varying numbers but always in low proportions. Immunofluorescing antigen was also observed in the trophoblastic epithelium of embryonic tissue but not in the ova of one pregnant mouse. In four of six animals some immunofluorescence was detected in leptomeninges, choroid plexus, arterial endothelia, perivascular connective tissues, and, on occasion, in astrocytes and neuroglia. In only one mouse were neurones involved. MIMS (1966) investigated by the same method the antigen distribution in WE strain carriers — unborn, newborn, suckling, young adult, old adult — from a colony initiated by LEHMANN-GRUBE (1964b) two to three years previously and arrived at results which differed qualitatively and quantitatively. In embryos most cells of all tissues contained small, sparsely distributed cytoplasmic and nuclear particles. With the development after birth the quantity of antigen per individual cell enlarged, although the number of positive cells in some tissues, such as muscle and cartilage, decreased significantly. Old carriers showed a considerable increase in the number of infected neurones and in the amount of antigen contained in these cells. Of great significance is the finding that in adult female carriers germinal epithelia, follicles, and an occasional ovum were infected. In various inbred mouse strains persistently infected by neonatal infection with the CA 1371 strain of LCM virus, OLDSTONE and DIXON (1969) demonstrated antigen by immunofluorescence in all tissues with greatest concentrations in brains (neurones of cortex, thalamus, hippocampus, cerebellum), livers, and kidneys.

DALTON *et al.* (1968) had difficulties in detecting virus particles by electron microscopy in organs of congenitally infected mice. None were found in liver, pancreas, or uterus, but a small number was located in the kidneys.

For many years it was thought that carrier mice do not respond at all immunologically to the viral antigen(s). It now has become clear that in neonatal and probably also in congenital carriers circulating antibody is present together with the virus (OLDSTONE and DIXON, 1967; BENSON and HOTCHIN, 1969). This aspect of the persistent infection will be more extensively discussed when dealing with the pathogenetic mechanisms of the LCM disease in the mouse (see Section V. A. 4. b).

For experimental purposes carriers are most often produced by neonatal infection. Surviving mice are, with few exceptions, carriers (HAAS, 1941; TRAUB, 1960b; LEHMANN-GRUBE, 1964b; VOLKERT and HANNOVER LARSEN, 1965a). All mothers are immediately infected, which may lead to illness and consequent loss of the offspring due to neglect, thereby simulating high pathogenicity of the virus for the newborn mice. Another important aspect of the transmission of the virus to the mother has to be mentioned. As early as ten days after infection the infants had circulating antibody detected by immunofluorescence method which was shown to originate in the mother, being transmitted with the milk. It disappeared on weaning and was replaced by low levels of indigenous antibody weeks later (BENSON and HOTCHIN, 1969).

VOLKERT and HANNOVER LARSEN (1965a) determined the kinetics of virus multiplication in newborn mice as reflected by the levels of infectivity attained in the blood and found no significant differences after intraperitoneal inoculation of 10, 100, or 1000 LD_{50} into mice less than 18 hours old. Within three days the titers in the blood had risen to $10^{4.5}$ LD_{50} per ml or more and on the sixth day all titers were $\geq 10^9$ LD_{50} per ml where they remained for a few days. They then declined rapidly to reach $10^{5.5}$ LD_{50} per ml by day 14, a concentration which was maintained more or less constant for many months. PETERSON and MAKSUDOVA (1969) followed the virus contents for up to 90 days in the organs of mice infected intracerebrally at age four hours or two days, four days, six days, or twelve days. Infectivity titers in brains and spleens remained essentially constant over the period of observation; in contrast, the virus concentration in the blood varied markedly. It may be considered a significant finding that the age of the mouse at inoculation did not demonstrably influence the virus titers.

In this laboratory, multiplication of the WE and E-350 strains was followed in newborn mice for 14 days after infection (HEUWINKEL and LEHMANN-GRUBE, unpublished). Mice, less than 24 hours old, were inoculated intraperitoneally with 1000 ID_{50} (mouse). At daily intervals, three animals from at least two litters were killed. They were skinned and eviscerated, the whole carcasses were ground with sand in a mortar and a ten per cent suspension was prepared and titrated in L cell tube cultures. The results of two such experiments may be summarized as follows. The WE virus climbed rapidly and attained maximum levels within three days. Significantly slower multiplication took place with the E-350 strain, which reached its highest concentration not before the seventh day. However, essentially equal concentrations of approximately 10^9 ID_{50} (mouse) per g of mouse tissue were eventually reached by both these virus strains. After having arrived at maximal values, the virus titers did not decrease within the period of observation, which contrasts with Volkert's observation related above where viremia was found to decline in neonatally infected animals. In organs of adult carrier mice which had been infected by neonatal contact with established carriers, TRAUB (1938b) found significantly higher virus concentrations than in the blood. Apparently, in older mice or, alternatively, during the later stages of an infection, less virus is released into the circulation.

The evolution of the infection in mice inoculated intracerebrally when approximately 12 hours old with 10^5 ID_{50} of the WCP strain was investigated by BROWN (1968) with the help of fluoresceine isothiocyanate-coupled antibody. The virus was found to be distributed in three ways: (1) spread from the site of inoculation with the cerebrospinal fluid to meninges and plexus and from there to the brain; (2) dispersion *via* the subcutaneous tissue; (3) dissemination with the blood. A synopsis of the relationship between time and appearance of antigen in the organs may be found in Table 3. On the fifth day the antigen was ubiquitous. At this time

Table 3. *Distribution of Virus Antigen as Determined by Immunofluorescence in the Tissues of Mice Inoculated at Birth with LCM Virus*
From P. BROWN: Arch. ges. Virusforsch. **24**, 220 (1968)
(With Permission of the Author)

	Time after inoculation				
	12 hours	1 day	2 days	3 days	5 days
Site of inoculation	0	+	++	++++	++++
CNS	0	+	++	+++	++++
Liver	0	+	++	+++	++++
Spleen	0	0	++	+++	++++
Kidneys	0	0	+	++	++++
Blood	0	0	+	++	+++
Lymph nodes	0	0	0	++	++++
Thymus	0	0	0	++	++++
Other	0	0	0	++	++++

the fluorescent cells were found throughout the central nervous system and although it was usually not possible to distinguish between cell types the location indicated that neurones were heavily involved. In 20 months, neither intensity nor distribution of antigen had changed to any extent.

The outcome of the neonatal infection, *i.e.* death or survival with persistent infection, depends on various factors of which route of inoculation and mouse and virus strains will be reviewed here. Others, such as age of the mouse and dose of the virus, will be dealt with when discussing pathogenetic mechanisms (see Section V. A. 4. b).

The route of inoculation seems to make little difference. Intranasal, intraperitoneal, and intracerebral infections have been employed with similar results. HOTCHIN *et al.* (1962) saw a somewhat greater pathogenicity when the virus was inoculated intraperitoneally rather than intracerebrally; however, WAGNER and SNYDER (1962) noted that less pathogenicity was associated with either the intraperitoneal or the intranasal as compared with the intracerebral route. TRAUB (1960b) observed that more newborn mice developed persistent viremia after intracerebral (52 of 52) than after intranasal (26 of 54) infection.

WHITNEY (1951a; 1951b) found that less than 20 per cent of 84 mice one to three days of age died when inoculated intracerebrally with cerebrospinal fluid from an LCM patient or liver spleen suspensions from wild carrier mice, materials which had killed 49 of 50 mature animals. The results were similar when these fresh isolates had been passaged once in mice. By way of contrast, when newborn mice were injected with LCM virus, strain Armstrong, which had been transferred 380 times in mice, only 9 of 37 survived. She concluded that adaptation might have enhanced the virulence of the agent for infant mice. Traub (1960 b) observed significant differences of the pathogenicities for newborn mice of four strains of LCM virus. He also noted differences with regard to pathogenicity for adult mice. Significantly, these two viral properties were not linked with each other. When studying the effect of age (see Section V. A. 4. b), Hotchin and Weigand (1961 a) found a low mortality in two outbred mouse strains, "Albany" and "Swiss", infected with the UBC = WE virus. Later, Hotchin *et al.* (1962) observed close to 100 per cent mortality with UBC in Albany mice, the only difference with the previous experiments being that the virus had been transferred five times more in mouse brains, thereby reaching the seventh intracerebral passage level. When virus of the first intracerebral passage was employed or when sixth passage material was transmitted ten times intraperitoneally with liver homogenates, the ability to induce persistent infection with close to 100 per cent survival in newborn mice was restored. The proportion of survivors after infection with the Albany virus strain which had been previously passaged in fertile eggs and with strains 600290 and 600286 which had gone through mouse brains three and four times, respectively, was likewise high. In contrast, strain 600287 in its 11th mouse passage killed four of six one-day-old mice. From these data Hotchin and his colleagues concluded that virus strains are either "docile" or "aggressive" in newborn mice. Since passages through mouse brains seemed to confer aggressiveness while intraperitoneal passages apparently favored docility, it was said that "the docility of an LCM strain is associated with its viscerotropism, and the aggressiveness with neurotropism". It will be pointed out later (see Section V. A. 4. a) that the characterization of an LCM virus strain as viscerotropic or neurotropic lacks rationale. But even if this terminology were acceptable, the mere passage five times in the central nervous system cannot necessarily be expected to have conveyed neurotropism on a previously viscerotropic agent.

Be this as it may, the classification of a strain to belong to either the docile or the aggressive category is in itself of doubtful value. The WE strain, found to be docile by Hotchin when not passaged in the mouse brain and also by Traub (1960 b) after guinea-pig passages, was aggressive in Australian Walter and Eliza Hall Institute multicolored mice, even without prior intracerebral passages (Lehmann-Grube, 1964 b). The same strain after 16 and 17 mouse brain passages or after 15 mouse brain passages followed by two transfers through L cells or after 14 mouse brain passages followed by two transfers through guinea-pigs and three further transfers through BHK-21 cells *in vitro* killed 249 of 250 C3H mice which had survived the first four days after their infection at the age of 24 hours or younger, independent of route or dose (Lehmann-Grube, unpublished). The Traub strain, which had been found by Volkert (1963) to kill 20 to 25 per cent of infant AKA (= AKR) and by Hannover Larsen (personal communication) 31 per cent (452 of 1450) C3H mice in Copenhagen, was lethal for 75 per cent of C3H mice of the same age in Marburg, the only other difference being one further passage in mice, either intracerebrally or intraperitoneally. Of altogether 477 newborn animals, 120 died in the first four days, presumably due to trauma or neglect by the mother. Of the remaining 357 mice, 191 (54 per cent) died between days 5 and 35, 45 (13 per cent) between days 36 and 60, and 2 further mice when older than 60 days. [The corresponding figures for the Copenhagen C3H mice, kindly supplied by Dr. J. Hannover Larsen, are as follows; in the first four days 236 babies died. Of the remaining 1214 mice, 216 (18 per cent) died on days 5 to 35; none thereafter.] Thus, with the above terminology, the Traub strain would be called docile for AKR and C3H mice in Dr. Volkert's laboratory but aggressive for C3H mice in Marburg. In contrast to the high proportion of C3H mice which died in this laboratory after infection with the Traub virus, 200 of altogether 333 (60 per cent) CBA mice survived the intraperitoneal inoculation of 1000 ID_{50} of the same virus preparation; deaths occurred 12 times between days one and four, 106 times between days 5 and 35, 15 times between days 36 and 60, and none thereafter (LEHMANN-GRUBE, unpublished).

In an attempt to further elucidate the role of prepassages on the virulence for newborn mice, three standard strains, Armstrong's E-350, Rivers' WE, and Traub's T, which had been maintained in various hosts previously, were passaged ten times each, either intracerebrally with brain or intraperitoneally with liver-spleen-kidney homogenates under otherwise identical conditions. The final pools, stored in ampoules at —60° C, were titrated in mice three times each, to obtain accurate measures of their activities. Outbred albino mice were then inoculated intraperitoneally when less than 24 hours old with 100 or 10,000 ID_{50} and deaths were recorded daily for five weeks. Part of the survivors were then tested and all proved to be carriers. The results of this experiment (Table 4) clearly show that

Table 4. *Influence of Passage History on Virulence of LCM Viruses for Mice Infected when Less than 24 Hours Old*

Strain	Virus		Death in newborn mice		
	Ten passages in	Dosis (ID_{50})	Number		%
WE	Brain	100	5/64[1]	8/138	5.8
		10,000	3/74		
	Internal organs	100	4/46	9/138	6.5
		10,000	5/92		
E-350	Brain	100	14/101	24/157	15.3
		10,000	10/56		
	Internal organs	100	1/32	4/78	5.1
		10,000	3/46		
T	Brain	100	1/35	4/107	3.7
		10,000	3/72		
	Internal organs	100	4/53	7/114	6.1
		10,000	3/61		

[1] Number of mice dead between 5th and 35th day over number alive on fifth day after infection.

all six substrains were docile. Hence, prepassages in the brains or the viscera did not noticeably influence the virulence for newborn mice. It is to be stressed that the WE strain used in this experiment is the same as the one which was aggressive in Walter and Eliza Hall Institute and even more so in C3H mice and is presumably identical with the UBC strain used by Hotchin, and that T is the strain which was docile in AKR, C3H (Copenhagen), and CBA but aggressive in C3H (Marburg) mice (see above). Thus, whether a virus is docile or aggressive depends on its interaction with the host and varies from mouse strain to mouse strain; it has to be determined empirically in each combination. Inasmuch as the LCM virus carrier state may be regarded equivalent to actively acquired immunological tolerance, it is comparable to the prototype of this phenomenon, namely induction by neonatal inoculation of homologous spleen cells where successes or failures, likewise, depended on the donor-recipient combination (Billingham and Brent, 1958—60).

According to Sikora *et al.* (1968), yet other variables have to be considered. These authors observed a marked increase of lethality in newborn LCM virus-infected mice due to minor degrees of stress, *e.g.* exchange of mothers. The cause was thought to lie in decreased maternal care. In the same category falls the observation of M. Volkert (personal communication) that at the State Serum Institute in Copenhagen, where the mice were kept under optimal conditions, lethality for AKR mice had been 25 per cent (see above). After having moved to a new domicile where the animal quarters were not as well controlled, the overall lethality soared to 80 per cent. By improving the conditions it could be lowered but is still — at present — at 40 per cent.

The question to be answered next is whether the carrier state as described above signifies a latent infection which, as will be recalled, has been defined as being persistent and inapparent. There can be no doubt concerning the persistence. The chronic infection is, however, not without consequences for the host. Even with the most "docile" mouse-virus combination, a certain proportion of mice inoculated neonatally die (see above). All survivors are, at least initially, more or less affected; they grow slower and may go through a phase of runting. They then may develop normally but when approximately one year old some of them have been found to develop ruffled fur, frequently blepharitis, and a hunched posture followed by degenerative changes of eyes and skin and general wasting with early death (Traub, 1938b; Hotchin, 1962a; Hotchin *et al.*, 1963; Hotchin and Collins, 1964; Hotchin, 1965; Oldstone and Dixon, 1969; Mims, personal communication); as Traub (1938b) had pointed out, "on the whole, the animals appeared to age sooner than uninfected mice". Organs from neonatal carrier mice were weighed by Baker and Hotchin (1967) 10 to 16 months after infection and were found to be lighter than those from control animals. Histologically, a marked glomerulonephritis with involvement of the capillary tufts, hyaline thickening of the basement membranes of the capillary loops, and perivascular infiltrations and a hepatitis with scattered areas of focal necrosis and inflammatory infiltrates were the most prominent alterations. Other organs were affected to a lesser extent (Hotchin *et al.*, 1963; Hotchin and Collins, 1964; Baker and Hotchin, 1967; Oldstone and Dixon, 1969). The ability to clear urea and creatinine from the blood was impaired in these mice (Baker and Hotchin, 1967). It is to be stressed that the extent of this "late-onset disease" was found to vary considerably in neonatally LCM virus-infected mice (Hotchin and Collins, 1964; Oldstone and Dixon, 1968a; 1969; Oldstone *et al.*, 1969). In some virus-mouse strain combinations it did not develop at all (Volkert and Hannover Larsen, 1965c; Oldstone and Dixon, 1969; Mims, personal communication).

The situation is different with congenitally infected mice. Outwardly these animals appear to be quite healthy. Thus, POLLARD *et al.* (1968b) found neither growth rates nor litter sizes to be reduced, but most investigators noticed some changes. TRAUB (1938b) observed that mice, infected *in utero*, grew slightly slower than noninfected ones. WEIGAND and HOTCHIN (1961) noticed a slight retardation of the growth rate around the tenth day in infant mice born to neonatal carriers. SEAMER (1965a) recorded smaller litters and increased mortality in the 14 days after birth, as compared with controls. According to TRAUB (1941), more mice died in an established carrier colony from lymphomatosis and noninfectious diseases (no details given) during a 12 months' observation period as compared with non-infected controls kept in parallel. MIMS (1968) observed slower growth and a reduced reproductive capacity in congenital carrier mice. Recently, he summarized his observations on established WE virus carriers extending over a period of 600 days (MIMS, personal communication). The birth weights were normal, but the litter sizes were significantly smaller. Carriers grew slower and remained lighter than normal mice. Throughout their lives, the mortality was increased. Many mice were wasted when one year old. In 15 to 20 members of the colony muscular dystrophy developed at the age of three weeks to nine months, leading to paralyses, mainly of the lower part of the body. Signs and histopathology closely resembled those seen in inbred strain 129 mice with dystrophia muscularis, a hereditary myopathy described by MICHELSON *et al.* (1955).

These definite, if irregular, signs of retardation are reflected by pathological changes, first reported by TRAUB (1936b) more than 30 years ago. Enlarged spleens, interstitial inflammation of the lungs and livers, and hyperplasia of the reticuloendothelial system were irregular findings. However, seven of seven mice had kidney lesions which ranged from small inflamed areas to marked interstitial nephritis. (Traub did not specify at what time during their ontogenesis these mice had made contact with the virus; it may be inferred that at least some were congenital carriers.) In later studies, TRAUB and KESTING (1963) observed enlarged lymph nodes and spleens in congenital carriers after the third week of their life. A subacute glomerular nephritis, though not of the interstitial type, was also noted by WILSNACK and ROWE (1964) in mice from an established carrier colony. In his first report on established carrier mice, MIMS (1966) had emphasized that "pathological changes are almost absent". Later, however, he observed severe anemia, glomerulonephritis, and liver infiltrates in many of these animals (MIMS, personal communication).

POLLARD *et al.* (1968a; 1968b) described widespread lesions in brain and all internal organs, notably the kidneys, of gnotobiotically raised mice older than one month from an LCM virus carrier colony of long standing. In later life, some of these mice had tumors in lymphoid organs and lungs (see Section IV. B). In tumor free animals, the thymuses were depleted of cortical thymocytes and the medullary areas were swollen. Lymph nodes and spleens contained large germinal zones and numerous plasma cells. The infiltrates in the visceral organs had become extensive. The most characteristic changes in the kidneys were extensions of swollen cytoplasms of endothelial cells into the capillary lumina which were greatly reduced. More recently, Pollard and his collaborators reported on an extension of this work. POLLARD and SHARON (1969) found the organs of these germ free carrier mice free of lesions up to the age of four months although lymph nodes and spleens were enlarged and had prominent germinal zones. With increasing age, immuno-proliferative changes became extensive. Numerous plasma cells, many of which contained Russell bodies, accumulated in the organs. In the viscera perivascular lymphoid infiltrations were so extensive as to replace portions of the parenchyma. Lymphoma-like changes were noted in some of the mice (see Section IV. B). In 2 of 20 "apparently healthy" mice and in an additional animal which had died at the age of three months, Kajima and Pollard (1969) detected mild to severe degenerative vascular alterations indicating the presence of necrotizing arteritis of small and medium sized arteries and arterioles in various tissues, especially in kidneys and spleens. In fully developed lesions complete obliteration was associated with extensive fibrinoid necrosis of the entire thickness of the vessel wall which extended occasionally beyond the adventitia. Varying numbers of nuclei, nuclear debris, and erythrocytes were embedded in large PAS positive eosinophilic fibrinoid masses which, on occasion, showed a lamellar pattern.

Undoubtedly, the changes as seen by Pollard and his colleagues are much more severe than the ones seen by all other investigators. Since the mice came from a carrier colony established 30 years ago, no uninfected animals from the same origin were available for comparison, and control mice had to be taken from an entirely different stock. It would have been preferable if a carrier colony had been established anew by neonatal infection. In this case alterations in the first few generations of congenitally LCM virus-infected mice could have been compared with uninfected controls raised and maintained in parallel.

In conclusion, while the pathological signs differ quantitatively between neonatally and congenitally induced carriers, none are entirely free and hence neither qualifies as a true example of latent infection.

As will be discussed later (see Section V. A. 5) virus was frequently found to persist up to months in the organs or even the blood of mice infected after maturation. Whether this is the rule is not known but seems doubtful. In contrast to Volkert and Hannover Larsen (1965c) we shall not consider such mice true carriers.

A question of great practical importance is how a laboratory mouse colony may be controlled for infestation with the LCM virus. Traub (1935a; 1935b; 1936a) had reported that persistent infections could be made clinically apparent by the intracerebral inoculation of inert material such as bacteriological broth. This observation was confirmed by Findlay *et al.* (1936) and Lépine and Sautter (1936). In spite of the fact that Traub (1936c) soon withdrew his statement, intracerebral provocation for the detection of the LCM virus carrier state has become a widely recommended procedure (Dingle, 1941; Maurer, 1958; 1964; Trum and Routledge, 1967).

It is no longer possible to find out why in early reports nonspecific irritation of the brain should have led to overt disease. Traub (1936c) thought that these mice were in the process of undergoing a contact infection and that the damage of the brain merely precipitated the clinical signs. Hotchin and Cinits (1958; Hotchin, 1958) provoked cerebral signs by injection of broth two to six days after an intraperitoneal infection, but Lépine *et al.* (1937a) never induced a typical disease in mice by intracerebral inoculation of broth after peripheral infection, and Lehmann-Grube

(1964a) did not see typical LCM signs develop in mice infected intraperitoneally and inoculated at the same time intracerebrally with 0.03 ml of gelatin saline. Whatever the reason, it is to be stressed emphatically that there is no known way to induce an acute LCM disease in a carrier mouse (HOTCHIN and CINITS, 1958; HOTCHIN, 1958; WILSNACK, 1966; PETERSON and MAKSUDOVA, 1969; HANNOVER LARSEN, personal communication; LEHMANN-GRUBE, unpublished), with the possible exception of the injection of endotoxin which was found by HOTCHIN (1962a) to cause typical LCM disease in neonatal carriers when ten months but not when five weeks old. Infection of neonatal carriers with *E. coccoides* had insignificant consequences (HOTCHIN, 1965). MIMS and SUBRAHMANYAN (1966) tried, without success, to alter the pattern of immunofluorescence in mature carrier mice by various stimuli, such as inoculation of cortisone or endotoxin, exposure to cold, starvation, pregnancy.

The most simple way to check a mouse stock is by intracerebral inoculation of, say, 1000 LD_{50} of a strain which is known to be 100 per cent lethal, *e.g.* the E-350 strain of Armstrong. If all inoculated mice succumb, the colony may be regarded free. Otherwise, organ homogenates are inoculated into virus free mice. If typical signs develop five or more days later, the causative agent is identified serologically by standard procedures (SMADEL and WALL, 1941).

4. Pathogenesis

a) *Multiplication and Distribution of the Virus*

The multiplication of the LCM virus in the mouse and its distribution throughout the body have been frequently described (LÉPINE and SAUTTER, 1936; RIVERS and SCOTT, 1936a; TRAUB, 1936a; LÉPINE *et al.*, 1937a; YAMADA, 1940a; MILZER, 1942; HAAS, 1954; ROWE, 1954; TRAUB, 1960b; SEAMER *et al.*, 1963; LEHMANN-GRUBE, 1964a; GLADKIJ, 1965). According to HAAS (1954), ROWE (1954), and TRAUB (1961a), the intracerebral inoculation is followed by a marked eclipse. The rates of intracerebral multiplication are rather uniform and do not vary between strains as different as E-350 and WE (see Fig. 7). HAAS (1954) removed brains

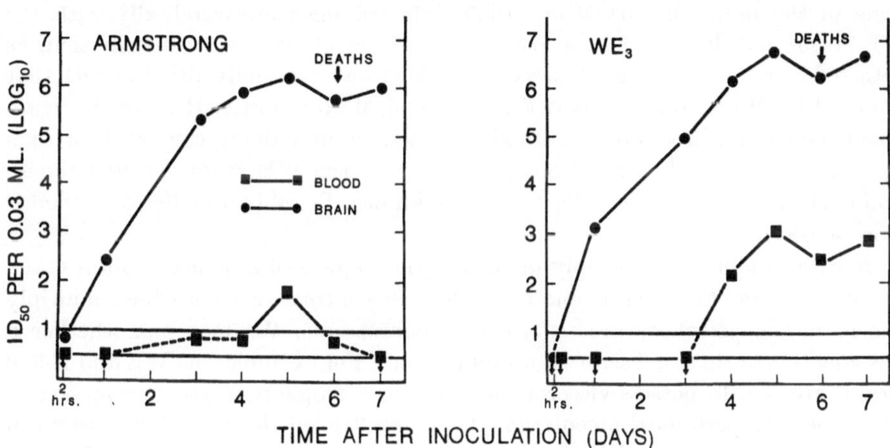

Fig. 7. Multiplication of LCM virus strains Armstrong (E-350) and WE in the mouse brain. From F. LEHMANN-GRUBE: Arch. ges. Virusforsch. 14, 344 (1964)

after infection and kept them at 36° C in saline or mouse serum. No eclipse occurred and the infectivity decreased slowly, which is what one would expect if, after intracerebral inoculation, the LCM virus multiplied predominantly in nerve cells which may be expected to lose their viability quickly under such conditions.

Many LCM virus strains multiply well in tissues other than the central nervous system. Indeed, some of them reach higher titers in livers or spleens than in brains. SHWARTZMAN (1946) determined the ability of strains WE, FA, and WWS after many serial intracerebral passages in mice or intracerebral and subcutaneous passages in guinea-pigs (mouse or guinea-pig substrains, respectively) to multiply in the organs of the mouse. After the intracerebral inoculation, all substrains multiplied well in the brain, but only those which had been passaged in guinea-pigs reached high concentrations in liver, spleen, and lungs and lower ones in the blood. In contrast, the mouse substrains did not make their appearance in the blood and were found irregularly in the viscera. After the intraperitoneal inoculation no significant differences were found among the strains. Shwartzman failed to detect any of the substrains — which included WE — in the brain after the intraperitoneal administration. This contrasts with my own data which show that the WE virus appeared in the mouse brain and multiplied there to a high titer after intraperitoneal infection (LEHMANN-GRUBE, 1964a).

REMEZOV and TOPLENINOVA (1961) determined immunofluorescing antigen in brains and spleens. In the former, it appeared 24 hours after intracerebral or intranasal infection, either focally or in single cells, with increase in the following days. After subcutaneous infection, it made its appearance in the brain after three to five days. In the spleen, first immunofluorescing antigen was detected three, one, and four days after intracerebral, subcutaneous, and intranasal infections, respectively.

WILSNACK and ROWE (1964) infected mice intracerebrally with the CA 1371 strain and found immunofluorescence as early as 24 hours later in meninges, choroid plexus, and ependyma but — significantly — never in neurones. After the intraperitoneal infection with strain WCP, immunofluorescing antigen appeared after 72 hours in liver parenchyma, bronchi, alveolar cells, and in the reticular cells of the red pulp of the spleen. Little antigen was detected in the kidneys and none in the brain. BENDA *et al.* (1965) infected mice intracerebrally with the WE strain and determined the pattern of intracerebral antigen distribution, as detected by indirect immunofluorescence, which was essentially identical with that reported by WILSNACK and ROWE (see above). More recently, HRONOVSKÝ *et al.* (1969) employing the direct method detected immunofluorescing antigen in a certain number of neurones from the cortex of the WE strain-infected mouse brain. The reason for these differences is unknown. Possibly, the direct method is more sensitive.

A strain's ability to multiply in the internal organs of a mouse is often taken as evidence for its viscerotropic character; in contrast, strains which multiply poorly in the periphery are regarded as neurotropic. We may ask whether a classification of this kind serves a useful purpose. For example, the WE and E-350 strains are said to possess viscerotropic and neurotropic properties, respectively. After the intraperitoneal inoculation, E-350 multiplied slower to lower titers in livers and kidneys than WE (LEHMANN-GRUBE, unpublished); little E-350 virus appeared for short periods of time in the brain, whereas the WE strain reached high intracerebral levels. Whatever the route of inoculation, a low viremia of short duration was observed with E-350, whereas WE could be detected in the circulation at high levels for long periods. In contrast, after intracerebral inoculation no differences were observed (Fig. 7); both strains multiplied equally well in the brain (LEHMANN-GRUBE, 1964a). We conclude that, if the WE strain is to be characterized, invasiveness is the criterion which stands out, and, although it is descriptive too, it has the advantage of not being misleading.

An important question is whether LCM virus is capable of multiplying in cells belonging to the immune apparatus of the host, *i.e.*, the lymphoid system. That it may do so in lymph nodes was shown by TRAUB (1964) who followed the virus multiplication in regional nodes after subcutaneous infection. Titers increased rapidly, reached their maxima around the fifth day and declined thereafter. HANAOKA *et al.* (1969) followed the virus concentration in spleens, lymph nodes, and thymuses of mice after intracerebral infection of the WE strain and found steep increases with maxima around the fifth day; serum titers were always lower. Participation of lymphoid cells may be deduced from the observation reported by MIMS (1966) that many such cells in spleens, lymph nodes, and thymuses of mice from an established carrier colony contained LCM-specific antigen as determined by immunofluorescence. Later MIMS and WAINWRIGHT (1968) mentioned that in mice, infected after birth or after maturation, lymphoid cells contained immunofluorescing antigen. By the same method, WILSNACK and ROWE (1964) detected antigen in "a few" lymphocytes in the white pulp of the spleen in intraperitoneally infected weanling mice. BROWN (1968) followed the distribution of antigen by immunofluorescence after neonatal infection. A few circulating lymphoid cells with specific fluorescence were first seen two days after infection. Their number increased and was high on the fifth day. By the same method BARATAWIDJAJA *et al.* (1965) saw viral antigen in "leucocytes" of mice from the seventh day after infection until death. On the ninth day the buffy coat was found to be infectious.

Whereas these observations seem to indicate that at least some lymphoid elements become infected and produce detectable amounts of immunofluorescing antigen, experiments performed *in vitro* have failed to prove that such cells are infectable. SCHWENK, SLENCZKA, and LEHMANN-GRUBE (to be published) separated circulating lymphocytes from mouse blood by means of a glass bead column according to RABINOWITZ (1964) and brought them into contact with LCM virus, strains WE or E-350. Although the cells could be shown by dye exclusion tests to have retained their viability, they neither became immunofluorescence positive nor produced infectious progeny in up to five days. In contrast, after transformation by phytohemagglutinin, virus was readily made which may be regarded as further proof that these cells were functionally intact. Furthermore, the virus content of lymphocytes separated from the blood of persistently LCM virus-infected mice was so low [*ca* 10^{-3} ID_{50} (mouse) per cell] as to exclude the possibility that these cells might have participated in the replication of the virus. Finally, peripheral lymphocytes from carrier mice were readily stimulated by phytohemagglutinin as detected by both morphological transformation and increased incorporation of tritium-labeled thymidine. It may be mentioned in passing that this latter finding reveals a probably profound difference between the persistent infection of the mouse with LCM virus and the prolonged infection of human babies born with the rubella syndrome where the peripheral lymphocytes exhibit marked functional abnormalities (Olson *et al.*, 1968). Thus, the answer to the question whether potential immune cells of the mouse participate in the infectious process may not be given with confidence and has to be deferred until more information has become known.

In the case of macrophages the situation is clearer. Seamer (1965b) infected mouse macrophage cultures and found that both the WHI and the UBC (= WE) strains multiplied to high titers without cytopathic effects. Mims and Subrahmanyan (1966) detected immunofluorescence in 95 per cent of mouse macrophages infected *in vitro* with the WE virus. These observations were confirmed in this laboratory by Schwenk *et al.* (to be published). There is no reason to assume that macrophages in the mouse should behave differently. This supposition is strengthened by the finding of Gledhill *et al.* (1965) that infection of the mouse with the WE strain of LCM virus led to depression of the phagocytic activity which was assayed by measuring the clearance rate of carbon particles from the circulation. As compared with virulent mouse hepatitis "3" and ectromelia viruses the depression was moderate.

b) Pathogenetic Mechanisms

The prominent feature of the interaction between LCM virus and the mouse is that intracerebral inoculation of the adult mouse with the virus is followed by overt disease and death, while the introduction of the virus before or soon after birth leads to a virtually nonpathogenic lifelong carrier state. The immunological significance of this apparent paradox was recognized by Burnet and Fenner (1949) who postulated that the virus becomes part of the animal's antigenic composition when introduced during immunological immaturity, being treated as "self", *i.e.* as nonantigenic, thereafter. This concept implies that the virus itself is quite harmless for the mouse (Burnet, 1955) whose fate is determined solely by an interaction between the virus as antigen and the host's immune mechanisms. Accordingly, the overt disease following the intracerebral inoculation is seen to result from an immunological conflict (Hotchin, 1958; Hotchin and Cinits, 1958) and the carrier state is made possible by a specific immunological hyporesponsiveness known as immunological tolerance. Additional manifestations of the interaction between virus and mouse are the subclinical course which often follows peripheral infection and the late-onset disease which may appear late in the life of a persistently infected mouse. Since the nonpathogenicity for the host cell may be regarded an essential prerequisite for the immunological events to take their course, this aspect will be discussed first.

Ideally, the congenital infection of the mouse with LCM virus may be expected to be latent. This, however, is not the case; pathology does develop (see Section V. A. 3). The question then is, whether these signs are due to direct effects of the virus upon the infected cells and tissues, or whether they represent an abortive immunological conflict in an animal whose immunologic response is specifically reduced. In the mouse cellular events are inevitably confounded with the complex response on the part of the whole animal, be this immunological or otherwise. Therefore, an *in vitro* model was sought and was found in Earle's L cells (Lehmann-Grube, 1967a; Lehmann-Grube *et al.*, 1969; see Section III. C). After infection, L cells and virus attained an equilibrium whereby the cells were morphologically and functionally not distinguishable from the noninfected controls although continuously producing virus. In his review on viral carrier states in cells *in vitro*, WALKER (1964) singled out four different types of carrier cultures: (I) infections of genetically resistant cells; (II) infections of genetically susceptible cells protected by antiviral factors in the medium; (III) infections of genetically susceptible cells protected by interference and interferon; (IV) regulated infections.

According to Walker, regulated infections of cells in culture have the following characteristics: (1) antibody or other antiviral factors need not be supplied in the culture medium in order to maintain an equilibrium; (2) the culture is not cured by addition of antiserum to the medium; (3) the culture is resistant to superinfection by the infecting virus and may show some resistance to related and little or no resistance to unrelated viruses; (4) all or most of the cells are infected when the culture is stable; (5) single infected cells divide and grow into colonies, most of which are infected. By comparing these criteria with our experimental results (see Section III. C), it is apparent that the LCM virus-L cell carrier cultures belong in this category.

The term "regulated infections of cells in culture" stresses the role the cell plays in maintaining the equilibrium. FERNANDES *et al.* (1964) have characterized the persistent infection of rabbit endothelium cells with rabies virus as "endosymbiosis" which places the emphasis on the mutuality of the virus-cell relationship. For our understanding of the phenomenon, this approach of thought appears to be essential. The virus must contribute to this coexistence by not introducing the information for either a block of cell-directed metabolism or the destruction of the infected cell, as is known for many other viruses. The cell, on the other hand, must exert a regulatory control on the synthesis of viral material. Speculations as to the underlying mechanisms are hardly justified with the present knowledge. One even cannot be quite certain that the part of the metabolism of LCM virus-infected cells which is directed towards the cells' own functioning is unaltered in the mouse, as it appears to be the case in L cells. What may be true in transformed cells *in vitro*, may be altogether different with highly differentiated parenchyma cells *in vivo*. However, at the present time there is no cogent reason to deny the applicability of the knowledge gained *in vitro* to the situation pertaining to the mouse and, hence, we may conclude that the infection of the cell in the animal is likewise self-regulated, being nonpathogenic by itself, and that the pathological signs in neonatally as well as congenitally infected mice are caused indirectly by, probably, the host's immune response to the virus infection (see below).

There is one observation which does not fit into our notion that the virus itself is essentially harmless for the cells it has invaded. Before an equilibrium is attained, some cells infected persistently *in vitro* go through an initial stage of morphological and functional alterations (see Section III. C). In order to answer the obvious question, whether this applies also to mouse cells *in vivo*, the following experiment was performed (LEHMANN-GRUBE, unpublished) which was based on the assumption that no allergic reactions would interfere during the first days of life in neonatally infected mice. Litters of outbred laboratory mice were brought to equal size, *i.e.* eight animals each. (No litter was included which lost more than one member during the observation period.) The mice were inoculated intraperitoneally when less than 24 hours old with 10,000 ID_{50} (titrated intracerebrally in weaned mice) of virus, strains E-350 or WE, and their growth was followed by weighing, usually twice daily. From Figure 8 it is obvious that the rate of growth was not

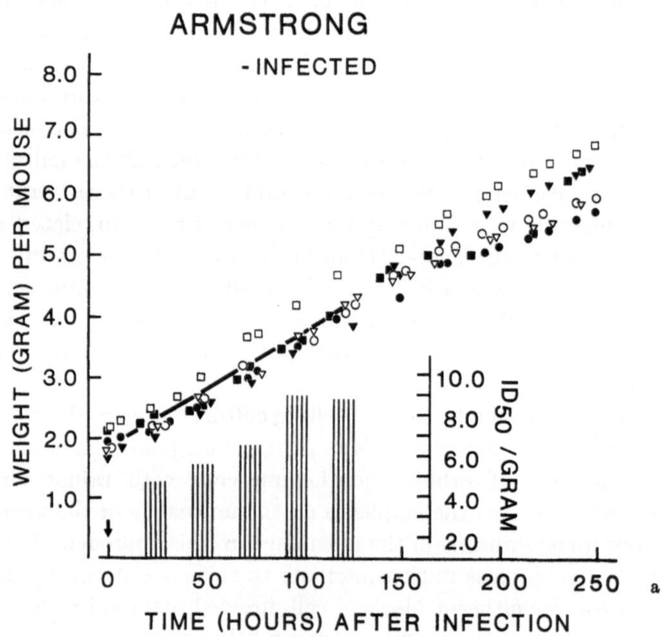

a

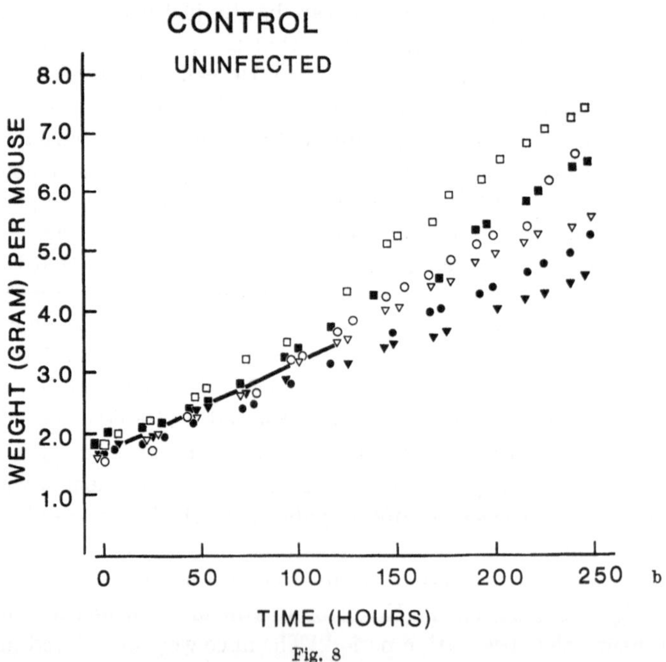

b

Fig. 8

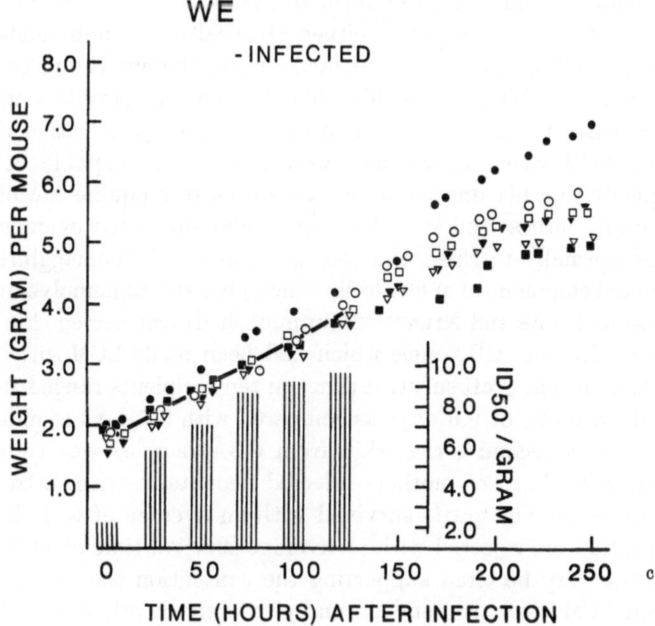

Fig. 8. Growth (as determined by weight measurements) of mice infected with LCM virus when less than 24 hours old. Differently shaped symbols represent different litters and bars denote infectivity (mouse ID_{50}) per gram of tissues

affected at all by the virus infection for at least five days. The visual impression is confirmed by the results from a mathematical analysis. The regression coefficients, weight (gram) on time (hour) after infection, are 0.017, 0.019, and 0.015 for strains WE- and Armstrong-infected and normal mice, respectively. Thus, we may conclude that the early cytopathic effect in carrier cultures is a peculiarity of some persistently infected cultivated cells and has no analogy *in vivo*.

After having shown that the virus is harmless for the cell it has invaded, the question has to be asked, why is it not eliminated by the host's immune mechanisms? The answer is that the host is incapable of doing so because it has acquired a state of immunological tolerance to the virus (BURNET and FENNER, 1949; HOTCHIN, 1961; VOLKERT, 1965; VOLKERT and HANNOVER LARSEN, 1965c; HANNOVER LARSEN, 1968a).

Immunological tolerance (BILLINGHAM *et al.*, 1953; 1955/56) has been extensively described and its biological significance discussed recently by DRESSER and MITCHISON (1968) and HRABA (1968). The main characteristics are as follows: it is a "state of indifference or nonreactivity towards a substance that would normally be expected to excite an immunological response" (MEDAWAR, 1961); the host is altered and not the antigen; tolerance is specifically directed towards the antigen which has induced it; it is systemic; it is central in the sense that the immunologically competent cell is affected. Of these criteria, the first three have been shown experimentally to apply to the LCM virus-mouse system.

It was clearly demonstrated by TRAUB and SCHÄFER (1939) and has been confirmed many times since that carrier mice, besides their inability to eliminate the virus, have reduced ability to form antibody. VOLKERT *et al.* (1964) demonstrated that the virus from carriers was neither physically nor immunologically different from the usual mouse to mouse passage virus, thereby ruling out the hypothesis put forward by HERRIOTT (1961) that the nonresponsiveness in LCM virus carrier mice is due to the appearance of naked nucleic acids rather than of complete virions. LCM virus carrier mice were found fully capable of responding immunologically to other unrelated viruses, *e.g.* eastern equine encephalomyelitis (TRAUB, 1961b). MIMS and WAINWRIGHT (1968) presented evidence that such mice reacted normally to sheep red cells as measured by hemagglutinin production and the development of spleen cells which give rise to hemolyzing plaques in agar. LEHMANN-GRUBE and NIEMEYER (unpublished) transferred skin grafts from normal AKR mice onto CBA mice which had been made LCM virus carriers by neonatal infection. The graft survival times in ten recipients ranged from eight to ten days with a mean of 9.6 days as compared with 9.4 days in nine uninfected control mice. In a second series, skin from CBA/Ca mice was transplanted to 13 AKR recipients born of mothers infected neonatally with LCM virus (first generation carriers). The grafts survived with an average of 10.1 days, whereas 14 control grafts were rejected with an average survival time of 11.4 days. Thus, ample evidence may be cited supporting the contention that mice, persistently infected with LCM virus, respond normally to antigens other than those of viral origin.

Adoptive immunization (MITCHISON, 1953; 1954) is known to terminate tolerance (BILLINGHAM *et al.*, 1953; 1955/56). In the case of LCM virus carrier mice this has been studied extensively by Volkert and Hannover Larsen. After the inoculation of lymph node and spleen cells from LCM-immune AKR donors into AKR recipients, which had been made carriers by neonatal infection, the virus concentration in the blood, which normally varied between $10^{4.7}$ and $10^{6.8}$ LD_{50} per ml, was reduced by more than 1000-fold, reaching lowest levels six weeks after transplantation. At least 50 times 10^6 cells were needed for optimal effects, but even with smaller numbers virus titers dropped significantly although later and less regularly. Cells from nonimmunized donors irregularly caused some virus reduction. No effects on viremia were obtained when donor cells had been frozen once or when they came from allogeneic (C3H) donors. Nor was the virus level in the carriers reduced by plasma from hyperimmunized syngeneic donors. The cells functioned equally well when given intravenously or intraperitoneally (VOLKERT, 1962; 1963).

VOLKERT (1963) having worked with AKR mice had emphasized that sex differences between donors and recipients did not noticeably influence the results, but recently HANNOVER LARSEN (personal communication) — using C3H mice — demonstrated that male to female transplantation led only to a temporary abolition of persistent infection; viremia returned after about four weeks and antibody levels slowly fell.

Cells from the buffy coat of the blood from immune mice likewise suppressed viremia and induced antibody, although significantly less vigorously than spleen and lymph node cells. Up to 10^8 thymus cells and 10^7 peritoneal exudate cells, consisting of 90 per cent macrophages, had only slight effects (HANNOVER LARSEN, personal communication).

The low levels of virus titer in carrier recipients were found to be permanent. After the transplantation of excessively high numbers of cells, blood and most organs were found to be entirely free of infectivity. Traces, however, were always detected, particularly in the kidneys (VOLKERT and HANNOVER LARSEN, 1964). Since even in mice actively immunized by infection virus was detected many months later (see Section V.A. 5), the incomplete virus elimination in LCM-immune mice is not unique for carriers which have acquired their immunity adoptively.

Marked quantitative differences were noted by VOLKERT and HANNOVER LARSEN (1965c) between mouse strains. Under otherwise identical conditions both virus reduction and appearance of antibody was faster and more pronounced in C3H as compared with AKR mice.

Lymphoid cells from recipient carriers had little effect on other carriers when sub-transplanted one day after primary inoculation. However, cells harvested one week later effectively suppressed viremia in the new host. This quality of cells in transplanted carriers remained unaltered for at least two months (VOLKERT *et al.*, 1964). Large numbers of allogeneic immune cells, *i.e.* cells from other mouse strains, depressed the virus titers for short periods only. Undoubtedly, the donor cells were immunologically destroyed by the recipients, thereby preventing their prolonged activity. Additional transplants from mice genetically different to the first donor had no effect. Presumably, common antigens among the donors caused an accelerated second-set response (VOLKERT and HANNOVER LARSEN, 1965b). As many as eight times 10^8 immune lymphoid rat cells were without consequences (HANNOVER LARSEN, personal communication). These observations further underline the specificity of the immunological suppression in LCM virus carrier mice (see above). UPHOFF and HAAS (1960) were not able to terminate the carrier state in X-irradiated recipients by transfer of bone marrow from hyperimmunized nonsyngeneic donors, which may be explained by the low immunologic capacity of marrow cells and the use of a histoincompatible donor-recipient combination. It is not clear why HOTCHIN (1965) did not succeed in demonstrating a depression of viremia in persistently infected mice up to six weeks after an intravenous inoculation of three times 10^7 lymphoid and thymus cells from histocompatible LCM-immune donors.

A most interesting observation with adoptively immunized carrier mice is the production of antibody with concentrations never seen in hyperimmunized mice and, indeed, hardly ever seen in any host-antigen combination. Complement fixation titers, which at best come to 256 after hyperimmunization, soared to almost 10,000 and neutralizing antibody, which appears in low concentrations in infected mice (see Section V.A. 5), reached indices of up to 10^4. In contrast to the depression of virus, however, these antibodies slowly disappeared (VOLKERT *et al.*, 1964). Passive transfer of large amounts of such high titered antisera alone or in combination with transplantation of allogeneic immune cells only incompletely and temporarily depressed the levels of viremia in the recipient carriers (VOLKERT and HANNOVER LARSEN, 1965b). Implantation into carrier mice of Millipore chambers containing syngeneic immune lymphoid cells had hardly any effect on virus titers, although neutralizing activities were much higher than, and complement fixation activities about as high as, in mice free of virus due to active immunization (Hannover Larsen, 1968a). These observations indicate that the antibody is not responsible for the disappearance of virus (see below). Since in mice not carrying the virus transplantation of syngeneic immune lymphoid cells induced antibody in titers such as are seen after ordinary immunization procedures, Volkert and Hannover Larsen (1965c; Hannover Larsen and Volkert, 1967) explain the development of excessively high antibody levels — fully confirmed by Slenczka and Lehmann-Grube (unpublished) — as being caused by the constant contact of the transplanted cells with high concentrations of antigen in the carrier host. I favor another explanation. In essence, the same observation was made by Möller (1968) who inoculated spleen cells from mice immunized with sheep red blood cells into syngeneic X-irradiated recipients, together with the antigen. The number of hemolytic plaque-forming cells recovered from the recipients was much higher than in the hyperimmunized donors. Hemagglutinin and hemolysin titers were likewise increased. Since the number of antibody-producing cells was much lower when the recipients had been immunized before irradiation or were given specific antibody passively, Möller concluded that the mechanism responsible for the excessive immune response in the immunologically incapacitated recipient of the transplanted immunologically activated cells plus antigen was absence of regulatory effects by early specific antibody. An analogous mechanism may be held responsible for the high antibody titers in transplanted carrier mice. Certainly, this very interesting phenomenon deserves further exploration.

An entirely different picture evolved when the persistently infected recipients were transplanted with 10^8 to 10^9 cells from syngeneic nonimmune donors. Although in a few mice virus concentrations were permanently reduced to trace levels, in many the virus titers did not change at all, while in still others transient drops occurred. Since antibody titers likewise showed variations, altogether five patterns of response were distinguished, and we encounter here another example of the already mentioned fact that antibody and virus concentrations in LCM virus-infected mice vary independently of each other (Hannover Larsen and Volkert, 1967).

As the great number of infected house mice show (see Section X. A. 1), the LCM virus carrier state is a natural phenomenon in mice. By way of contrast, this cannot be said of the LCM disease, which may be expected to occur under natural conditions only when a carrier infects a normal animal by contact. This, from the behavior of *M. musculus* (Freye and Freye, 1960), undoubtedly is a rare event. Lymphocytic choriomeningitis of the mouse is essentially an artificial disease produced in the laboratory.

The concept that clinical signs and death in mice infected as adults are allergic phenomena was first clearly stated by Hotchin and Cinits (1958; Hotchin, 1958). Reviews have been published by Hotchin (1961; 1962a). It is a peculiar but characteristic property of the LCM virus never to cause signs of disease in the nonsensitized mouse before the fifth day after infection irrespective of the dose inoculated, even though, after large inocula, maximum titers in the tissues might have been reached as early as on the second day. It is to be stressed that the characteristic convulsions in mice following the intracerebral inoculation are seen also with other viruses, *e.g.* influenza (Henle and Henle, 1946). However, the sudden onset, not before the fifth day, in animals which had appeared to be quite healthy a few hours previously is unique for the LCM virus. Histopathological changes, likewise, were found to make their appearance long after maximum virus concentrations had been reached (Rowe, 1954). These observations indicate that indirect mechanisms are responsible for the development of pathology; their immunological nature is strongly suggested by the early observation made by Traub (1938b) and confirmed by Rowe (1954) that some time after an immunizing infection, *i.e.* during a period of waning immunity, signs but usually not death follow the intracerebral infection after a significantly reduced latent period, which was interpreted by Traub (1938b; 1939a) as signifying an allergic state. Such accelerated reactions could be elicited by Traub (1962a) as early as 46 days after the immunizing subcutaneous infection. Rowe (1954) studied the pattern of intracerebral infectivity in these mice after challenge. It was indistinguishable from the one in control mice for three days. Thereafter, the titers declined more rapidly. Moderate to severe meningitis was present as early as the second day (Traub, 1938b; Rowe, 1954). Of interest is Rowe's finding that in the few animals which demonstrated signs of an accelerated response for six or seven days the titers in the brains had already markedly declined, indicating that the antigen responsible for the immune conflict is not identical with the fully infectious virus.

Comparable in significance to the accelerated response is the shortening of the latent period relative to the intracerebral inoculation by a prior peripheral infection which, by itself, is of low pathogenicity (Haas, 1954; Rowe, 1954). This phenomenon was confirmed and quantitatively elucidated by Seamer and his colleagues (Seamer and Hotchin, 1961; Seamer *et al.*, 1963) who used the UBC (= WE) strain. Shortening of the latent period relative to the intracerebral inoculation was not accompanied by an altered pattern of virus multiplication in the brain. When the WHI strain was employed, peripheral sensitization was less effective. The authors interpreted their results as indicating the development of sensitivity to the virus, causing illness and death when coinciding with a high virus concentration, especially in the brain. Haas (1954) found the latent period to be shortened if intracerebral or intraperitoneal infection was followed by repeated intraperitoneal inoculations. For this there exists no ready explanation; possibly, the development of allergy was hastened under these circumstances.

The immunological responsiveness of the mouse matures quickly after birth, and there is a limited time period during which a critical level of antigen must be reached to block effectively the immunological apparatus. Thus, whether immunological tolerance or immunity, as defined here (see Section I. A), to the antigen ensues will depend on the age of the animal and the rate of its immunological maturation which is known to differ significantly between strains of mice (Hechtel *et al.*, 1965; Playfair, 1968), as well as on the dose of the virus and its rate of multiplication. Of these, only the age factor has been studied adequately. The early finding by Traub that mice infected shortly after birth become carriers while adults respond with disease or active immunity was later extended by Hotchin and Cinits (1958; Hotchin, 1958), Hotchin and Weigand (1960; 1961a), Traub (1960b), Hotchin *et al.* (1962), and Peterson and Maksudova (1969) who all showed that the ability to respond clinically to the infection was age dependent and was established within a few days after birth. As Figure 9 shows, the curve which relates age with proportion of mice surviving intracerebral inoculation (Lehmann-Grube, unpublished data) has a striking similarity with the curve relating age with proportion of mice responding with tolerance following the

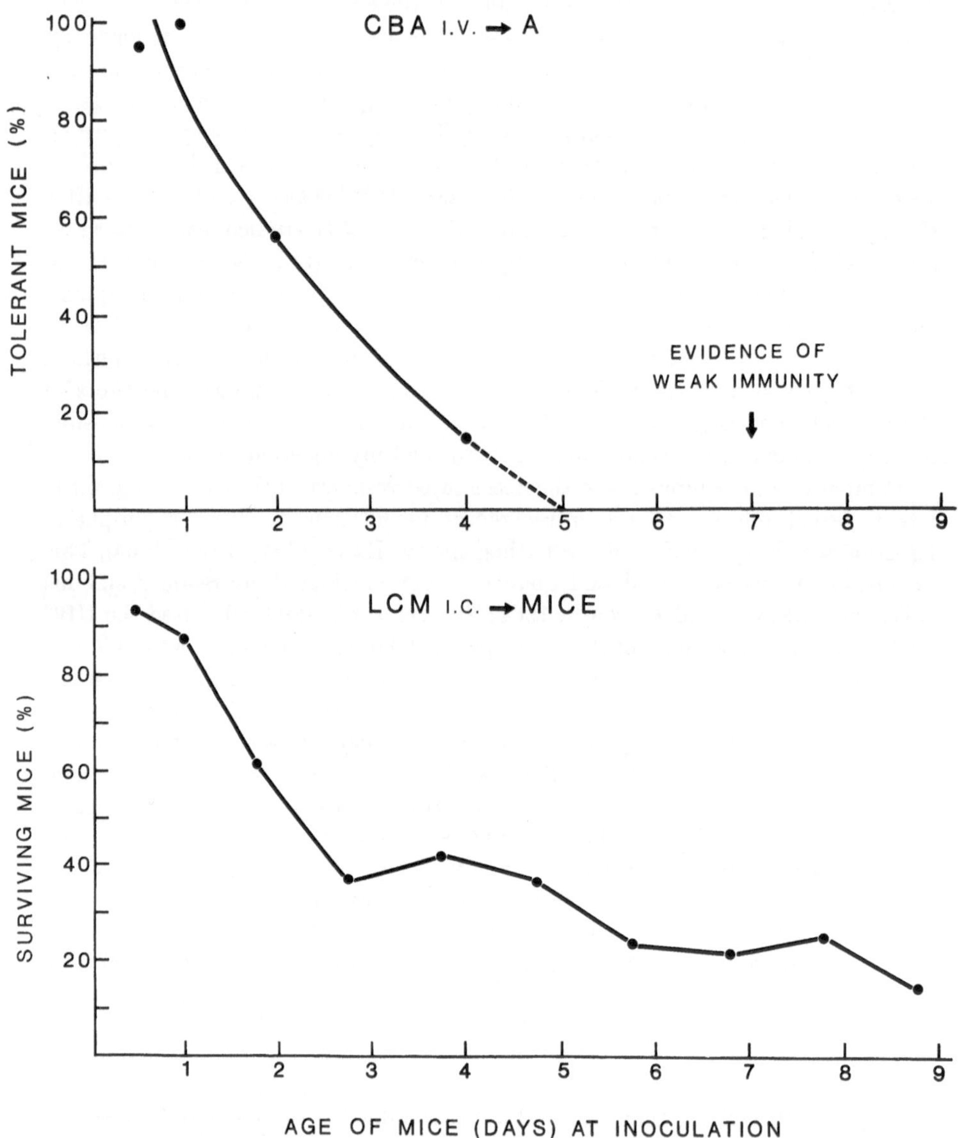

Fig. 9. Relationship between age of mice at time of intracerebral infection with LCM virus, strain E-350, and death rate in comparison with relationship between age of mice at inoculation of allogeneic spleen cells and occurrence of immunological tolerance. Upper part of the figure from R. E. Billingham and L. Brent: Transplant. Bull. 4, 67 (1957). (With permission of the authors and of the Williams and Wilkins Co., Baltimore.)

intravenous inoculation of allogeneic spleen cells (Billingham and Brent, 1957), lending further support to the idea that the LCM virus carrier state in mice represents true immunological tolerance. In older mice, higher doses of the WE strain virus were found necessary to cause signs and deaths (LEHMANN-GRUBE *et al.*, 1960). It is not known whether old animals are less susceptible to the infection or whether they are less prone to develop an immunological conflict.

An influence of the dose on the outcome of a neonatal infection was noted by HOTCHIN *et al.* (1962) who found large amounts of the UBC virus to be somewhat more effective in inducing persistent infection in Albany albino mice than small ones. A more pronounced effect was observed by LEHMANN-GRUBE (1964b). The proportion of Walter and Eliza Hall Institute mice, surviving the neonatal infection with strains Armstrong or WE, could be significantly increased by increasing the dose. Whether this effect was only dose dependent may be questioned, however, because together with the amount of virus the route was changed from intracerebral to intraperitoneal. No dose effect can be deduced from the data on Table 4.

VOLKERT and HANNOVER LARSEN (1965a) studied the opposite, *i.e.* the effect of low virus doses. After the intraperitoneal inoculation of one LD_{50} many newborn mice became persistently infected without responding serologically. A few had virus in their blood at concentrations as high as were found in typical carriers but also produced antibody, as after active immunization of mature mice, attaining complement fixation titers up to 256. Later all these animals lost the virus, but for some time before this high virus titers coexisted with high antibody concentrations. Apparently, in these mice sufficient antigen was not available initially to suppress the quickly developing immunological apparatus of the host.

Neither the rate of immunological maturation of the mouse nor the rate of viral multiplication have been studied in respect to their influence on the virulence of LCM virus in newborn mice. From the above considerations it may be expected that a virus which, under otherwise identical conditions, causes a high mortality in newborn mice multiplies at a slower rate than a strain of low pathogenicity. This conclusion may also be reached from the observation of HOTCHIN (1962a) that a concomitant inoculation of equal doses of two strains being of high and low pathogenicities, respectively, induced persistent infection rather than LCM disease in newborn mice.

Over the years a great variety of treatments have been shown to protect the adult mouse from death due to LCM virus infection (Table 5). Their common denominator is immunosuppression. None is specific in the sense that it inhibits exclusively the immunological response and, with the exception of neonatal thymectomy and treatment with antilymphocytic serum, none seems to act preferentially on the humoral or the cell-mediated mechanisms (BERENBAUM, 1967; GABRIELSEN and GOOD, 1967).

The sparing effect of X-rays in LCM virus-infected mice is well documented. Significantly, pretreatment with irradiation all but abolished the usual histopathological alterations in infected mice (ROWE, 1954; 1956; SCHLEIFSTEIN and COLLINS, 1960; COLLINS *et al.*, 1961), although virus multiplication was not affected (ROWE, 1954; 1956; HOTCHIN and WEIGAND, 1961b) or even augmented (MAKSUDOVA, 1967).

BENSON *et al.* (1960; HOTCHIN and WEIGAND, 1961b) counted the leukocytes after X-irradiation of LCM virus-infected and noninfected mice; the numbers were depressed to the same extent in both groups. MAKSUDOVA (1967) reported

Table 5. *Protection of Adult Mice from Disease due to Infection with the LCM Virus*

Treatment	Reference
X-Irradiation	ROWE (1954; 1956), HOTCHIN and CINITS (1958), HOTCHIN (1958), SCHLEIFSTEIN and COLLINS (1960), HOTCHIN and WEIGAND (1961b), COLLINS *et al.* (1961), MAKSUDOVA (1967), HANNOVER LARSEN (1969c)
Methotrexate (= Amethopterin)	HAAS and STEWART (1956), HAAS *et al.* (1957b), LERNER and HAAS (1958), LEVI and HAAS (1958), BARLOW and HOTCHIN (1961; 1963), SIDWELL *et al.* (1965), FURUSAWA *et al.* (1967), HANNOVER LARSEN (1969c)
Folic acid deficient diet	HAAS *et al.* (1957b)
8-Azaguanine (= Guanazolo)	HAAS and STEWART (1956)
5-Fluorouracil	LEVI and HAAS (1958)
Chlorambucil (= Leukeran)	BARLOW (1962)
1,3-Bis(2-chloroethyl)-1-nitrosourea	SIDWELL *et al.* (1965)
Azaserine	LEVI and HAAS (1958)
6-Diazo-5-oxo-nor-l-leucine (DON)	LEVI and HAAS (1958)
Thymectomy of the newborn	ROWE *et al.* (1963), LEVEY *et al.* (1963), EAST *et al.* (1964), HOTCHIN and SIKORA (1964), SIKORA (1964), MORI *et al.* (1964), FÖLDES *et al.* (1964; 1964/65; 1967), SZERI *et al.* (1966/67)
Antilymphocytic serum	GLEDHILL (1967), HIRSCH *et al.* (1967; 1968), HIRSCH and MURPHY (1967; 1968), MIMS (1969), MIMS and TOSOLINI (1969)
Graft *versus* host disease	KOLTAY *et al.* (1968; 1969)
High virus dosis	BENGTSON and WOOLEY (1936), HOTCHIN and BENSON (1963), HANNOVER LARSEN (1967; 1968b), LEHMANN-GRUBE (1969b; 1969c)

that with BALB/c mice the leukopenia following irradiation was even more marked in virus-infected animals as compared with noninfected (irradiated only) controls.

REMEZOV and YAKOVLEVA (1960) assayed the levels of properdin in the sera of mice after X-irradiation and LCM virus infection and found them to be reduced and increased, respectively. When both measures were combined, lower than normal concentrations were found after irradiations corresponding to 400 and 300 r, but higher than normal concentrations after 200, 100, or 10 r. Unexplained is the observation of HOTCHIN and CINITS (1958) that mice died in convulsions when intraperitoneal infection was preceded by X-rays.

The consequence of the injection of cortisone is more difficult to assess. Usually, this hormone enhances susceptibility of mice to viruses, such as West Nile, Ilheus, Bunyamwera (SOUTHAM and BABCOCK, 1951). HOTCHIN and CINITS (1958; HOTCHIN, 1958) observed extended survival times in LCM virus-infected mice treated with cortisone, but the controls died early from the drug alone. LEHMANN-GRUBE (unpublished) saw no prophylactic effect from doses below those which were highly toxic. HANNOVER LARSEN (1969c) treated mice with toxic doses of cortisone and observed a slight though not significant effect. In the treated group, 25 out of 60 mice survived 14 days while among the controls 5 out of 20 survived. Cortisone had no effect on duration of viremia and formation of antibody in intraperitoneally infected animals. Similar difficulties of interpretation were encountered by BARLOW and HOTCHIN (1961) who assayed the effects of 6-mercaptopurine and nitrogen mustard. Colchicine in nontoxic doses was also tried but did not exert protection.

Of further substances tested, the folic acid antagonist methotrexate (amethopterin) seems to have some effect on LCM disease. HANNOVER LARSEN (1969c) found it to be superior to cortisone or X-irradiation, but according to other authors, little protection is achieved (SIDWELL *et al.*, 1965; FURUSAWA *et al.*, 1967). In other systems, too, the efficacy of this compound is limited (HUMPHREYS *et al.*, 1963; BERENBAUM, 1960). Its action could be reversed completely by citrovorum factor (HAAS *et al.*, 1957b) but only partially by nucleic acid precursors, such as adenine, guanine, orotic acid, thymine, cytidine, and uridylic acid (LEVY and HAAS, 1958). Again, in spite of prevention of disease, virus multiplication was not inhibited (HAAS and STEWART, 1956; HAAS *et al.*, 1957b; LERNER and HAAS, 1958; BARLOW and HOTCHIN, 1961). BARLOW and HOTCHIN (1963) found that timing of treatment relative to infection depended on dose of virus. For optimal effects, peak of infectivity and maximum drug concentration must coincide. For instance, in the brains of mice, infected intracerebrally with 10^6 LD_{50}, the highest titers were reached after 48 hours; when infected with 10^2 LD_{50}, the same level was obtained a further 24 hours later. Thus, mice infected with 10^6 or 10^2 LD_{50} were best protected when amethopterin was given 48—72 or 96 hours, respectively, later. The histopathology in spared mice was ameliorated but not abolished (LERNER and HAAS, 1958).

Folic acid deficient diet, known to inhibit the formation of antibodies to various antigens (AXELROD and PRUZANSKY, 1955), was shown to reduce death due to LCM virus infection. Of the purine analogues, 8-azaguanine (guanazolo) and of the pyrimidine analogues, 5-fluorouracil have been found active although less so than amethopterin.

The alkylating agent chlorambucil (= leukeran) selectively reduces the number of lymphocytes in the circulation. In contrast, myleran has little diminishing power on the lymphocyte population but produces a fall in the neutrophils. The two compounds together produce alterations which are very similar to those produced by a single whole body X-irradiation (ELSON, 1955). In view of the marked effect of whole body irradiation on the LCM disease, it is of interest to note that of these two substances only the lymphocyte-affecting chlorambucil and not myleran protected LCM virus-infected mice. Chlorambucil acted in a two-fold fashion (BARLOW, 1962): (1) it spared a portion of the mice, although virus multiplied; (2) mice which died did so usually within 24 hours after drug administration, irrespective of time of intracerebral infection. While this latter result is not understood, the prevention of LCM disease may be seen as another example of effects due to immunosuppression. The compound 1,3-bis(2-chloroethyl)-1-nitrosourea is in its action related to the alkylating agents. It significantly prolonged the lives of infected mice but spared a significant number in one of many experiments only; virus multiplication was unaffected (Sidwell *et al.*, 1965). The two antibiotics, 6-diazo-5-oxo-nor-l-leucine (DON) and azaserine, both direct inhibitors of enzyme activities (Berenbaum, 1967), only moderately influenced LCM disease in mice for the better (Levy and Haas, 1958).

For our understanding of the role immunosuppression plays in preventing the development of LCM disease, it is noteworthy that mice treated with X-rays, amethopterin, azaserine, DON, or folic acid deficient diet, failed to eliminate at the normal rate the virus after peripheral infection (Haas *et al.*, 1957a; Levy and Haas, 1958; Hannover Larsen, 1969c).

Removal of the thymus soon after birth considerably influences the course of the LCM disease in the adult mouse. When mice, so treated, are infected intracerebrally in later life, they are usually well protected. They respond with virus-specific antibody, although multiplication of virus is not inhibited (Rowe *et al.*, 1963; East *et al.*, 1964; Hotchin and Sikora, 1964; Sikora, 1964; Földes *et al.*, 1964; 1964/65; 1967; Szeri *et al.*, 1966/67). Brains of neonatally thymectomized mice, which had survived intracerebral infection with LCM virus, were essentially free of pathological alterations (Rowe *et al.*, 1963; Földes *et al.*, 1964; 1964/65). Again, after peripheral infection virus continued to multiply for prolonged periods (Mori *et al.*, 1964). The effects of neonatal thymectomy on the pathogenicity of LCM virus could be partially reversed by intraperitoneal implantation of diffusion chambers containing thymus tissue (Levey *et al.*, 1963). This was interpreted to mean that the thymus produced a humoral factor, a notion which was further advanced in other studies (Miller and Osoba, 1967).

The events following the treatment of mice with antilymphocytic or antithymocytic sera are, *cum grano salis*, identical with those after thymectomy. Mice were protected against intracerebral infection although virus multiplied (Gledhill, 1967; Hirsch *et al.*, 1967; 1968; Hirsch and Murphy, 1968). Complement-fixing antibody appeared and histopathology was absent (Hirsch *et al.*, 1967; 1968). Upon discontinuation of serum treatment, characteristic LCM disease and histopathology developed in many mice; infectious virus gradually disappeared (Hirsch *et al.*, 1967). Of 65 serum-treated mice, 12 developed severe wasting with loss of weight, alopecia, facial edema, and stiff tail three to seven weeks after infection. The other mice of this group appeared outwardly to be healthy, although they were lighter than the controls most of which remained completely free of signs. All protected mice developed glomerulonephritis with deposition of mouse γ-globulin in the glomerular tufts. In the wasted animals, the most prominent findings were hyperplasia of reticular cells which infiltrated the tissues throughout the body (Hirsch *et al.*, 1968).

Mims (1969) treated WE virus-infected pregnant mice with antilymphocytic serum, thereby normalizing the gestation period and saving a few of the offspring which, without treatment of the mother, would all have died. Thus, fetal death probably resulted from an immunologic conflict, presumably in the mother.

Inasmuch as the graft *versus* host reaction is accompanied by marked immunodepression (Koltay *et al.*, 1965), the altered LCM disease in such animals may be considered related to the sparing effects of other immunosuppressive treatments such as have been discussed above. KOLTAY *et al.* (1968) inoculated (C 57 BL $\times$ CBA)F_1 hybrids intravenously with spleen cells from adult C57BL donors, which resulted in loss of weight, reduction of lymphocytes, and early death. Seven days after the transplantation, 300 LD_{50} of LCM virus were inoculated intracerebrally. While control mice were dead within eight days, transplanted animals lived up to 44 days with few exhibiting neurological signs typical of LCM; most died with runting. Later, KOLTAY *et al.* (1969) described the histopathology in these mice. In 12 (C57BL $\times$ CBA)F_1 hybrids with marked graft *versus* host disease due to the inoculation of C57BL spleen cells which had received 300 LD_{50} of LCM virus typical graft *versus* host histology was found, but neither neurological signs nor meningeal alterations characteristic of infection with the LCM virus were present. In these animals "a virus carrier state could be demonstrated" (no details). In another group of 13 animals with less marked clinical or histological evidence of graft *versus* host reaction, "a peculiar leukocytic meningoencephalitis" was found, the nature of which remained uncertain. Two further mice which had failed to develop a graft *versus* host reaction exhibited signs typical of LCM.

Neither illness nor histopathology of the brain due to inoculation of 100 LD_{50} of LCM virus was altered in strain A inbred mice by intraperitoneal treatment with phytohemagglutinin. It was concluded that phytohemagglutinin does not possess immunosuppressive properties in mice (BÁNOS *et al.*, 1969).

Those who work with LCM viruses are well aware of the fact that at high doses often more mice survive the intracerebral inoculation than at lower ones. To my knowledge, this phenomenon was first described by BENGTSON and WOOLEY (1936) who, aptly, called it a "pre-zone". Although a nuisance for the titration of the virus (see Section XI. A. 1), this high zone inhibition (see Fig. 10) is of considerable theoretical interest. In spite of multiplication of the virus to high titers these mice survive. HOTCHIN and BENSON (1963) suggested that the "high dose inhibitory phenomenon" — later called "high dose immune paralysis" (HANAOKA *et al.*, 1969) — was caused by development of immunological tolerance to the virus. It should be stressed, however, that persistent infection of long duration does not ensue. LEHMANN-GRUBE (1969b) searched for infectivity in the brains of mice which had survived $10^{6.7}$ or $10^{2.7}$ ID_{50} (mouse) of WE virus; 80 days after intracerebral challenge with 10^3 ID_{50} of Armstrong virus, the central nervous systems of five of altogether 26 mice were free from infectivity; most of the remaining mice had little virus, *i.e.* ten ID_{50} or less, per brain.

An interesting contribution concerning this phenomenon has come from HANAOKA *et al.* (1969). After the intracerebral inoculation of 1000 LD_{50} of the WE strain virus, changes of the lymphoid organs developed which were interpreted as being due to selective destruction of the thymus-dependent lymphocytes. The authors inferred that the high dose survival was caused by a reduction of the intensity of the cellular immune response being in principle identical to survival with persistent infection after neonatal thymectomy or treatment with antilymphocytic serum. There are several reasons why this hypothesis does not satisfy, of which the following is most obvious. Two substrains of WE were used, one passaged eight times in the mouse brain (called "neurotropic") the other passaged six times in the brain followed by eleven passages in the mouse liver (called "viscerotropic"). Only the latter caused a persistent infection with survival at high doses; the former was 100 per cent lethal with the same inocula. According to the above hypothesis, one would have expected differences between these strains in their effects on the lymphoid organs. In fact, these were all but absent. Neither histopathology nor weight measurements revealed significant dissimilarities; only the degrees of viremia differed with the substrains used, being lower in the case of the brain-passaged variant.

Experimental proof that the thymus-dependent lymphocytes are not selectively destroyed in these mice has been obtained by Lehmann-Grube and Raff (details to be published). LCM virus, strain WE, was passaged 11 times in the abdominal organs (liver, spleen, kidneys) of mice and 1000 ID_{50} (mouse) were

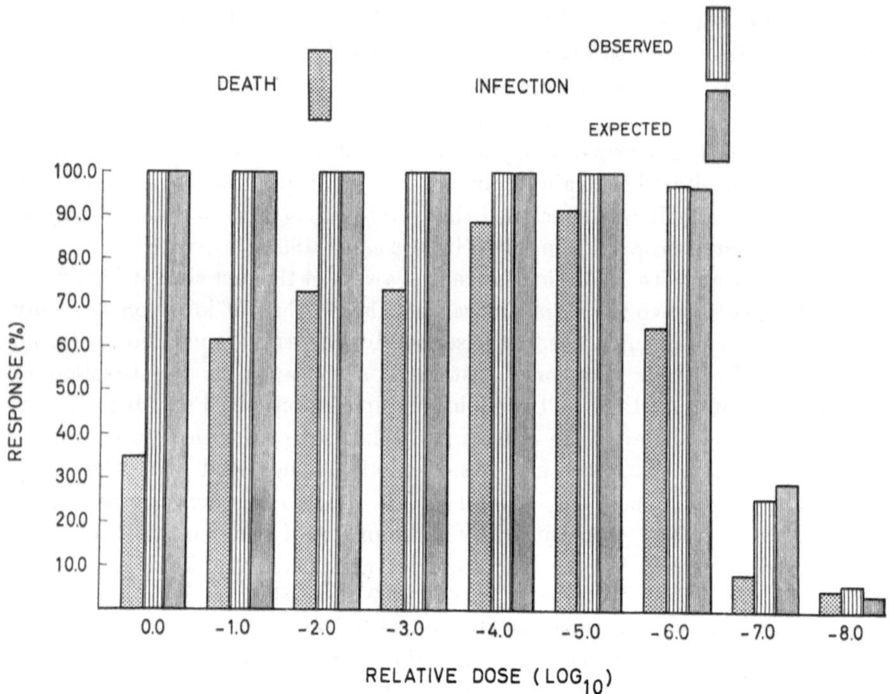

Fig. 10. Dose-response relationship of LCM virus, strain WE, in mice. From F. Lehmann-Grube: J. Hyg. (Lond. **67**, 269 (1969). (With permission of Cambridge University Press, London.)

inoculated intracerebrally into outbred albino mice or inbred CBA mice. In repeated experiments and at various intervals after infection, theta antigen-bearing cells of spleens were enumerated on the basis of their selective destruction by anti-theta antiserum raised in AKR mice (Raff, 1969). In no case was the proportion of theta positive cells reduced. On the contrary, most assays revealed relative increases of their numbers, indicating that cells other than T-cells were predominantly affected.

It is known that not all strains of LCM virus exhibit this high dose survival. For instance, the classical strain E-350 of Armstrong causes 100 per cent lethality with highest inocula (Lehmann-Grube, 1969b). No explanation is at hand and speculations are possible but with our present knowledge unrewarding. It should be mentioned that high dose survivors are unlike neonatal carriers in at least one important aspect; adult mice, surviving intracerebral injection of large amounts of virus, do not exhibit the characteristic renal histopathology (BAKER, 1969) of mice made carriers by neonatal infection. Possibly, this is related to the fact that high dose survivors produce significantly more antibody than do neonatal carriers (BENSON and HOTCHIN, 1969).

HANNOVER LARSEN (1967; 1968b) induced persistent infection in adult mice by intraperitoneal inoculation of the virus. Repeated injections of excessive amounts of virus were required, contrasting with the experience just related. The cause of this difference — which could be sought in route of inoculation, virus strain, mouse strain — is unknown. The viremia found in a few normal mice which survived prolonged parabiotic union with carriers (HOTCHIN, 1965) may represent a further example of induction of persistent infection in adult mice.

LUNDSTEDT and VOLKERT (1967) demonstrated that induction of long-lasting persistence of the virus after intraperitoneal infection was facilitated if the mice were treated with rabbit anti-mouse lymphocytic serum. Complement-fixing antibody appeared in some of these mice but only for short periods. It is noteworthy that two rabbit control sera also prolonged viremia and delayed antibody response although to a lesser extent.

All the examples cited above, where freedom from clinical signs in spite of unimpeded virus multiplication was achieved, may be best interpreted as being due to immunological tolerance — with or without prior general immunosuppression — although in a restricted sense. In contrast to neonatal or congenital carriers which, at the most, produce traces of antibody and, as a rule, maintain constant virus levels until death, significant concentrations of antibody were detected in the blood of the majority of these mice and most of them eliminated the virus after delays. There was never a consistent correlation between elimination of virus and concentration of circulating antibody, and we note again that these seem to have no causal relationship with each other. Undoubtedly these mice were only partially tolerant, for, besides producing specific antibody, they had retained some of their ability to reject the virus, though slowly.

If the disease in adult mice which follows an intracerebral infection is the result of an immune response to the virus, one would expect that the injection of LCM-immune lymphoid cells to a carrier should result in convulsions and death of the recipient. This, however, is not the case. In hundreds of such transfers, neither Volkert (VOLKERT *et al.*, 1964; VOLKERT and HANNOVER LARSEN, 1965c) nor LEHMANN-GRUBE and SLENCZKA (unpublished) have ever noticed anything which would resemble the LCM disease. HOTCHIN (1959) did see convulsions in two of six carriers in consequence of the transfer of lymph nodes from convalescent donors, but this was not confirmed later (HOTCHIN, 1962a; 1965). More recently, LUNDSTEDT (1969b) reported that a few C3H carrier mice developed hypokinesia, conjunctivitis, and ruffled fur 10 to 30 days after they had received an intraperitoneal injection of lymphoid cells from LCM-immune C3H donors. Since this observation contrasted markedly with "hundreds of adoptive immunizations carried out in this laboratory", the significance of the finding was questioned. Apparently, for clinical signs to develop, both antigen and immune response must be in a critical functional or quantitative relationship to each other, which is usually not attained after inoculation of immunologically prepared cells. I cannot agree with Volkert and his colleagues (Volkert *et al.*, 1964; Volkert, 1965; Volkert and Hannover Larsen, 1965c) who maintain that lack of signs following the inoculation of immunologically activated cells speaks against the assumption that an allergic reaction causes the LCM illness in mice.

Before the possible mechanisms of the virus-induced immunological conflict can be discussed, we have to answer the question, what antigens are involved in the development of specific tolerance or responsiveness? Persistence of virus and lack of antibody leave no doubt that in established LCM virus carrier mice immunological tolerance is directed towards the virus. This, however, does not necessarily imply that the viral antigens are also the cause for the allergic reactions in the adult mouse. Other possibilities have to be considered (Table 6). New antigens may develop comparable to the ones which appear on

Table 6. *Hypothetical New Antigens in LCM Virus-Infected Mice which may be Responsible for Pathologic Immune Phenomena or Tolerance*

I. Cell-associated	II. Soluble
1. Coded by virus	1. Coded by virus
a) Viral (structure)	a) Viral (*e.g.* capsomers, s-Antigen)
b) Cellular (*e.g.* transplantation, cytotoxicity)	b) Cellular
2. Coded by cell	2. Coded by cell
c) Alteration	c) Alteration
d) Induction	d) Induction
e) Demasking	e) Demasking

virus-induced tumor cells (Habel, 1967) and possibly on other virus-infected nontransformed cells (Wiktor *et al.*, 1968). The antigens may be part of the cells appearing after alteration, induction, or unmasking in consequence of the virus infection. If this is the case, the immunological conflict in LCM virus-infected mice could be regarded as an example of an auto-immune disease. The possibility has also to be considered that the antigens are present in a soluble form, precipitating an anaphylactic shock by forming antigen-antibody complexes much in the same way as it is known to occur with other soluble antigens (Weiser *et al.*, 1941; Tokuda and Weiser, 1958). The available evidence, though only circumstantial, favors the assumption that new antigens appearing on LCM virus-infected cells may be held responsible and that they are of viral origin as exemplified by measles virus-infected HeLa (Mannweiler and Smerdel, 1968) and mumps virus-infected human conjunctiva cells (Speel *et al.*, 1968).

Lehmann-Grube (unpublished) did not observe cytolysis of LCM virus-infected cells *in vitro* after the addition of viral antisera with or without complement, and Lehmann-Grube *et al.* (1969) were not able to detect new antigens on cells, persistently infected with LCM virus, by means of cytotoxic antibody in sera of immunized mice. (Since these experiments were done at a time when the carried virus had changed its properties, it cannot be excluded that cells releasing fully infectious virus might have responded differently.) Hotchin (1962a) claimed to have obtained cytolysis *in vitro* of cells from testes of persistently LCM virus-infected mice by spleen lymphocytes of normal or LCM-immune mice. Experiments performed by BENSON (1963b) would indicate that such results are of little meaning for our question. She found that LCM-immune spleen cells caused about equal destruction of both normal and LCM virus-infected mouse testis cells; spleen cells from nonimmunized donors caused this effect, again in both types of target cells, to a lesser degree. With lymphoid cells from LCM-immune mice, LUNDSTEDT (1969a) demonstrated some cytotoxic activity against LCM virus-infected L cells. Unfortunately, his data are not as consistent as one would like them to be for the drawing of definite conclusions. OLDSTONE *et al.* (1969) observed cytopathologic alterations of LCM virus-infected mouse embryo cells when they were brought into contact with LCM-specific antibody plus complement or with splenocytes from LCM-immune mice without complement (no details).

More recently, the search for antigens which are responsible for immunological responsiveness or paralysis has taken on a new dimension by the observation of Holtermann and Majde and, independently, of Lehmann-Grube that LCM virus carrier mice have acquired new histocompatibility antigens. The experimental evidence is as follows. HOLTERMANN and MAJDE (1969) transferred skin grafts from SWR neonatal carriers onto normal recipients. Rejection, commencing on the tenth day and proceeding to completeness by day 14, occurred in 13 of 13 trials. Second-set responses were seen when transplantation was repeated. The results obtained by myself were similar, although differences were noted. First attempts were made with transplants from carrier mice grafted onto normal syngeneic recipients. Of 18 such mice (ten C3H and eight AKR) 15 died with loss of weight, hunched back, and conjunctivitis between days 5 and 14. Two more C3H mice were killed when moribund on days 22 and 38. In all these mice evaluation of the grafts was uncertain. A single AKR recipient was only temporarily ill. Its graft from a zero generation syngeneic carrier mouse became hemorrhagic on the tenth day. Three more normal AKR mice which had received intraperitoneally five times 10^7 spleen cells from AKR carriers died between days 10 and 17.

Initially it was suspected that these mice suffered from the dual stress of a peripheral LCM virus infection combined with the trauma of transplantation. This, however, could be ruled out when it was found that mice, which had received allogeneic grafts before, together with, or after intraperitoneal virus infections, almost always remained outwardly healthy. Since LCM-immune mice never died or showed signs when transplanted with syngeneic carrier grafts, recipients of skin grafts were made immune by a subcutaneous virus infection followed, two weeks before transplantation, by an intracerebral challenge inoculation.

In several large-scale experiments performed with AKR, CBA, and C3H mice it was found that not all grafts from persistently infected donors were rejected by syngeneic LCM-immune recipients, but that a few were accepted without apparent alterations while others underwent partial rejection. In these latter cases a typical homograft reaction set in at the expected time, *e.g.* ten days after transplantation, but rather than leading to complete necrosis, a slow recovery took place. The final result was a graft with a reduced size and an altered texture. In such cases evaluation was often difficult and final interpretation was dependent on histological examination. It was furthermore found that the graft survival times varied considerably between and within experiments, even with otherwise identical donor-recipient combinations, and that this variation might simulate second-set responses. It is noteworthy that such results were obtained irrespective of whether the persistently infected donors had been infected neonatally or were born of carrier mothers (details to be published).

The present knowledge does not permit making a final statement concerning the basic mechanism, but the interpretation given by HOLTERMANN and MAJDE (1969) is plausible. These authors think that the antigens, which manifest themselves by a homograft type reaction in syngeneic recipients, are due to virus which is being assembled in close contact with the cell membrane. Observations very similar to the ones described were reported by BREYERE and WILLIAMS (1964) who found that a proportion of skin grafts from BALB/c mice suffering from virus-induced leukemia were rejected by syngeneic recipients; other grafts were rejected partially. Here, too, the most likely interpretation is that the new histocompatibility antigens were identical with the budding virus.

Whereas these observations do not prove that new transplantation antigens — be they viral or cellular in nature — are responsible for the observed immune phenomena, they nevertheless have opened up a new path which may be followed profitably to answer this important question. This, however, may turn out to be a difficult task. The scarce clinical signs after peripheral infection which, as the studies with immunosuppressive measures show (ROWE, 1954; HAAS and STEWART, 1956; ROWE *et al.*, 1963; MIMS and TOSOLINI, 1969), are not less caused immunologically than death following intracerebral inoculation, and the quick and complete recovery indicate that either few cells are antigenically altered and then eliminated or, else, the alterations of the cell surfaces are slight and reversible. It should be remembered that persistently infected mouse cells *in vitro* were slowly cured by antibody to the virus, which was not due to preferential elimination of infected cells (see Section III. C). POTTER and HAAS (1959) rendered an LCM virus-infected and apparently highly infectious transplantable mouse ascites-tumor free of virus by passing it five times through LCM-immune mice. No difficulties were reported and it may be assumed that the cells' viability had not markedly suffered during this process (see Section IV. A). The dramatic disease following the intracerebral inoculation of the adult mouse should not be construed as proof of the existence of qualitatively or quantitatively strong antigens. Nerve cells with even minor new surface antigens may be expected to be affected by cellular or humoral immune reactions leading to functional disorder, even without morphologic damage. It should be kept in mind that nerve cell destruction in mice which had died after intracerebral infection is all but absent (see Section V. A. 4. c).

There are no data to support the hypothesis put forward by HANNOVER LARSEN (1969d) that tolerance in mice persistently infected with LCM virus is a consequence of virus multiplication in the specifically immune reactive cells, thereby suppressing their immunological responsiveness, rather than a specific block of immunological reactivity due to exposure of the immune apparatus to the antigens in question.

Since the antigens which are responsible for immunological responsiveness and tolerance have not yet been identified, it is not surprising that we do not fully understand the nature of the immune processes involved. The experimental data which have direct bearing on this problem have all been obtained with the whole virus. The following discussion is therefore presented with the reservation that the identification with the virus of the antigen "X", which is responsible for the immunological conflict, is so far not much more than a working hypothesis. The situation is further complicated by the fact that the relationship between virus and s-antigen is virtually unknown (see Section II. F). In particular, these may differ antigenically, and since all tissues produce the soluble antigen, the data obtained with the virus may apply to the soluble component as well. In order to facilitate our discussion, we shall make the most simple assumption, namely, that the s-antigen is part of the virus structure and antigenically not different from it.

On the previous pages we have encountered a number of examples which indicate that antibody formation and virus elimination are causally not related. These will be summarized here together with additional illustrating examples. Neonatal thymectomy as well as treatment with antilymphocytic serum spared mice from LCM disease, although virus multiplication was unaltered and antibody was produced. This is not an unexpected result from such procedures, particularly if both signs of the disease and virus elimination were dependent on cellular rather than humoral mechanisms (METCALF, 1966; MILLER and OSOBA, 1967; MEDAWAR, 1969). Antibody appeared in mice which survived the intracerebral or intraperitoneal infection of high doses of virus and developed persistent infection (HANNOVER LARSEN, 1967; 1968b; BENSON and HOTCHIN, 1969; HOTCHIN, 1969). Antibody was also produced in a few mice which became carriers in consequence of the inoculation at birth of one LD_{50} (VOLKERT and HANNOVER LARSEN, 1965a) as well as in carriers which retained the virus after having been transplanted with syngeneic nonimmune lymphoid cells (HANNOVER LARSEN and VOLKERT, 1967), or with syngeneic immune lymphoid cells contained in Millipore chambers (HANNOVER LARSEN, 1968a). HANNOVER LARSEN (personal communication) transplanted syngeneic lymphoid cells from immune male donors into persistently infected female C3H mice. The resulting adoptive immunity was of short duration; virus reappeared and antibody disappeared from the circulation. However, whereas viremia was essentially restored after four weeks, the disappearance of antibody took much longer. Thus, for many weeks, virus and antibody were found to coexist. When residual virus in noncarrier immune mice was activated by antilymphocytic serum, viremia developed in spite of constant or even increased concentrations of complement-fixing antibody (VOLKERT and LUNDSTEDT, 1968). TRAUB (1960b) and VOLKERT and HANNOVER LARSEN (1965a) showed that the development of circulating antibody and the ability to eliminate the virus may be separated from each other simply by varying the time interval between birth and infection. A thorough study of this phenomenon was presented by HANNOVER LARSEN (1969a) who showed that all possible combinations could be obtained: (1) high antibody, low virus; (2) high antibody, high virus; (3) low antibody, low virus; (4) low antibody, high virus titers (see Fig. 11). It is unexplained why other investigators failed to detect complement-fixing activity in sera from mice infected as late as seven days (WEIGAND and HOTCHIN, 1961) or even 12 days (PETERSON and MAKSUDOVA, 1969) after birth. LUNDSTEDT (1969b) incubated spleen cells from LCM-immune C3H mice for 75 minutes at

37°C in antilymphocytic serum (no complement added) and inoculated 30×10^6 viable cells into syngeneic LCM virus carriers. In seven of ten mice thus treated, complement-fixing antibody concentrations rose to variable levels but virus titers were unaffected. In three further mice virus disappeared—though significantly slower than in the controls—and antibody titers were high. HANNOVER LARSEN (1969c) determined the kinetics of viremia and complement-fixing antibody in the

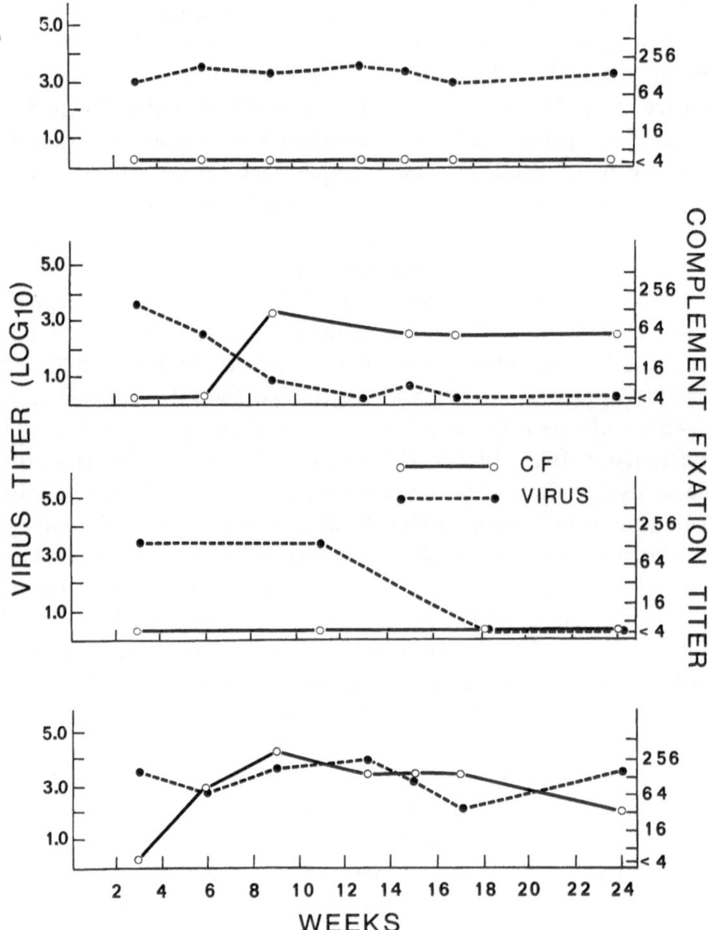

Fig. 11. Independence of viremia and complement-fixing antibody in mice infected with LCM virus, strain Traub, when two to nine days old.
At intervals, mice were bled and concentrations of virus (mouse LD_{50} per 0.03 ml) and complement-fixing antibody were determined in parallel. Adapted from J. HANNOVER LARSEN: Immunology **16**, 15 (1969). (With permission of the author and of Blackwell Scientific Publications Ltd., Oxford.)

blood after intraperitoneal infection of immunologically suppressed mice and found both to pursue quite independent courses. This was particularly striking in the case of X-irradiated animals.

All these data strongly suggest that virus elimination is not due to the activity of circulating antibody, but rather is accomplished by cellular mechanisms, a conclusion which was reached by TRAUB (1936b) more than 30 years ago. It would therefore be logical to consider that cell-mediated immune tolerance prevents virus elimination leading to the carrier state and that the opposite of immunological tolerance, immunity leading to allergic reactions, is also cell-mediated. The following observations may be interpreted as indicating that delayed-type hypersensitivity is involved.

Mice inoculated intracerebrally with LCM virus were 10,000 times as susceptible as controls to endotoxin from Gram-negative bacteria. The latent period, relative to the intracerebral infection, could be considerably shortened; mice dying within 24 hours after endotoxin injection did so with typical LCM signs, even when the entire sequence of endotoxin injection and death occurred during the first 30 hours after intracerebral inoculation of the virus. After subcutaneous inoculation of the virus, mice were 500 times more sensitive to endotoxin (Barlow and Fairley, 1963). Hyperreactivity to endotoxin has been repeatedly demonstrated in animals, including mice, which had been infected with tubercle bacilli (Bordet, 1936; Freund, 1936; Packalén, 1951; Suter and Kirsanow, 1961) and *Brucellae* (Abernathy *et al.*, 1958) which have in common the ability to elicit marked delayed-type hypersensitivity. Stetson (1959) has drawn attention to the great similarity between endotoxin and delayed-type hypersensitivity reactions, be they local or generalized. The mutual enhancement of LCM virus and endotoxin in mice may thus be seen as being due to a summative effect of generalized hypersensitivity and related effects. Whether the same explanation holds true for the aggravating effect of pretreatment with *Eperythrozoon coccoides* on peripheral infection with LCM virus (Gledhill and Seamer, 1961; Seamer *et al.*, 1961) is doubtful. Seamer and Gledhill (1965) measured the virus concentrations in blood, livers, and brains of mice infected peripherally with the UBC virus and found traces only; the lethality was low. If *E. coccoides* was inoculated prior to virus infection, virus titers increased by several logs: *e.g.* in the brain, 10^5 to 10^7 LD_{50} per g were present as compared with none in the virus-only controls. Thus, the enhancing effect of infection with *E. coccoides* on the pathogenicity of LCM virus appears to be the consequence of enhanced virus multiplication, leading to concentrations in the brain high enough to imitate the effects of intracerebral inoculation.

It seems pertinent to mention that the relationship between *E. coccoides* and mouse hepatitis virus is closely similar to the one between *E. coccoides* and LCM virus; the susceptibility to mouse hepatitis virus is increased by infection with *E. coccoides*, apparently due to the same mechanism, *i.e.* enhancement of virus multiplication. Furthermore, infection with the mouse hepatitis virus increases the action of endotoxin in mice (Gledhill *et al.*, 1955; Gledhill, 1958). The relationship between mouse hepatitis and LCM viruses (Gledhill *et al.*, 1961) needs clarification. The mechanism of the endotoxin-like effect of chlorambucil on LCM virus-infected mice (Barlow, 1962) is unknown.

Further evidence for the role cell-bound immunity plays in the disease of the mouse following the infection with the LCM virus may be seen in the fact that for clinical signs to develop the full activity of complement is not required (Lehmann-Grube, 1969d). The same was found to apply to the prototype of a cell-mediated immune reaction in the mouse, *i.e.* the homograft response following skin grafting (Caren and Rosenberg, 1965).

The most direct evidence for a generalized reaction of delayed-type hypersensitivity in mice infected with LCM virus may be obtained from the development of a local foot pad reaction (see Section V. A. 2). The concept of hyperergic allergy was exemplified by von Pirquet (1907) with the skin reaction to vaccinia virus which he considered to be due primarily to an interaction between antigen (the virus) and cell-bound or circulating antibody. The similarity of a local vaccinia reaction and the LCM foot pad response is not superficial. Von Pirquet's finding that the course of the individual lesion was dose dependent has its analogy in the local response to LCM virus (Roger and Roger, 1964d; 1964e). What is more important, von Pirquet's observation that the skin lesions due to vaccinia virus inoculated at different sites at intervals of two days within a certain period of time reached their maxima together was found by Roger and Roger (1964b) to apply to the LCM foot pad response as well. The suppressive effects of whole body — but not local — X-irradiation (Benson, 1963a), neonatal thymectomy (Mori *et al.*, 1964), and treatment with antilymphocytic serum (Mims, 1969; Mims and Tosolini, 1969) on the foot pad response are further indications of its immunological basis. Amethopterin, likewise, suppressed the local foot pad response but the majority of these mice died, which has not been explained (Sikora and Hotchin, 1963). Furthermore, just as the interval between intracerebral inoculation and cerebral disease may be shortened by a prior sensitizing infection (see above), appearance of the foot pad reaction may be hastened in the same way (Roger and Roger, 1964g). The resemblance of the phenomena associated with the foot pad reaction with those associated with the signs after intracerebral infection (see above) is striking and probably indicates similar pathogenetic mechanisms. Unexpected and unexplained is the finding that the latent period of the foot pad response may be shortened by one to two days if antiserum is given less than four days after local inoculation of the virus. In contrast, signs due to intracerebral or intraperitoneal inoculation of virus were not accelerated by antiserum (Roger and Roger, 1964g). While all these phenomena leave little doubt as to the major role immunologically active cells play in the LCM disease, at least one observation is on record which may be interpreted to mean that antibody may also take part. Infant mice born of immune mothers were found to respond more often with disease to the infection with LCM virus than did mice of equal age from normal animals (Traub, 1961a).

The outwardly unimpeded subsequent development of those mice which had survived the first two to three weeks after neonatal infection was generally taken to mean that immunological responses in neonatally infected mice eventually were suppressed, leading to complete immunological tolerance. This notion became doubtful when evidence accumulated that many of these mice developed clinical and pathological signs when a few months old (see Section V. A. 3). The assumption that this "late-onset disease" was also due to an immunological interaction between host and virus-induced antigen though different from the acute response (Hotchin, 1962a; 1965; 1967), was strengthened by the results obtained in experiments in which persistently infected mice were joined in parabiotic union to LCM-immune partners. Late-onset disease developed faster and was more severe than in single mice and had the additional feature of being associated with severe anemia (Hotchin, 1962a; 1965). As with the late disease in carriers, wasting and anemia following parabiosis is not a general phenomonon. HANNOVER LARSEN (1968a) joined C3H carriers to immune animals and did not observe pathological effects in 30 weeks. OLDSTONE and DIXON (1968a) noted that parabiosis of C3H virus carriers with C3H hyperimmune mice did not have detectable consequences for the two mice but that a similar type of parabiosis with SWR mice caused early death of the carrier and injury to the immune partner.

OLDSTONE and DIXON (1967; 1968a) presented evidence for the existence of low concentrations of LCM-specific antibody in carriers which had survived neonatal infection, thereby confirming the long neglected finding of TRAUB and SCHÄFER (1939; TRAUB, 1939a; 1960b) that the sera of a few carrier mice contained complement-fixing antibody at low concentrations. Recently, BENSON and HOTCHIN (1969) detected antibody by means of immunofluorescence in neonatal carriers, first about two months after infection, but HOTCHIN (1969) failed to elute antibody from the kidneys of such animals.

These studies were extended by OLDSTONE *et al.* (1969; OLDSTONE and DIXON, 1969). Using the CA 1371 strain of LCM virus, inbred mice were made carriers by neonatal infection. As determined by immunofluorescence, LCM virus antigen was found in all tissues, notably in the brain, the liver, and the kidneys. By the same method the glomeruli of carrier mice as well as the hepatic lesions were shown to have accumulated host cell γ-globulin and the third component of complement; all other tissues were free of host plasma proteins. In the kidneys, host γ-globulin was found in traces as early as ten days after infection. On days 14 and 21 the deposits had become considerable. In eluates from such kidneys, LCM-specific complement-fixing antibody was detected, the amount of which increased with the animals' age. Monkey kidney cells infected with LCM virus, but not uninfected control cells, absorbed 50 per cent of the γ-globulin contained in the kidney eluates. Antiglomerular basement or antinuclear activities were not demonstrated. Labeled guinea-pig complement, component three, was faster eliminated from carriers than from controls; by direct immunofluorescence it was found to have accumulated in the glomeruli. After repeated precipitation of carrier serum with rabbit anti-mouse γ-globulin the infectivity was reduced 1000-fold. A correlation was found between virus plus antibody concentrations in the mouse strains on the one hand and the extension of their late disease on the other. There can be no doubt that the findings of Oldstone and Dixon prove the ability of mice infected at birth with LCM virus to respond with specific antibody through most of their lives. There is likewise little room to deny the existence of antigen-antibody complexes, and the conclusion that these are probably responsible for the late glomerulonephritis (see also UNANUE and DIXON, 1967) and possibly also for the alterations in other organs seems justified.

While the significance of these findings is not to be questioned, it should nevertheless be pointed out that the experiments were done with mice inoculated after birth and that they did not take advantage of the unique opportunity offered by the LCM virus to study the effect of a foreign antigen on a host which was presumably immunologically at zero level on first contact. It is *a priori* likely and has been well documented experimentally by HOWARD and MICHIE (1962) and BRENT and GOWLAND (1963) that newborn mice are capable of responding immunologically. We remember that newborn mice react — initially at least — with retardation of development, and many die. There are hints, however, indicating that even mice which were infected congenitally, *i.e.* presumably at the very beginning of their ontogenetic development, also are capable of producing antibody. Retardation during later development and the histopathology in some instances (see Section V. A. 3) are not necessarily the result of an immunological interaction. However, Traub and Schäfer (1939; Traub, 1939a; 1960b) had detected low concentrations of complement-fixing activity in some mice from an established carrier colony. Pollard *et al.* (1968b) measured the total globulin and γ-globulin concentrations in the sera of established carriers and found them to be higher than in control mice. Lehmann-Grube, Hirsch, and Allison (unpublished) demonstrated immune complexes in the kidneys of C3H carriers of the first and second congenital generations but not in controls (Fig. 12) which is highly suggestive of the presence of circulating antibody to the LCM virus in congenital carriers.

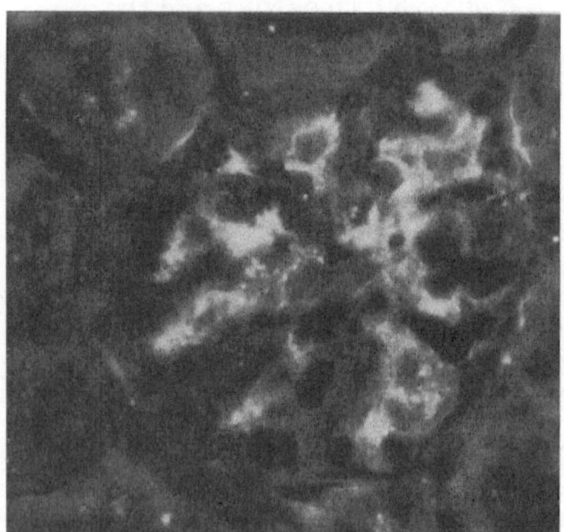

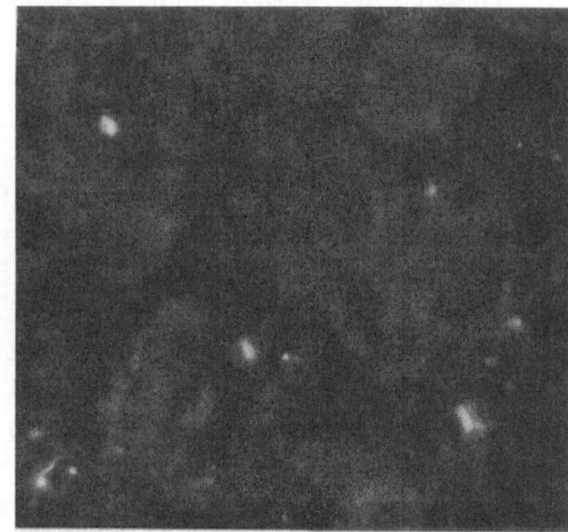

Fig. 12. Sections of kidneys from C3H mice stained with fluorescein-conjugated antimouse gamma globulin. Left: Mouse congenitally infected with Traub strain of LCM virus (second carrier generation). Right: Normal mouse of the same age

Immunological tolerance is not an all-or-none phenomenon but rather an "impressed diminution in immunologic responses below those which normally occur after known antigenic excitation" (Chase, 1959) and it is difficult to follow Oldstone and Dixon (1969; Oldstone, 1969) who challenge the notion that the LCM virus carrier state is the expression of a true example of immunological tolerance. These mice do not respond with clinical signs and they are incapable of eliminating the virus, which leaves no doubt that the cell-mediated response towards the viral or virus-induced antigens is greatly diminished though not abolished. Lehmann-Grube (1964b) observed that in a few mice, made carriers by injection of high doses of virus when younger than 24 hours, the virus which had been present 50 to 80 days after the infection had disappeared when tested for again at days 180 to 190, indicating development of ability for virus elimination which is probably cell-mediated.

There is another consideration which merits our attention. As we have seen, antibody concentrations in LCM virus-infected mice occur at two levels (if we disregard in this context the high titers reached after adoptive immunization of carrier mice), and both the minute amounts which are just barely detectable in mice infected neonatally as well as the comparatively high concentrations, such as are found after nonlethal infections of adult mice, may be associated with virus concentrations characteristic of carrier mice. If, as OLDSTONE and DIXON (1969) suggested, the low concentration of antibody in carrier mice were a peripheral phenomenon in the sense that "this antibody cannot be detected free in the circulation because of an excess of antigen or virus", then normal antibody concentrations in carrier mice could only be due to less efficient masking, representing merely the other extreme of the same phenomenon. If this were true, carrier mice with intermediate levels of antibody concentration should be found more frequently than either or both of the two extremes. This, however, is definitely not the case. Although conversions take place, as may be seen in Figure 11, intermediate grades of antibody concentrations are not known to occur and it appears reasonable to assume that true differences exist and that the trace amount present in a typical carrier mouse results from central failure of production rather than from masking by antigen whereas the comparatively high antibody response — with or without virus at carrier level — is the expression of the opposite reaction, *i.e.* immunity. One would like to know whether the classes of antibody that participate in the two responses differ qualitatively as well as quantitatively.

After having once again emphasized that the existence of virus-specific immunological tolerance in LCM virus carrier mice is not at variance with our present knowledge, we are still confronted with the fact that, although the virus is integrated into the antigenic pattern of the host, antibody is nevertheless produced. The ever increasing body of data which demonstrate the existence of autoantibody — sometimes associated with clinical or pathological signs, but often completely free of them — (KIDD and FRIEDEWALD, 1942a; 1942b; MILGROM *et al.*, 1957; BOYDEN, 1964; HACKETT and THOMPSON, 1964; LAFFIN *et al.*, 1964; NORINS and HOLMES, 1964; BURGIO and SEVERI, 1965; SCHLESINGER, 1965; HILDEMANN and WALFORD, 1966; ELSON and WEIR, 1969) indicates that the presence of antibody to self may be the rule rather than the exception. Furthermore, the ease with which auto-antibody may be induced is remarkable (HRABA, 1968). Indeed, it has been postulated that auto-antibody has a physiological function by aiding in the removal from the body of normal catabolic products (GRABAR, 1957; BOYDEN, 1964). The data of ROWLEY and FITCH (1965) indicate that antibody may be necessary to inhibit the transformation of potential to antibody-producing cells. WALFORD (1964; 1967) has collected observations which may be interpreted to mean that aging is associated or even caused by an increase of auto-immune phenomena. Taking this view, pathological alterations in congenital carriers are nothing else but pathological auto-immune phenomena. It is not known and should be determined whether abnormalities in mice born to carrier mothers are the rule or whether they occur only in certain virus-mouse strain combinations.

The clear demonstration in the case of infection of the mouse with LCM virus that immunological tolerance consists of at least two separable components, one related to circulating antibody and the other to cell-bound immunity, confirms previous reports with other antigens (TURK and HUMPHREY, 1961; BATTISTO and

Chase, 1965; Borel *et al.*, 1966) and may turn out to be a general phenomenon. We have become acquainted with several observations which are best interpreted by assuming that the cell-mediated ability to eliminate the virus may be specifically suppressed, although, at the same time, the ability of forming antibody is left intact, which is reminiscent of the phenomenon of "immune deviation" (Asherson, 1967).

Recent evidence suggests that at least two populations of lymphocytes participate in the immune response, one being thymus dependent (T-cells) and the other thymus independent (B-cells). Both T- and B-cells appear to cooperate in the humoral response though only the B-cells secrete antibody (Mitchell and Miller, 1968). Cell-mediated immune responses, on the other hand, depend primarily on the functional activity of T-cells (Miller and Osoba, 1967). It is also becoming clear that immunological tolerance may affect these two cell types independently (Isaković *et al.*, 1965; Smith *et al.*, 1966; Staples *et al.*, 1966; Taylor, 1968; Playfair, 1969). Thus it would seem that for a given antigen T-cells may be tolerant while B-cells remain immunologically competent. This consideration may apply to all self antigens as well as to the viral antigens in LCM virus carrier mice, and, indeed, it may be hypothesized that the biological role of immunological tolerance, namely prevention of self destruction, applies only to its cell-bound component and that its "failure" with regard to the production of circulating antibody is the rule rather than the exception.

Whether the cell-associated suppression is likewise incomplete in mice infected congenitally with LCM virus is unknown. One 20-month-old mouse from an established carrier colony was observed by Mims (personal communication) to tremble spontaneously and to undergo tonic convulsions after spinning, as is typical for mice inoculated intracerebrally, indicating participation of cellular immune mechanisms in at least this one animal. The experimental elucidation of this question may be difficult but worth every effort. Be the answer yes or no, it is bound to broaden our knowledge of the mechanism of immunological tolerance and at the same time deepen our understanding of its biological significance.

c) Pathology

Many descriptions are on record (Armstrong and Lillie, 1934; Findlay *et al.*, 1936; Findlay and Stern, 1936; Lépine and Sautter, 1936; Rivers and Scott, 1936a; Traub, 1936a; 1939c; Kasahara *et al.*, 1939; Yamada, 1940a; Alice, 1945b; Alice and McNutt, 1945; Shwartzman, 1946; Lerner and Haas, 1958; Collins *et al.*, 1961) of which the one given by Lillie and Armstrong (1945) is the most extensive. In the central nervous system they found slight meningeal infiltrations on the third day after intracerebral inoculation which increased to a maximum between the sixth and ninth day, being more intense on the base than dorsally. At about the same time, inflammation of the choroid plexus was at its height, with greater involvement in the third and fourth than in the lateral ventricles. The picture was strikingly similar after peripheral inoculation, although it developed slightly slower. Ventricular exudates were only seen after intracerebral inoculation and were thought to result from the introduction of foreign matter into the brain. During the period of greatest meningeal, plexal, and ventricular involvement, lymphocytic infiltrations often extended into the Virchow-Robin spaces. Sometimes distinct edema of the corona radiata next to the lateral ventricles was observed. Occasional foci of cellular gliosis were found in a few mice. Irrespective of the route of inoculation, encephalitis was conspicuously absent. FINDLAY and STERN (1936) also emphasized that the nerve cells, even those in close proximity to the meningeal or ventricular exudates, remained unaffected. An occasional Purkinje cell was necrotic.

More involvement of the brain tissue was seen by TRAUB (1936a). In some mice he found the brain stems to be infiltrated. Small collections of oligodendroglia cells were seen in a few mice in the cortex at the base of the brain. In many mice a proportion of the cerebellar Purkinje cells were pyknotic and shrunken. In the spinal cord, an occasional ventral horn cell was degenerated and surrounded by oligodendroglial and microglial cells. Traub too concluded that "on the whole, nerve cell degeneration and neuronophagy were not frequent, and the changes in the nervous tissue proper were few". In contrast to most investigators, COLLINS *et al.* (1961) found a "well-marked meningoencephalitis and myelitis" on days seven and eight after intracerebral inoculation of the WE virus; the plexus were free of alterations.

The visceral reactions were infrequent after intracerebral inoculation but became more prominent when peripheral routes were employed.

Because of the immunologic implications of the LCM virus infection of the mouse, the alterations in its lymphoid organs are of particular interest. After intracerebral infection the circulating leukocytes fell slightly on the third day from 7,000 per mm^3 to 5,000 per mm^3, followed by a rise to 9,000 or 10,000 per mm^3 and a further decline prior to death; lymphocytes were relatively reduced all the time (BENSON *et al.*, 1960). Diminished numbers of leukocytes were also counted by MAKSUDOVA (1967) in BALB/c mice after the intracerebral inoculation of 100 LD_{50} of LCM virus. According to LILLIE and ARMSTRONG (1945), the spleens were enlarged to two or three times their normal sizes. The follicles were moderately active, being hyperplastic on the sixth to eighth day. Sometimes there was accumulation of nuclear fragments either free in the lymph clefts or in the phagocytes. In mice which had died early this graded into frank karyorrhectic necrosis of follicular substance, but more often there were hemorrhagic disruption and replacement of follicles as part of perifollicular hyaline thrombosis and hemorrhage. The splenic pulp was moderately congested in most animals and contained variable amounts of myeloid cells. Again, in animals that died early there were focal to patchy hyaline thrombosis and karyorrhectic necrosis of the pulp. TRAUB (1936a) noted enlargement of the spleens; after intravenous infections they were up to six times larger than normal. Microscopically, the Malpighian bodies were increased in size and the red pulp was infiltrated with mononuclear cells. According to FINDLAY and STERN (1936), the spleens were congested with "slight enlargement of the malpighian bodies".

In intracerebrally infected mice, LERNER and HAAS (1958) noted that the lesions in the lymphoid organs were not consistent. Involved spleens contained numerous phagocytic cells. The follicles were hyperplastic but were sometimes obliterated by reticuloendothelial hyperplasia. The pulp was occasionally congested or hemorrhagic with necroses and follicle destruction. RIVERS and SCOTT (1936a) saw "nothing particularly characteristic of the disease" in the spleens.

In lymph nodes, Lillie and Armstrong (1945) distinguished two types of changes, one involving the follicles, the other the pulp and the sinuses. Sometimes they occurred together, but more often nodes showed either the one or the other process. Follicular changes comprised swelling and hyperplasia, dilatation of lymph clefts, and accumulation of nuclear fragments in these and in the swollen and phagocytic littoral cells. The lesions of pulp and sinuses consisted of serum and fibrin exudation in focal areas, often subcapsular, accompanied by more or less cellular depletion, hemorrhage, karyorrhexis, erythrophagia, and frank coagulation necroses. As was mentioned in connection with the spleen, alterations were most marked in mice that had died early. In Traub's series (Traub, 1936a) some of the normally sized lymph nodes had "reticuloendothelial hyperplasia". In his later studies on the multiplication of the W strain of LCM virus in cells from lymph nodes cultivated *in vitro*, Traub (1962b; Traub and Kesting, 1963) noted that in subcutaneously infected mice the regional lymph nodes were invariably swollen on the fourth day, the other nodes and the spleen one to three days later. They became frequently "as large as in animals sacrificed at an early stage of lymphatic leukemia". During this time cultivation *in vitro* of such nodes was not possible. After intracerebral infection, Lerner and Haas (1958) saw hyperplastic follicles and phagocytic cells. Reticuloendothelial hyperplasia was occasionally "so extensive as to obliterate follicular architecture". The lesions were not consistent and varied in frequency and severity. Apparently, no changes were noticed by Rivers and Scott (1936a).

Alterations found by Lillie and Armstrong (1945) in the thymuses of intracerebrally or intraperitoneally infected mice consisted essentially of karyorrhexis and necrosis of cortical lymphocytes accompanied by dilatation of lymph spaces in both the cortex and the medulla and accumulation of nuclear debris which was taken up by the swollen littoral cells. Cell necrosis soon resulted in extensive depletion of the cortex, and the expansion of the littoral cells led to an "epithelioid replacement". After intraperitoneal inoculation this process became apparent on the fourth day and after intracerebral inoculation two or three days later.

A thorough account of the changes in lymphoid organs of multicolored W.E.H.I. mice after the intravenous inoculation of 10^5 LD_{50} of the WE virus was given by Mims and Tosolini (1969). In the spleens perifollicular lesions consisting of large pale cells, some infected as evinced by immunofluorescence, some pyroninophilic, with areas of amorphous extracellular eosinophilic material appeared on days four to five. With time more cells degenerated and on day six the lesions were severe extending into the follicles. The authors noted the similarity of these alterations with those seen in spleens during homologous disease, parabiotic intoxication, and other graft *versus* host reactions. Similar changes developed in lymph nodes. After subcutaneous infection, the local nodes underwent extensive irreversible necroses. In the thymus, changes were first noted on the fifth day with depletion of lymphocytes in the cortex. In the medulla the cell density was increased, the veins were dilated, and karyorrhectic nuclear fragments were seen lying inside reticular cells.

Changes in all lymphoid organs were noted by Hanaoka *et al.* (1969) who followed the events in spleen, lymph nodes, and thymus after the intracerebral inoculation of 1000 ID_{50} (mouse) of the WE strain. Virus propagation was accompanied by a marked depletion of the "thymus-dependent areas", in both spleen and lymph nodes, of small lymphocytes commencing as early as two days after infection and a similar disappearance of small cells in the thymus three to five days later. In this period the weights of the thymuses dropped significantly as compared with noninfected controls; the weights of spleen and lymph nodes were said to be likewise affected although not significantly. These alterations bear a striking similarity to those seen in mice treated with cortisone or subjected to severe stress (DOUGHERTY, 1952; ISHIDATE and METCALF, 1963). It is conceivable that the WE strain which is known to multiply in most if not all organs of the mouse assumes the role of a stressor acting through the release of adrenocortical hormones rather than by destroying selectively the small lymphocytes in a more direct way.

Neither the findings of Hanaoka and his colleagues nor my interpretation may be generalized. A comparison of the various accounts given above reveals differences which probably depend on virus strains, doses, routes of inoculation, and even the host. Thus, the marked changes in WE virus-infected mice did not show up when the Armstrong strain was used. In C57BL, Bagg, CBA, and A mice splenic lesions were all but absent, although virus titers in C57BL mouse spleens were higher and immunofluorescence as extensive as in stock mice (MIMS and WAINWRIGHT, 1968; MIMS and TOSOLINI, 1969).

As regards the other organs and tissues, generalized lymphocytic infiltration, sometimes including larger lymphoid and plasma cells, macrophages, and polymorphonuclear leukocytes involved pleura and peritoneum, kidney cortex and pelvis, liver, pancreas, lungs, heart, adrenal glands, salivary glands. Fatty degenerations were found in liver and kidneys as early as the third day after infection. Focal necroses occurred in the liver; in the bone marrow these were more diffuse (LILLIE and ARMSTRONG, 1945).

In the cytoplasm of mononuclear cells from infected mice, monkeys, and rats FINDLAY and STERN (1936) detected "small collections of minute granules only just within the power of resolution of the microscope"; none in the controls. These granules were even better recognized if the smears were first stained with Giemsa's stain and then examined with dark field illumination. REISS-GUTFREUND *et al.* (1961) observed two types of cell inclusions in mice and guinea-pigs after infection with human isolates of uncertain identity (see Section XII). POLLARD *et al.* (1968a) saw by means of the electron microscope cytoplasmic inclusions containing small electron-dense "virus-like" particles in spleen cells from established carrier mice. They were considered to be of LCM virus origin.

5. Immunologic Response

TRAUB (1936b) observed a rapid development of protection in adult mice. Intracerebral challenge of mice one day after intraperitoneal inoculation of virus led to typical convulsions, whereas, if intracerebral challenge was delayed until day five, a few mice were protected. On day eight no disease developed. LYON (1940) found that three days after subcutaneous infections, a significant proportion of mice were capable of withstanding intracerebral challenge, and on the fifth day protection was complete. Similar results were reported by ROWE

(1954) and Haas (1954). With the WE virus, Seamer *et al.* (1963) observed partial and almost complete resistance, respectively, four and five days after the subcutaneous infection. When the WHI strain was employed, resistance developed faster.

Uphoff and Haas (1960) lethally X-irradiated nonimmune and LCM virus-hyperimmunized (BALB/c $\times$ DBA/2)F_1 hybrids and protected them with bone marrow and spleen cells from normal and hyperimmunized donors. As a rule, the immune state of the recipient mouse determined the response to intracerebral virus challenge 21 and 33 days later. In contrast, Volkert (1963) achieved adoptive immunization by the inoculation of spleen and lymph node cells from LCM-immune syngeneic donors. Recipients were protected against 100 LD_{50} when transplantation was done at least two weeks and against ten LD_{50} when transplantation was done at least one week before intracerebral challenge.

It is noteworthy that in spite of the absence of clinical signs after intracerebral challenge in mice immunized by peripheral infection the virus multiplies. Rowe (1954) studied the relationship between the time after immunizing infection and the virus' ability to multiply in the brain. With short intervals, the multiplication was reduced though not abolished. At nine months, titers on the second day were as high as in the nonimmunized control mice, but they fell rapidly. Surprisingly, many of the mice which remained free of clinical illness nevertheless histologically had meningitis. It developed at an accelerated rate, appearing at least three days earlier than in nonimmune mice. Haas (1954) measured the rate of virus multiplication in the brains of subcutaneously immunized mice and found it to be indistinguishable from multiplication in nonimmune animals for the first three to five days. In contrast, virus did not multiply if immunity had resulted from an intracerebral infection but was rapidly eliminated (Rowe, 1954; Haas, 1954; Traub, 1961a). Multiplication in the viscera after intraperitoneal inoculation was more effectively suppressed, irrespective of whether immunity followed intraperitoneal or intracerebral infection (Rowe, 1954).

Traub and Kesting (1963) and Traub (1964) noted some delay of virus multiplication in lymph node cell cultures immediately after dispersal of the cells, if the organs had come from actively immune mice. In infected L cells, the virus titers were not affected by the addition ot spleen cells from immune C3H mice to the culture (Lundstedt, 1969a).

Infants born of actively immunized mothers were not measurably protected when challenged by intracerebral inoculation (Traub, 1961a; Weigand and Hotchin, 1961).

Hannover Larsen (1969b) followed the development of the ability of lymphoid cells to adoptively immunize syngeneic carrier mice (see Section V. A. 4. b). On days zero, two, and four after intraperitoneal infection of the donor mice no effect was obtained. With cells from the eighth day a proportion of the recipients was freed of the virus and developed antibody, signifying specific immunologic activity of the donor cells. At about the same time the infected donor mice had lost the virus from the blood and had begun to produce measurable amounts of complement-fixing antibody.

The rapid development of solid immunological protection contrasts with the slow and weak response in respect of circulating antibody. After nonlethal infection, complement-fixing antibody is regularly demonstrated (TRAUB and SCHÄFER, 1939; SMADEL and WALL, 1940; WEIGAND and HOTCHIN, 1961; VOLKERT *et al.*, 1964; HANNOVER LARSEN, 1968b; 1969b). It appears between the 6th and 12th day, reaches moderate titers of 64 to 128 and persists unaltered for many months, presumably lifelong. Booster effects following repeated virus inoculations are not obtained. At no stage is the complement-fixing activity affected by 2-mercaptoethanol (HANNOVER LARSEN, 1969b). According to LEWIS and CLAYTON (1969a), antibody titers determined by indirect immunofluorescence are, on the whole, somewhat higher than complement fixation titers.

SINKOVICS and MOLNÁR (1955) searched for antibody in homogenates prepared from retromediastinal lymph nodes after intranasal infection. Complement-fixing antibody was occasionally detected at low concentrations; neutralizing antibody was consistently absent. After intranasal instillation of a vaccine, prepared from LCM virus-infected mouse brain, again neutralizing activity was not found. In marked contrast, complement-fixing antibody attained high titers (64—128) which by far exceeded the titer in the serum (four). Probably lack of antibody formation in the regional lymph nodes is the functional expression of their severe pathological alterations after infection with LCM virus (see Section V. A. 4. c) which may be expected to be absent after vaccination. Sinkovics and Molnár observed cellular activation in lymph nodes from both groups of mice. Hemorrhages and edema, however, were only seen after infection with native virus.

Until recently, neutralizing antibody in mice, even after repeated infections, could either not be demonstrated at all (TRAUB, 1936b; TRAUB, 1937; TRAUB and SCHÄFER, 1939; SMADEL and WALL, 1940; HAAS, 1954; SINKOVICS, 1955; SINKOVICS and MOLNÁR, 1955; SMORODINTSEV, 1957; WEIGAND and HOTCHIN, 1961; VOLKERT *et al.*, 1964; PETERSON and MAKSUDOVA, 1969) or at low levels (ROWE, 1954; TRAUB, 1959; TRAUB, 1960b; TRAUB, 1961a; TRAUB, 1964). HOTCHIN *et al.* (1969) used a refined assay and claimed to have detected considerable amounts of neutralizing antibody which appeared many months after infection. The data are as follows; antibody was detected in one of four sera from pairs of carrier and immune mice joined in parabiosis which is comparable to adoptive immunization. One of two high dose survivors (see Section V. A. 4. b) had neutralizing antibody which, again, is a special case. Altogether two mice were tested which had been immunized in the usual way, *i.e.* by peripheral infection. Of these one had neutralizing antibody, the other did not.

Two explanations could account for the failure of detecting neutralizing activities in LCM-immune mice; either mice are essentially incapable of producing such substances, or, alternatively, neutralizing antibody is present but is missed because of inadequacies of the employed techniques. By means of a quantal assay of the virus in L cell tube cultures (LEHMANN-GRUBE and HESSE, 1967), LEHMANN-GRUBE and SLENCZKA (to be published) proved the second alternative to be correct; after infection, mice produce neutralizing antibody which can readily be demonstrated. The results of several experiments may be summarized as follows. Neutralization becomes detectable during the fourth week after infection with LCM virus, WE strain. The titer — defined as the reciprocal of that serum dilution which reduces 100 ID_{50} down to one ID_{50} — rises slowly, reaching maximum values between days 50 and 100 after infection. Complement-fixing activities appear earlier and climb faster. Figure 13 illustrates a representative experiment. Control sera were free of either activities.

As compared with other virus infections, the neutralizing titers are low; their maxima range between 30 and 50. It has been repeatedly argued that the poor neutralizing antibody response indicates "weak" antigenicity of the LCM virus. Whereas this may be true with respect to the humoral response, it cannot be accepted in a general form. The virus is fully capable of inducing a specific protection which, again, indicates that circulating antibody is not concerned with either the removal of the virus or the prevention of the illness of the mouse (see Section V. A. 4. b). Nor has evidence come to light which would support the hypothesis, sometimes stated to explain the ease with which immunological tolerance is established (see Section V. A. 3), that the virus is antigenically related to the mouse.

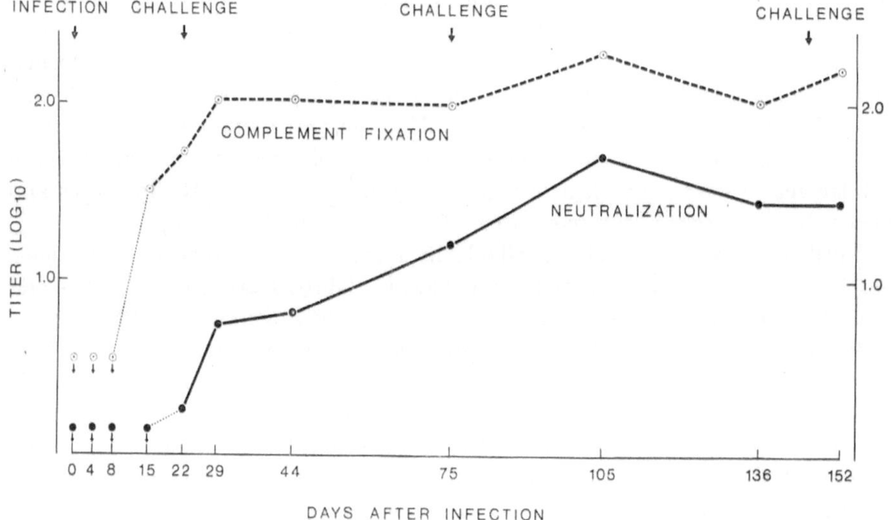

Fig. 13. Development of neutralizing and complement-fixing antibodies in mice infected with the WE strain of LCM virus.

At intervals after subcutaneous infection with 10^3 ID_{50} (mouse) and intracerebral challenge inoculations with the same dose of virus, groups of mice were bled and the neutralizing strengths of the pooled sera determined. Neutralizing titer is the reciprocal of that serum dilution which reduces 100 ID_{50} of LCM virus, strain WE, down to one ID_{50}. The complement fixation tests were performed with the microtiter system according to Sever (1962)

It may be added here that in mice which had been infected as adults and which were fully immune as far as protection is concerned infectivity was frequently detected in the organs — notably the kidneys — and even the blood up to many months after infection (Traub, 1938b; Haas, 1954; Rowe, 1954; Smorodintsev, 1957; Traub, 1961b; Lehmann-Grube, 1964a; Volkert and Hannover Larsen, 1965c; Hannover Larsen, 1969c). Also, virus was activated in such mice by treatment with antilymphocytic serum (Volkert and Lundstedt, 1968). Traub (1962b) demonstrated infectivity in lymph nodes 14 and 30 but not 41 days after *in vivo* infection by cultivation *in vitro*. In a later study he detected virus by this method up to two months after infection but not thereafter (Traub, 1964).

It could be argued that LCM virus-infected mice never completely eliminate the virus. The confirmed observation that immunity wanes as time passes by (see Section V. A. 4. b) speaks against this possibility. Probably, virus multiplication and the host's elimination mechanisms are delicately balanced with the weights on either side dependent on factors such as virus strain, infecting dose, mouse strain, route of inoculation, *etc.*

MIMS and WAINWRIGHT (1968) investigated the effect of peripheral virus infection on the ability of Walter and Eliza Hall Institute mice to respond to other antigens. After inoculation of the WE strain of LCM virus into the foot pad of the mature mouse, the development of hemagglutinating antibody was reduced when sheep red cells were inoculated 11, 15, and 20 but not 5 or 56 days later. Intravenous infection resulted in a similar antibody depression. Other immune reactions, *i.e.* the development of antibody to human serum albumin and the anaphylactic response to ovalbumin were likewise depressed. In mature C57BL mice, infected intravenously with WE strain virus and immunized seven days later, the number of plaque-forming spleen cells was greatly reduced. In neonatally WE virus-infected mice antibody responses were reduced when sheep red cells were given ten days later. In contrast, the ability to respond to antigens was not affected in established neonatal or congenital carriers.

When mice which had been immunized with sheep erythrocytes 15 days after infection were bled again four months later, the antibody titers did not differ significantly from those of the controls. The secondary immune responses upon challenge in both groups were equal. However, if the booster inoculation of red cells was preceded by an LCM virus infection, the secondary response was significantly depressed. No immunosuppression was observed after the infection of the mouse with the Armstrong (E-350) strain of LCM virus.

Ectromelia virus was much more lethal for mice which had been inoculated a week earlier with the WE strain, and ectromelia-immune mice showed reduced foot pad swelling due to ectromelia virus and failed to control virus multiplication when infected with LCM virus before challenge with ectromelia virus.

Other virus infections of the mouse are known to affect the immune response to a variety of antigens. The lactic dehydrogenase-elevating agent resembles the LCM virus, inasmuch as pathology in infected cells is absent (NOTKINS, 1965). Infection of mice with this virus prolonged skin homograft survival (HOWARD *et al.*, 1969) but enhanced the humoral response to human γ-globulin (NOTKINS *et al.*, 1966). Agents causing mouse leukemia, *e.g.*, Gross' passage A virus (PETERSON *et al.*, 1963; DENT *et al.*, 1965), Friend virus (SALAMAN and WEDDERBURN, 1966; ODAKA *et al.*, 1966; CEGLOWSKI and FRIEDMAN, 1967), and Rauscher virus (SIEGEL and MORTON, 1966a; 1966b), usually suppressed both types of immunity, even if the immunizing antigens were given before any signs of leukemia had developed. OSBORN *et al.* (1968) analyzed the depression of humoral antibody responses in mice inapparently infected with murine cytomegalovirus.

In all these examples of virus-induced incapacity of immunological responsiveness, little is known of the basic mechanisms. FRIEDMAN and CEGLOWSKI (1968) presented evidence indicating that in the case of Friend virus, antigen-responsive precursor cells are affected by the infection, an explanation which does not account satisfactorily for the observations made with the LCM virus.

With the present knowledge it cannot be excluded that, after peripheral infection, cells of the immunological system are destroyed directly or indirectly by the multiplying LCM virus — as it seems to be the case after intracerebral inoculation (see Section V. A. 4. c) — thus lowering the host's immunological capacity. Circumstantial evidence, however, militates against this possibility. No suppression of response to other antigens was apparent on the fifth day after virus infection, although at this time the virus multiplication might be assumed to have been at its peak. Immunosuppression occurred independently of follicular lesions in the lymphoid tissues of WE virus-infected mice (Mims and Wainwright, 1968). Furthermore, Schwenk, Slenczka, and Lehmann-Grube (see Section V. A. 4. a) have obtained no evidence that lymphoid cells of the mouse, either from the blood or from the spleen, participate in the infectious process. It should also be kept in mind that infected mice respond immunologically quite vigorously to the virus (see above). Nor is immunologic competition an explanation which accounts for the facts; why should the effect of Armstrong virus, which is undoubtedly as strong an antigen as WE, be different? It appears likely that immunosuppression by different viruses is mediated by different mechanisms, and a final interpretation of the effects the LCM virus has on the immunological capacity of the infected host cannot be given at the present time.

B. Guinea-Pig

1. Signs of the Disease

In the earliest reports on the LCM virus, its pathogenicity for guinea-pigs was noted (Armstrong and Lillie, 1934; Rivers and Scott, 1936a; Traub, 1935a; 1935b; 1936a). Later it turned out that many strains do not cause overt disease in guinea-pigs, although they are — with few exceptions (Ackermann *et al.*, 1964; Scheid *et al.*, 1966) — infectious for them. All grades of virulence may be encountered. At one end of the spectrum is found the WE strain of which one infectious unit kills the guinea-pig, independent of the route of inoculation (Smadel and Wall, 1940; Shwartzman, 1946; Jochheim *et al.*, 1957; Benda *et al.*, 1964; Lehmann-Grube, unpublished). At the other end we may place Armstrong's strain E-350 which hardly ever is lethal for these animals.

The disease following subcutaneous or intraperitoneal infection with the WE strain virus may be described as follows. Three to six days after the infection, depending on the dose, the temperature becomes elevated often reaching 41.5° C. The animal rapidly loses weight and develops marked prostration, weakness, conjunctivitis, salivation, and labored breathing. Shortly before death, which with high doses occurs six to seven days after infection, the temperature drops to subnormal levels. The disease picture does not differ whether the virus is administered peripherally or by way of the central nervous system except that the course is more acute after the intracerebral inoculation. With less pathogenic strains transient fever may be the only objective sign of an infection.

Using the UBC (=WE) strain, Roger (1963a) elicited a local inflammatory reaction by intradermal inoculation which was neutralized by LCM-specific antibody. As compared with a similar phenomenon in rabbits (see Section V. E) guinea-pigs required three to four $\log_{10}$ less virus. The reaction following an intradermal injection was usually accompanied by a fatal systemic disease. On occasion, the local reaction preceded the generalized disease by several days.

2. Pathogenesis

a) *Multiplication and Distribution of the Virus*

After subcutaneous injection of the highly virulent J. P. strain, Milzer (1942) detected infectivity in the blood 24 hours later; it persisted until the animal's death. Nikolitsch and Fenje (1959; Nikolitsch, 1959) determined the infectivity of blood and brain after intramuscular infection. It was present in the circulation on the second day (no earlier test) and in the brain on the fourth to fifth day. At the site of inoculation the results were too variable to permit the conclusion that the virus had multiplied locally. Using the Paris strain of LCM virus, Mendoza (1937) studied its distribution after the intraperitoneal infection. The highest virus concentration was attained in the spleen; next came the lymph nodes. Of the other organs, only the suprarenal glands contained enough virus to indicate local multiplication. Lungs and livers, though highly infectious, could not be titrated because of bacterial contaminations. Benda *et al.* (1964) followed the development with time after subcutaneous, intranasal, and inhalation infection of the weakly pathogenic K strain in various organs and found early and high titers in lymph nodes and spleens, low titers in the lungs, and traces in the blood. After subcutaneous or inhalation infection with the highly virulent WE strain, most virus was found in spleens and lymph nodes, equalled only by the lungs, with peak titers around the fifth day. All other organs had less virus although always more than the blood, indicating multiplication throughout the body. Traub (1936b) searched for virus in blood and urine of subcutaneously infected guinea-pigs and found it in the urine for up to 44 days after infection even though, at the same time, tests performed with the blood were negative. It is not known whether there was no virus or whether it was present in a neutralized form. The consistent finding that the LCM virus multiplies preferentially in the spleens and lymph nodes of guinea-pigs is of considerable interest because it may indicate a propensity of this virus to multiply in lymphoid cells. However, as in the case of the mouse (see Section V. A. 4. a) direct proof is lacking.

Data concerning the distribution of virus in guinea-pigs after infection by inhalation may also be found in papers by Benda (1964) and Benda and Činátl (1964).

b) *Pathology and Pathogenetic Mechanisms*

In spite of the marked differences of virulence among the strains, the pathology they produce in the organs of infected guinea-pigs is rather uniform and only differs quantitatively between strains and also routes of inoculation (Findlay *et al.*, 1936; Findlay and Stern, 1936; Rivers and Scott, 1936a; Traub, 1936a; Kasahara *et al.*, 1939; Yamada, 1940a; Lillie and Armstrong, 1944; Alice, 1945b; Alice and McNutt, 1945; Benda *et al.*, 1964). A mild chiefly basilar meningitis and inflammatory alterations of the plexus chorioidei are often found. The brain is never involved to any extent. Among the other organs, the lungs are mainly affected, with areas of inflammatory consolidation in many parts. All other organs may or may not show similar changes. In spleens and lymph nodes follicle hyperplasia and intrafollicular phagocytosis of nuclear fragments and in the splenic pulp early polymorphonuclear infiltration and later reticuloendotheliosis and lymphoid cell infiltration have been described. On the whole, the pathology of

LCM virus infections in guinea-pigs is rather uncharacteristic, and claims that the identity of a new LCM virus isolate was established on the basis of its pathology in guinea-pigs should be regarded with caution.

Traub (1935b; 1936a) discovered intranuclear inclusions in the cells of the pia mater and the meningeal vessels as well as in monocytes lining the meninges and in glia cells in 8 of 14 guinea-pigs. Since they were not present in mice or in the lungs of guinea-pigs, he considered their etiological significance to be doubtful.

Little can be said concerning the pathogenetic mechanisms. Data obtained by Benda *et al.* (1964) indicate that the virus multiplies in the local lymph nodes before it spreads throughout the body. One wishes to know whether, as in the mouse, an immune conflict is involved. The observation by Rowe (1954; 1956) that the course of the disease is not affected by X-irradiation makes such an assumption unlikely, although more data are needed before this question may be answered.

3. Immunologic Response

It has been said before that many strains of LCM virus are weakly pathogenic for guinea-pigs; but they do induce solid protection to virulent strains. The details of this conversion are not known. It seems to be a rapid process; ten days after a subcutaneous infection with E-350 the guinea-pigs resisted challenge with the otherwise invariably lethal WE strain (Hesse and Lehmann-Grube, unpublished).

The development of complement-fixing antibody is strain dependent. Smadel and Wall (1940) infected guinea-pigs with the WWS strain. Antibody was found 14 days later with peaks at five to six weeks after infection and quick disappearance thereafter. With the RES strain antibody formation was delayed. After repeated inoculations of LCM virus isolated by C. Armstrong, Howitt (1937) found marked complement-fixing activity in one of six guinea-pigs only. Jochheim *et al.* (1957) experienced great difficulties employing the highly virulent WE strain. The animals either died or had not been infected at all as was established by their death following challenge. A few guinea-pigs could be immunized with heat, ultraviolet light or formalin vaccines, or with partially neutralized virus. Complement-fixing antibody, however, appeared irregularly and usually — though not always — in low titers. Lépine *et al.* (1938a; 1938b) found complement-fixing antibody in none of 12 infected guinea-pigs.

After the subcutaneous infection with the weakly pathogenic E-350 strain on days zero and ten, Hesse and Lehmann-Grube (unpublished) did not detect complement-fixing antibody on day 17; on day 21 low concentrations had appeared, which did not increase further. When the booster inoculation on the tenth day was done with the highly virulent WE strain, again complement-fixing antibody did not become demonstrable before day 21; it climbed higher, however, reaching moderate titers on days 28 and 34 but began declining five days later. Significantly higher concentrations of complement-fixing antibody with titers of up to 512 were obtained by Hronovský *et al.* (1969) who had adopted a similar regimen; four and seven weeks after an intraperitoneal infection with the A strain of LCM virus the animals were challenged with WE. No systematic study seems to have been done to investigate the reason for such discrepancies. From what we know, the cause could lie either with the guinea-pigs or the virus strains. The above mentioned observation, that antibody appeared later following infection with RES than with WWS strain in apparently the same stock of guinea-pigs, indicates that differences of the serologic responses between virus strains do exist.

In contrast, neutralizing antibody appeared more regularly and significantly later, *i.e.* five to eight weeks after infection; it also persisted longer (SMADEL and WALL, 1940). The failure of BENDA and ČINÁTL (1964) to detect neutralizing activity in guinea-pigs after infection with the avirulent strain "K" is unexplained. In a more recent study reported from the same laboratory, moderate concentrations of neutralizing antibody were detected in the sera of three of three guinea-pigs four weeks after the intraperitoneal inoculation of the same virus strain. At seven weeks the neutralizing indices had climbed to about $\log_{10}$ two. At the same time the complement fixation titers ranged from 256 to 512 and the immunofluorescing titers were 128 in all three animals (HRONOVSKÝ *et al.*, 1969). The duration of persistence of neutralizing activity in guinea-pig sera seems to be unknown.

C. Monkeys

1. Signs of the Disease

In many reports, "monkey" is used without qualification regarding the species, though it may be assumed that either *Macaca mulatta (M. rhesus)* or *M. cynomolgus (M. irus)* was employed in most cases. There is general agreement that the LCM virus is pathogenic for both these species and also for cebus monkeys (ARMSTRONG and LILLIE, 1934). After inoculation into the brain, fever developed and remained high for from three to ten days. It fell to subnormal levels at the time of death, but recovery was the rule (ARMSTRONG and LILLIE, 1934; RIVERS and SCOTT, 1936a). After peripheral infection, the clinical course was found to be less severe (ARMSTRONG and WOOLEY, 1937). However, LILLIE (1936b) reported that of 51 monkeys inoculated by various routes, 42 had died or were killed *in extremis*. This higher pathogenicity was also observed by FINDLAY and STERN (1936) who employed the American strain of Armstrong as well as their own isolates. Only one of nine rhesus monkeys inoculated intracerebrally, and one of two inoculated intraperitoneally, survived. All four crab-eating macaques *(Macaca irus)* succumbed after intracerebral or intraperitoneal inoculations. Death was preceded by a sudden fall in temperature; neurological signs were minimal.

ARMSTRONG and LILLIE (1934) investigated the cerebrospinal fluid from infected monkeys and counted increased numbers of cells ("almost entirely lymphocytes"). They noted that the disease induced in monkeys closely resembled Wallgren's syndrome in man.

The French strain of virus caused a benign infection in monkeys, including chimpanzees, even after intracerebral inoculation (LÉPINE and SAUTTER, 1936; LÉPINE *et al.*, 1937b). Fever developed in rhesus monkeys infected with the Japanese isolate. In the majority of cases, no nervous system signs were seen but an occasional animal became "paralytic and lethargic" (KASAHARA *et al.*, 1939). (The identiy of the "red-haired monkeys", mentioned by KASAHARA *et al.*, 1937a;

1937b as being susceptible, is uncertain.) No clinical signs at all were elicited by WIKTOR *et al.* (1966) who inoculated rhesus monkeys intracerebrally or intraperitoneally with three strains isolated from inadvertently infected cell cultures.

The description given by DALLDORF *et al.* (1938a) for the disease produced in rhesus monkeys by the distemper virus may be cited here because it was later shown to be most probably due to an LCM virus contaminant (DALLDORF and DOUGLASS, 1938). Independent of the route of infection, an acute febrile disease followed which in half the cases was distinctly biphasic. Besides fever, the predominant signs were weakness, diarrhea, and emaciation. In the early phases, rhinitis and conjunctivitis were sometimes found. Of 63 monkeys, three died with encephalitis and one with pneumonia. In five rhesus monkeys infected intracerebrally or intraperitoneally with LCM virus, strain M, by WENNER (1948) tremulous movements, hyperexcitability, marked clumsiness, and a stiff gait developed, accompanied by moderate fever, prostration, and inappetence. All animals recovered. A sixth monkey showed no signs of disease after intravenous inoculation.

In later reports, a decidedly higher virulence was noted, even when the same strains were employed. MILZER and LEVINSON (1949) reported that *M. mulatta* uniformly succumbed to subcutaneous infection with as few as about 100 intracerebral mouse LD_{50} of strain J. P. virus. DANEŠ *et al.* (1963) injected Rivers' WE strain into *M. cynomolgus* and *M. rhesus*. Both species succumbed to the disease, apparently with a high lethality. The effects of infection by inhalation were more precisely determined. In *M. cynomolgus* less than 200 mouse LD_{50} caused viremia and clinical signs and more than 350 LD_{50} were lethal. *M. rhesus* was found to be even more susceptible, death ensuing after the inhalation of as little as 12 mouse LD_{50}. Clinical signs in these monkeys consisted of loss of appetite with reduction of weight and fever which subsided shortly before death. X-rays, taken at different times after inhalation, revealed bronchopneumonia in one animal only. COGGESHALL (1939) reported on a highly virulent infection among the rhesus monkeys in his laboratory. The disease was characterized by dependent edema, serosanguineous nasal discharges, prostration, and a high lethality. This has remained a unique observation and it is to be regretted that the identification of the agent was not documented in greater detail.

2. Pathogenesis

a) Multiplication and Distribution of the Virus

After infection, the virus appears in the organs and in the blood stream (ARMSTRONG and LILLIE, 1934; ARMSTRONG, 1936; ARMSTRONG *et al.*, 1936; FINDLAY and STERN, 1936; DALLDORF, 1939b; YAMADA, 1940a). The kinetics of viral infection were followed in some detail by DANEŠ *et al.* (1963) after infection by inhalation. In cynomolgus monkeys which had inhaled high or low doses the virus was found in the lungs and hilar lymph nodes on the second day and two days later in the blood. The same sequence was seen in rhesus monkeys, except that the delay in appearance of virus in the blood was as long as six days. Undoubtedly, virus multiplied locally before it was distributed into the circulation.

b) *Pathology and Pathogenetic Mechanisms*

Alterations of tissues and organs in infected monkeys have been frequently described (Armstrong and Lillie, 1934; Rivers and Scott, 1936a; Kasahara *et al.*, 1939; Yamada, 1940a; Daneš *et al.*, 1963). The most extensive investigation was conducted by Lillie (1936b). It will be recalled that the name given to this virus was derived from the alterations it caused in monkeys and mice, and a lymphocytic choriomeningitis has remained the most conspicuous lesion in experimentally infected monkeys. Apart from some infiltration associated with the vessel sheaths and a few foci of cellular gliosis, the brain was usually free from lesions. The same was found in the spinal root ganglia. Only Daneš *et al.* (1963) reported meningoencephalitis in *M. cynomolgus* and, less severe, in *M. rhesus* after inhalation infection with the WE strain. The lungs were often involved, with congestion, serous exudation, interstitial edema, hemorrhages, and perivascular lymphocytic infiltrations. Some animals had pyelitis and a cystitis which was sometimes hemorrhagic. Liver changes were seen in a proportion of the monkeys. These consisted of coagulative to fibrinoid hemorrhagic necroses, which could also be found in the adrenal and parathyroid glands. Spleen, lymph nodes, and bone marrow usually showed hyperplasia. All organs had focal interstitial or perivascular lymph cell infiltrations, notably the kidney, epidydimis, uterus, Fallopian tube, parathyroid, heart, tracheal mucosa, and, less often, the esophageal mucosa, pancreas, adrenal, testis, ovary, and skeletal muscle.

In monkeys which had become infected accidentally and by an unknown route during work with strains from fatal human cases, Armstrong (1942) saw "a marked destruction of liver tissue beyond anything seen with any of the many mouse strains". Kersting and Lennartz (1955) described encephalitis characterized by inflammatory glial nodules which were distributed throughout the brains of rhesus and cynomolgus monkeys after infection with LCM virus, strain WE, but later it was found that the inoculum had consisted of a mixture of LCM and rabies viruses (Lennartz, personal communication).

3. Immunologic Response

After having survived an infection, monkeys are specifically protected when challenged. The details of this immunologic conversion remain obscure. Wooley *et al.* (1937) infected monkeys and assayed their sera for neutralizing antibody two or more weeks later. One of 17 was without measurable protective substances, a finding which may be ascribed to the short interval between infection and bleeding. This may also be the explanation for the failure of Benda and Činátl (1964) to detect neutralizing antibody by means of a mouse test in monkeys rendered immune by infection with a nonpathogenic variant. No details were given, but apparently sera were collected three or four weeks after the immunizing infection.

Smadel and Wall (1940) reported that high titers of complement-fixing antibody developed in monkeys during the epizootic disease described by Coggeshall (1939). The tests were performed with the isolate and not with a prototype strain. Jochheim *et al.* (1957) detected complement-fixing antibody in a rhesus monkey up to two years after infection.

D. Syrian Hamster *(Mesocricetus auratus)*

1. Signs of the Disease

Smadel and Wall (1942) infected hamsters intracerebrally or intraperitoneally with the WE strain of LCM virus. Of 54 animals three became ill and died. In two of these *Klebsiella capsulatum* was found, making the real cause of their death uncertain. The authors concluded that "while it cannot be said that hamsters never die as a result of infection with the virus of choriomeningitis, it is evident that such an occurrence is rare". Neither Wenner (1948) who inoculated eight hamsters intracerebrally with an isolate from mice, nor Lewis *et al.* (1965) who transplanted an inadvertently LCM virus-infected hamster tumor, nor Wiktor *et al.* (1966) who infected hamsters intraperitoneally or intracerebrally with cell culture isolates saw clinical signs develop. Inapparent infection was also observed by D. Armstrong *et al.* (1969) who found their apparently healthy hamsters to be infected with LCM virus. In contrast, Rhodes and Chapman (1949) observed a characteristic illness after the intracerebral inoculation of an LCM virus which they had "obtained from Dr. Smadel". Six to eight days after infection, the animals became ruffled, incoordinated, and jerky and lost weight. With large doses, death occurred after 8 to 17 days. The intraperitoneal infection was followed in most hamsters by flaccid paralyses of the hind legs; up to ten per cent died. Volkert and Hannover Larsen (1965a) infected newborn hamsters intraperitoneally with 10^5 LD_{50} of the Traub strain virus; of 33 animals 22 died during the second and third week.

2. Pathogenesis

a) Multiplication and Distribution of the Virus

Five days after the intracerebral or intraperitoneal inoculation, Smadel and Wall (1942) detected large amounts of virus in blood and organs (no test performed earlier). During three weeks the concentration in the blood lay between 10^3 and 10^5 lethal doses (per ml?) and in brain and spleen titers of 10^6 and 10^8, respectively, were reached. On occasion, virus was found in the brain as late as eight weeks after the infection. Large amounts of virus were excreted with urine and feces. The infection could be transferred five times by cerebral passages. Further details were worked out by Rhodes and Chapman (1950). After the intracerebral inoculation, viremia became apparent at 24 (not at 2, 6 or 12) hours. High titers of 10^5 LD_{50} (per 0.03 ml?) were reached and maintained until the end of the experiment on the 12th day. In brain and cord virus multiplication commenced 24 to 36 hours after infection, attaining maxima of more than 10^6 LD_{50} (per 0.03 ml?) from two to five days; on the 12th day approximately 10^5 LD_{50} were still present. When newborn hamsters were infected intraperitoneally, the virus multiplied for about four weeks, but then the titers declined. At the age of three months, only traces were found in a few animals (Volkert and Hannover Larsen, 1965a).

b) Pathology and Pathogenetic Mechanisms

Pathology in infected hamsters was found to be all but absent. The spleens were moderately enlarged. In the brains mild meningeal reactions were observed consisting of a few scattered lymphocytes in the subarachnoid spaces (Smadel and

Wall, 1942). Normal histology of the brain was found by Wenner (1948) in a hamster seven days after intracerebral inoculation of virus.

Little may be said of the pathogenetic mechanisms. Rhodes and Chapman (1950) noted that infectivity was high in the organs before any signs of illness were recognizable, which is reminiscent of the infection of the mouse where the same phenomenon is interpreted as indicating that the disease is not caused directly by the virus but rather results from an indirect interaction between host and pathogen.

3. Immunologic Response

Complement-fixing antibody appeared around the 14th day after infection; at this time the complement-fixing antigen which had been present in the spleens disappeared. Circulating virus disappeared after the fourth week and neutralizing antibody appeared shortly thereafter. Both types of antibody persisted for at least several months (Smadel and Wall, 1942). After the infection of newborn hamsters no complement-fixing antibody was detected for up to three weeks. It then appeared and reached high titers at the age of six weeks. For some time both virus and antibody were found to coexist in the blood (Volkert and Hannover Larsen, 1965a).

E. Rabbit

As a rule, rabbits do not respond with overt disease after inoculation of LCM virus, irrespective of the route. Even newborn animals were not killed by very high virus inocula (Volkert and Hannover Larsen, 1965a). Whether minor alterations, such as elevation of the temperature, may ensue seems to be unknown. Armstrong (1942) noted that strains isolated from human fatal cases produced fever in rabbits. According to Smadel and Wall (1940), nursing rabbits are retarded in growth when inoculated intracerebrally.

Roger (1962) reported to have elicited a local inflammatory reaction in the rabbit skin by inoculation of infected mouse brain containing at least 10^4 LD_{50}. The response was not obtained by normal mouse brain. It was abolished by heating and by the addition of antiserum. This phenomenon is reminiscent of a virus-induced skin reaction in guinea-pigs (see Section V. B. 1) and the foot pad reaction in mice (see Section V. A. 2); its exact nature is not clear.

It is not known to what extent the LCM virus multiplies in this animal. Kasahara *et al.* (1937a) could not transmit the virus serially through rabbit brains but succeeded in the testes. According to Yamada (1940a), passages in the rabbit brain were possible after the virus had multiplied once in the central nervous system of the guinea-pig. The data presented by Overman and Friedewald (1950) leave no doubt that the WE virus may multiply in the rabbit eye — though not to high titers — after inoculation into the corpus vitreum. The infected eyes reacted with a mild hyperemia which disappeared within 24 hours. A severe alteration of the rabbit eye, consisting of conjunctivitis, iridocyclitis, and keratitis, following inoculation of a homogenate of WE virus-infected guinea-pig spleen into the anterior chamber was described by Blanc *et al.* (1951b). The potency of the virus inoculated was not specified, except that "a strong dose" was employed. Undoubtedly, the amount of foreign material thus inoculated must have been very high.

Jochheim *et al.* (1957) found virus in the blood from days 4 to 16 after subcutaneous inoculation. This, together with the rapid development of complement-fixing as well as neutralizing antibodies (see below) after a single inoculation makes it likely that a true infection is established.

Complement-fixing antibody became detectable 11 days after the intraperitoneal inoculation and reached peak titers of 64 to 128 around the fourth week; they were down again to 8 to 16 in as short a time as two weeks later (Smadel and Wall, 1940). After one subcutaneous inoculation Jochheim *et al.* (1957) found complement-fixing antibody on the eighth day followed by an increase with a peak after three weeks. Thereafter, the antibody levels decreased rapidly. The quick disappearance of complement-fixing antibody was found to be the rule in numerous rabbits which had been inoculated intravenously in this laboratory for the purpose of producing antisera. Booster injections did not halt the decline (Jochheim *et al.*, 1957). Neutralizing antibody was demonstrable four to six weeks after the intraperitoneal inoculation of the virus (Smadel and Wall, 1940).

No detailed study on the pathology seems to have been performed. Smadel and Wall (1940) noticed slight lesions in meninges and plexus after intracerebral inoculations in a few instances.

F. Embryonic and Hatched Chick

Bengtson and Wooley (1936) inoculated LCM virus (presumably the original strain of Armstrong and Lillie) in various dilutions onto the chorioallantoic membranes of 11- to 12-day-old fertile chicken eggs and found virus in both membranes and brains after seven days' incubation at 37.5° C. Material from the eighth alternating brain to chorioallantoic membrane passage contained virus in low concentrations. Tubaki (1940) worked with an isolate from a human case that he inoculated either onto the chorioallantoic membrane or into the allantoic sac of seven- to nine-day-old chicken embryos. After seven passages virus was detected in all embryonal organs, with concentrations of 10^4 mouse ID_{50} (per 0.03 ml?) in the chorioallantoic membrane, 10^5 ID_{50} in the brain, and 10^3 ID_{50} in liver, spleen, amniotic fluid, and blood. Milzer and Levinson (1942) cultivated an isolate from a laboratory infection for ten consecutive passages in the chorio-allantoic membrane of the developing chick embryo. Strain "T", which resembled WE in many respects, was found by Alice and McNutt (1945) to multiply in the tissues of chick embryos and their membranes after chorioallantoic membrane inoculation, but the concentrations remained low even after eight passages. High virus concentrations were found by Prick and Verlinde (1947) in the chorioallantoic membranes during the sixth egg to egg passage of a Dutch isolate.

Whitney *et al.* (1953) accomplished chorioallantoic membrane and yolk sac passages and claimed to have attained adaptation. When inoculated by either route, virus was found in the allantoic fluids, the membranes, and the embryos. Its concentration was approximately ten times higher in the chorioallantoic membrane than in the fluid. Transfer *via* the allantoic cavity failed.

A comprehensive study was reported by Tobin (1954). He inoculated the chorioallantoic membranes of 10- or 12-day-old fertile eggs with high or low doses of the WE strain and with low doses of the 84 B (own isolate) virus. After an initial drop and a latent period of at least 12 hours, multiplication was at least 10^4-fold. Five days after a chorioallantoic membrane infection, virus was found in low titers in all embryonic fluids and in higher titers in livers and brains. After amniotic infection, it was present in the amniotic fluid and in the brain (no other organs tested). No growth occurred after allantoic or yolk sac inoculation. In spite of the multiplication of the virus, passage experiments were not uniformly successful. The WE strain was easily transferred from embryo to embryo during April and May but not in October and November. Such fluctuation of susceptibility, whether determined by season of the year or not, might have been the cause for the failure reported by HAYES and HARTMAN (1943) to passage the virus — presumably the WE strain — in the egg by chorioallantoic membrane inoculation.

All these observations show that the LCM virus may multiply in the fertile egg but that it does so to a limited extent. However, the concentrations obtained are usually high enough to be of use as an immunizing antigen or for the production of complement-fixing antigen. KRAFT and GORDON (1947) transferred the virus *via* the yolk sac, the chorioallantoic membrane, and the allantoic cavity. Not much virus was found in the allantoic fluid, but the embryonal tissues contained "considerable amounts". Virus thus passaged was used by WHITNEY *et al.* (1952; 1953) for preparing complement-fixing antigen. Embryo and chorioallantoic membrane suspensions were equally good sources; the allantoic fluids contained no detectable complement-fixing antigen though infectivity was present. Antigens from the 10th and 57th chorioallantoic membrane passages and the 31st and 33rd yolk sac following 36 chorioallantoic membrane passages were of equal potency. In contrast, TOBIN (1954) found no complement-fixing antigen in chorioallantoic membrane, liver, or brain of chicks at any time after infection with high or low virus inocula.

In most studies, infection of chick embryos was found to kill few of the hosts; pathological alterations were all but absent (LILLIE, 1936a). In contrast, ALICE and MCNUTT (1945) observed a high mortality after inoculation onto the chorioallantoic membrane, with an increase following rapid transfers through the yolk sac, although the titers in embryos and membranes did not reach higher levels after as many as eight chorioallantoic membrane passages followed by 28 yolk sac passages. Presumably strain characteristics may be held responsible for these differences. Alternatively, the age of the embryo has to be taken into account. VOLKERT and HANNOVER LARSEN (1965a) found the Traub virus to be highly virulent for chick embryos 7 or 11 days old when infected *via* the yolk sac; but at age 15 days all of ten embryos survived 10^5 mouse LD_{50} and hatched normally.

In newly hatched chicks which had been infected as 13-day-old embryos, BENGTSON and WOOLEY (1936) saw illness with quick recovery; one was born with "a marked deformity of the leg". ALICE and MCNUTT (1945) failed to detect virus in hatched chicks which had survived the embryonal infection. In a more detailed attempt, TOBIN (1954) infected 16-day-old embryos *via* the chorioallantoic membranes with 10^5 ID_{50} and found infectivity in the brains two and four but not 10, 14, and 18 days after hatching. Similar results were reported by TRAUB (1955) who infected seven-day-old embryos with a strain, adapted by passages through chorioallantoic membranes, and detected virus before and one day after hatching but rarely thereafter. Neither TOBIN (1954) nor TRAUB (1955) demonstrated significant concentrations of circulating antibody after hatching in birds which had been infected during their embryonic stage. Since TRAUB (1955) found no neutralizing antibody in an adult rooster which had been inoculated repeatedly with virus, this observation is not very meaningful. In newborn chicks, the virus multiplied inapparently in brains and viscera after the intracerebral inoculation and could be detected in high concentrations after 21 days but was absent three weeks later (ALICE and MCNUTT, 1945).

G. Other Nonhuman Vertebrates

Besides those already mentioned, representatives of a variety of species were tested over the years for susceptibility to the virus. In most cases the intracerebral route was chosen. The response of rats varied; some authors found them to remain essentially free of disease (ARMSTRONG and LILLIE, 1934; LÉPINE and SAUTTER, 1936; KASAHARA *et al.*, 1937a; LÉPINE *et al.*, 1937a; KASAHARA *et al.*, 1939; BENDA *et al.*, 1955; GLADKIJ, 1965) whereas others saw signs of disease (TRAUB, 1935b; 1936a; FINDLAY *et al.*, 1936; FINDLAY and STERN, 1936; ALICE, 1945b; ALICE and MCNUTT, 1945; WENNER, 1948). VOLKERT and HANNOVER LARSEN (1965a) found newborn rats up to the age of five days to be highly susceptible. They then developed resistance and at the age of three weeks they survived very high virus doses given intraperitoneally. Rats inoculated intraperitoneally when one week old were viremic three weeks later indicating that the agent had multiplied. At the age of three months no virus was present. High titers of complement-fixing antibody developed. MIMS (1969) confirmed the high susceptibility of immature rats; after the intraperitoneal inoculation of 10^6 LD_{50} of the WE strain virus, all of 15 newborn animals were dead by day 11. After the intravenous inoculation of 10^6 LD_{50} into pregnant females, part of the offspring was infected, leading to death or runting, but most newborn animals were free of virus and healthy.

GLADKIJ (1965) followed the virus, strain 92, in rat organs for up to 26 days. His data indicate that multiplication might have occurred to a limited extent in the brain after intracerebral and possibly in the spleen after intraperitoneal infection. All other organs remained free or contained only traces of infectivity.

TRAUB (1936a) saw no signs of illness in intracerebrally inoculated pigeons. FINDLAY *et al.* (1936; FINDLAY and STERN, 1936) mentioned that dog, ferret, hedgehog, field vole *(Microtus agrestis)*, bank vole *(Evotomys glareolus)*, rabbit, hen, canary, pig, and parakeet did not respond with disease to the inoculation. No apparent disease was induced in dogs and ferrets by DALLDORF (1939a), although the virus was transmitted from one dog to a cage mate indicating that it had multiplied. In an extensive follow-up study, DALLDORF (1943) infected 65 adult dogs by intracerebral, subcutaneous, intraperitoneal, or combined inoculations and did not see signs of disease in any of them. In puppies, slight fever was observed for seven to ten days. In most, but not all, dogs infected subcutaneously complement-fixing antibody appeared. Neutralizing antibody developed "to a moderate degree", and, again, there was spread of virus to other dogs. Slight fever on the fifth and the 14th and viremia on the 11th day were observed by VER-

LINDE (1946) in a dog inoculated intracerebrally with an isolate from a patient in Holland.

DALLDORF (1939a) mentioned that the only alterations caused by the LCM virus in dogs and ferrets were intranuclear inclusions in the suprarenal cortex. They were also found in infected mice, guinea-pigs, and monkeys. Later, he characterized them as being acidophilic, corresponding to Cowdry's type B, and considered them to be of diagnostic value (DALLDORF, 1943).

The animals responding with unspecified clinical signs were listed by ARMSTRONG (1941) to include chimpanzees, monkeys, guinea-pigs, white rats, cotton rats, rice rats, white and gray mice, and dogs. Signs in the dog contrast with most other reports. Presumably, Armstrong's experience with this animal was based on experiments with isolates from three human fatalities, which were different in many respects from other known strains of LCM virus (ARMSTRONG, 1942). ALICE (1945b) found rabbits, cats, dogs, hens, pigeons, and newborn chicks to remain free of signs.

HOWITT and VAN HERICK (1941) tested the susceptibility of cotton rats *(Sigmodon)* and mice *(Microtus)* to the WE virus by intracerebral inoculation. Each were subdivided into three age groups: one to two, two to six, and over six months, respectively. All of 23 *M. californicus* survived, irrespective of age. Of 50 *M. montanus*, all nine of the old adults and all ten of the very young animals survived, while of 31 animals belonging to the immature adults 17 died. The cotton rats were on the whole less resistant; significant numbers died in all age groups, more in the case of *S. hispidus eremicus* than of *S. hispidus texianus*. WENNER (1948) reported that two of six cotton rats, inoculated intracerebrally with strain "M" died; four remained healthy.

LAWRENCE *et al.* (1943) inoculated an LCM virus preparation intracerebrally and intraperitoneally into two cats which did not develop apparent disease. Attempts to recover the virus from their spleens were unsuccessful. According to MAURER (1964), rabbit, hamster, squirrel, ferret, horse, and dog could be infected, while cattle, pig, cat, and chick appeared to be resistant; no details were provided.

With strain "T" — isolated in a guinea-pig which had been inoculated with brain material from a sick cow — ALICE and MCNUTT (1945) found that intracerebral inoculation of baby pigs was followed by multiplication to high titers, leading to disease in one and death in a second of altogether three animals. Two further piglets which had received the virus *via* the conjunctival sac remained healthy. One bull, one pregnant cow, and four calves were inoculated by various routes but did not respond. In one calf, the tissues were found free of virus 30 days later; no lesions had developed.

H. The Human Disease

1. Clinical Features

Wallgren, in 1925, drew attention to a clinical syndrome characterized by (1) acute onset with definite signs of meningitis, (2) meningitic alterations of the cerebrospinal fluid with a moderate to high increase of mononuclear cells, (3) bacterial sterility of the cerebrospinal fluid, (4) short and benign course without secondary complications, (5) absence of any other demonstrable etiology, and (6) absence of an epidemiological relationship with other infectious diseases known to cause meningitis; he called it acute aseptic meningitis ("méningite aseptique aiguë") (WALLGREN, 1925). When RIVERS and SCOTT (1936a) presented evidence for an etiological relationship between the LCM virus and Wallgren's syndrome it was thought that this finding was generally applicable and that a new disease entity had been established. Hence, ARMSTRONG and DICKENS (1935; DICKENS, 1937) suggested that the term acute aseptic meningitis should be replaced by "acute lymphocytic choriomeningitis". In a comprehensive review of infectious diseases written at that time REIMANN (1937) expressed the view that acute lymphocytic meningitis was "established as a specific infectious disease caused by a filterable virus".

It was soon realized by many, including the original authors, that Wallgren's syndrome had a multitude of causes among which the LCM virus did not even play a major role (RIVERS and SCOTT, 1936b; ARMSTRONG and WOOLEY, 1937; DOMINICK, 1937; LUCCHESI, 1937; BAIRD and RIVERS, 1938; RIVERS, 1939); nevertheless, the term was retained for years and, by implying a definite etiologic relationship, caused considerable confusion in the literature (RASMUSSEN, 1947; STRAUSS, 1948). Even recent accounts have not always been thoroughly expurgated from such sources of spurious evidence. Thus, in the 24th edition of Dorland's Illustrated Medical Dictionary (printed in 1968) "acute aseptic meningitis" and "lymphocytic choriomeningitis" are used synonymously.

Our knowledge concerning disease caused by the LCM virus has come from (1) natural infections (ARMSTRONG and DICKENS, 1935; FINDLAY *et al.*, 1936; SCOTT and RIVERS, 1936; RIVERS and SCOTT, 1936b; ARMSTRONG and SWEET, 1939; ARMSTRONG *et al.*, 1940; ARMSTRONG, 1941; FARMER and JANEWAY, 1942; MILZER, 1943; TREUSCH *et al.*, 1943; PRICK, 1946; PRICK and VERLINDE, 1947; BROOKSALER and SULKIN, 1948; HAVENS, 1948; IVÁNOVICS *et al.*, 1948; GREEN *et al.*, 1949; MACCALLUM, 1949; DUNCAN *et al.*, 1951; ADAIR *et al.*, 1953; NIHOUL and LECOMTE-RAMIOUL, 1953; PINTO and FERREIRA, 1954; SCHEID and JOCHHEIM, 1956a; SCHEID and JOCHHEIM, 1956b; ACKERMANN and JANSEN, 1958; TRAUMANN *et al.*, 1962; SCHEID *et al.*, 1964; COHEN *et al.*, 1966), (2) accidental laboratory infections (LÉPINE and SAUTTER, 1938; ARMSTRONG, 1941; ARMSTRONG and HORNIBROOK, 1941; MILZER and LEVINSON, 1942; HAYES and HARTMAN, 1943; MILZER, 1943; AFZELIUS-ALM, 1951; SCHEID *et al.*, 1956a; POLJAK and BÁRDOŠ, 1958; BAUM *et al.*, 1966; COHEN *et al.*, 1966; D. ARMSTRONG *et al.*, 1969), and (3) infections induced for therapeutic purposes (LÉPINE *et al.*, 1937b; LÉPINE, 1939; BLANC *et al.*, 1951b). Of the numerous reviewing articles only a few will be mentioned: KREIS (1938), TRAUB (1939c), CARDOSO (1941/42a), FARMER and JANEWAY (1942), SMADEL (1942a), KREIS (1948), VAN ROOYEN and RHODES (1948), LACORTE (1953), SCHEID (1957), PANOV *et al.* (1963), LACORTE (1964), SHVAREV (1964a), SCHEID (1965), WARREN (1965), RHODES and VAN ROOYEN (1968).

The clinical signs are diverse. ARMSTRONG (1941) distinguished three major forms: the "grippal or non-nervous system", the "meningeal", and the "meningo-encephalomyelitic" types, in which should be included encephalitides and encephalomyelitides. A similar classification was proposed by SCHEID (1957) who considered further subdivisions attempted by others to be of little value.

Although Armstrong (1942) had regarded its occurrence as uncertain, much has been speculated on the "asymptomatic type", but not a single observation has become available which would make such cases probable, and while we cannot say definitely that they do not exist, subclinical LCM virus infections in man undoubtedly are rare.

The grippal type begins after an incubation time of 6 to 13 days. Fever, malaise, muscular pain, sometimes accompanied by coryza and bronchitis, are the predominant signs. It may run a remittent course with up to three spells. On occasion, the disease is rather severe and may be taken for typhoid fever. The significance of the grippal type is difficult to assess. Most of the reported cases followed laboratory or therapeutic infections; few have been observed under natural conditions. Milzer (1943) listed one case of "influenzal" disease among nine LCM virus infections, and Balek *et al.* (1954) 2 among 16. It is difficult to suppose that they would have been overlooked consistently if their occurrence were frequent and it seems safe to conclude that they are rare.

One extraordinary observation is to be mentioned here. In people who worked — unknowingly — with LCM virus-infected hamsters, Baum *et al.* (1966) saw an LCM epidemic which affected ten persons out of a total of 30 involved. All had severe "grippe-like" illnesses with fever, headache, myalgia, anorexia, aching pain in the chest. In none of the patients did meningeal signs develop. The cerebrospinal fluid, taken from one, was normal. During convalescence, unilateral orchitis developed in three of nine men in the series. Arthralgias were invariably experienced which, in two cases, led to frank arthritis of the hands. In two of the patients generalized alopecia was recorded. Although the diagnoses were convincingly based on virus isolations and antibody studies, the disease as well as its epidemiology must be considered unusual in many respects. The authors assumed that the virus had changed some of its properties in the course of passage in the hamsters.

By far the most frequent clinical manifestation of human infections with the LCM virus, be it transmitted naturally or in the laboratory, is the syndrome singled out by Wallgren (see above) which has been given various names in the past; none is entirely satisfactory (Scheid, 1948). I shall use the term abacterial meningitis or, perhaps even more appropriate, LCM meningitis. Often preceded by a prodromal stage which resembles the above-mentioned "grippe", the onset is acute with stiff neck, fever, headache, malaise, muscular pains. These signs may remain mild and of short duration, or may be quite severe leading to a considerable degree of prostration.

The demarcation between meningitis and meningoencephalitis is not sharp. In this latter category we find a diverse multitude of signs grouped together in all possible combinations. Findlay *et al.* (1936) reported two such observations; Treusch *et al.* (1943) one. In the patient with an abacterial meningitis described by Prick (1946; Prick and Verlinde, 1947) the sixth cranial nerve was involved indicating participation of structures other than the meninges alone. Scheid and Jochheim (1956a) saw a young woman who developed a severe encephalomyelitis accompanied by an organic type of psychosis of a few days' duration. One of the laboratory infections (H.-L. W.) documented by Scheid *et al.* (1956a) ran a severe course of long duration, leading to meningoencephalitis and myocarditis with involvement of liver and kidneys.

An unusual observation was reported by Scheid *et al.* (1968; Scheid and Ackermann, 1969). A 25-year-old man developed a disorder of the central nervous system which in all respects resembled classical encephalitis lethargica (von Economo). The isolation of the virus from the cerebrospinal fluid on the sixth day of the disease and the increase of LCM-specific neutralizing and complement-fixing antibodies leave no doubt as to the etiology.

Similar in some respects is the case of an encephalitis described in detail by Shvarev (1966). A 17-year-old girl from Leningrad fell ill during the latter part of January, 1955. She showed improvement three weeks later, but in March a relapse occurred which lasted until early in May. Throughout, psychopathological alterations were prominent and it was stated that the illness had some resemblance with encephalitis lethargica. Physical examination revealed few organic signs; the cerebrospinal fluid, taken twice, was practically normal. LCM virus was isolated in mice and guinea-pigs from blood and cerebrospinal fluid as late as 11 weeks after onset. At the same time LCM-specific complement-fixing antibody was present while neutralizing antibody could not be detected. One month later, antibody was demonstrated with both methods. (This is an interesting and unusual case and it may be regretted that the virological part of the report contains no details.)

Likewise insufficiently documented are the three cases of encephalitis described by Nayak *et al.* (1964) from India. In two of them the only virological information is complement fixation titers of 64, 29 and 39 days and 25 and 40 days after onset, respectively. In the third patient the titer rose from 16 on the fifth to 64 on the 14th day after onset.

Participation of the brain in the disease process is not rare. In a carefully controlled study, which will be further dealt with below, Meyer *et al.* (1960) proved that 58 cases of acute infectious diseases with involvement of the central nervous system were caused by the LCM virus. Twenty had been clinically diagnosed as encephalitis; of these, six had paralyses (no details).

None of the above syndromes is diagnostic of infection with the LCM virus, and this is even more so with a variety of clinical signs which have been found in association with LCM virus infections, usually with one of the major types. Sore throat, sometimes severe pain in the back and the extremities, pleural pain aggravated on respiration, constipation, skin rash, swelling of the lymph nodes, loss of weight do not give hints as to the etiology. Nor is the usual absence of an increase of the erythrocyte sedimentation rate of much help. Changes of the differential blood count are likewise not regularly observed, although they may occur. In 14 of 16 people infected subcutaneously, Mollaret *et al.* (1939) observed initial leukopenia and granulocytopenia followed by lymphocytosis and monocytosis and, finally, by eosinophilia and sometimes a transitory leukocytosis. During the second meningitic and/or fever phase the blood picture had usually returned to normal. The authors assumed that alterations are the rule but are overlooked because examination of the blood is usually not done before the onset of meningitis, by which time the blood has returned to its regular composition. An unusual case in many respects is the fatal illness of one of the laboratory workers described by Smadel *et al.* (1942) where leukopenia was a prominent finding. Baum *et al.* (1966) detected leukopenia in four out of four investigated cases of influenza-like illnesses due to laboratory infections (see above).

The combination of encephalitis with unilateral orchitis and unilateral parotitis in a proved case of LCM virus infection (LEWIS and UTZ, 1961) is so far unique. The identity of the virus which was isolated by WENNER *et al.* (1949) from a patient with meningitis and epididymitis is doubtful. It behaved unlike a true LCM virus, because mice were ill as early as four days after infection and rabbits developed signs of disease and died after intracerebral inoculation.

THIEDE (1962) reported on cardiac involvement in two patients. One had an abacterial meningitis, the other a nonspecific disease for weeks with malaise, fever, cough. Apparently no virus isolation was attempted, but the titer of complement-fixing antibody rose in one patient from negative on the second day of illness to eight in two weeks and fell again to nondetectable levels; it rose from four at six weeks to 32 two and three weeks later and became negative five months after onset in the other patient.

The great majority of infections with LCM virus in man run a benign course. *Sequelae*, even in severe cases of encephalitis, are scant or absent. All three of Scheid's patients with encephalitis, to whom we have already referred, recovered almost completely (SCHEID and JOCHHEIM, 1956a; SCHEID *et al.*, 1956a; 1968). TREUSCH *et al.* (1943) saw complete recovery in a case of severe acute encephalitis with deep coma, hemiparesis, and hemianesthesia. Among the 69 proved and ten probable infections with LCM virus described by RASMUSSEN (1947) and ADAIR *et al.* (1953), four had muscle weakness or paralysis, and two of these died. The fate of the two survivors was not documented. Of the 20 cases of LCM encephalitis etiologically diagnosed by MEYER *et al.* (1960) only one retained "severe *sequelae*" (no details). No further information was supplied by MILZER (1943) about the one case of paralytic poliomyelitis and two of the three cases of acute encephalitis which he listed as having been caused by the LCM virus. Patient B. D., with encephalitis, recovered completely (TREUSCH *et al.*, 1943). Of the three cases of encephalitis of NAYAK *et al.* (1964) two regained their health while one remained mentally deteriorated.

Of uncertain significance is the case of BARKER and FORD (1937). A woman had an abacterial meningitis in February, 1936. The LCM virus was isolated from her spinal fluid at the Rockefeller Institute. No serology was reported. Initially, the convalescence was uneventful, but in early summer, *i.e.* three to four months later, pareses and sensory disturbances developed from the fourth thoracic segment downward. Lumbar punctures, X-rays, and finally surgical exploration revealed that thick fibrous masses had completely obliterated the subarachnoid space. After a transient improvement, a complete paraplegia developed in November. KELIHER (1944) described an encephalitis with pronounced mental alterations lasting for more than eight weeks which was preceded by a "grippe". The virus was isolated by Dr. C. Armstrong in a ferret (!) but no serology was done to confirm the etiology. SHVAREV (1964b) described 12 cases of LCM virus infections with syndromes varying from paraplegia and polyradiculitis to arachnitis and similar affections, all indicating severe involvement of the spinal cord and its membranes. The etiological diagnoses were based on positive results from neutralization and/or complement fixation tests, but the description of the virological part of this study is not detailed enough to permit critical evaluation.

Other reports must be treated with even greater circumspection. The etiology of a disease in a dancer, clinically resembling poliomyelitis with lasting paralyses (MacCallum and Findlay, 1939), was not unequivocally identified. The virus was isolated under unusual circumstances and antibody did not develop. The alleged LCM virus etiology of one case with fever, pneumonia, a severe encephalitis, and an ascending transverse myelitis leading to paraplegia without improvement after seven months (Colmore, 1952) must likewise be questioned.

In several reports, the LCM virus has been accused of causing recurrent or chronic diseases with involvement of the central nervous system (Leichenger *et al.*, 1940; Baker, 1947; Bieling and Koch, 1952; Chang *et al.*, 1954). None may be considered as having been sufficiently documented, with the exception of case "B.D." described by Treusch *et al.* (1943).

The question remains as to how often LCM virus infections of man are lethal. In view of the fact that this virus often causes accidental infections in the laboratory, the answer is of prime importance for those who, either voluntarily or because of professional commitments, are in frequent contact with this virus. Fortunately, the answer may be given with confidence that death due to LCM virus is an extremely rare event. In fact, there is only one fatal case in which the diagnosis could be based on the demonstration of a significant increase of antibody (see below).

Smadel *et al.* (1942) reported the case of a laboratory worker who died after a nonspecific illness with high fever, generalized aches, sore throat, cough, and vomiting. There were no cerebral signs. The predominant laboratory finding was a leukopenia. A man who had assisted at autopsy fell ill eight days later and died with high fever, necrotizing pharyngitis, diffuse erythematous rash, bleeding from the mucous membranes, and hemorrhages. Again, there was no apparent involvement of the central nervous system. In both cases, LCM virus was recovered from various organs by inoculation into guinea-pigs as well as mice. Isolations were repeated from specimens which had been kept at —70° C. Furthermore, material from one of the cases was sent to another laboratory where the virus was again found. There can be no doubt as to the etiology in both cases; but they certainly represent unusual observations. The clinical features were not at all characteristic of an infection with LCM virus. The virus, too, differed from most isolates; in experimentally infected mice and guinea-pigs the histopathology was unusually severe with a true encephalitis besides the choriomeningitis which is seen as a rule. The source of this virus remains obscure, unless one assumes that both cases were included among the three fatalities reported by Armstrong (1942), two of whom had been engaged in the preparation of a distemper vaccine, and the third had assisted at autopsy. Armstrong also reported some unusual properties of these isolates; they produced fever in rabbits and white mice and caused a paretic disease in a dog besides being more potent for guinea-pigs and mice. (Both Drs. Armstrong and Smadel are deceased making it impossible to establish that the two cases of Dr. Smadel were identical with two of Dr. Armstrong's three fatalities, although it is almost certain that they were.)

In view of the scarcity of reliable information on the histopathology of human LCM diseases it is to be regretted that the virological part of the report by Mitchell and Klotz (1942) on what was initially a moderately severe meningitis in a 12 year-old child who later died is rather scant. Nevertheless, this may be considered one of the few proved cases. Adair *et al.* (1953) reported two fatalities among the 79 cases of diseases of the central nervous system which had been caused ("proved" or "probable") by the LCM virus. They died 14 and 19 days, respectively, after onset, one with a clinical picture resembling Landry's ascending paralysis, the other with bulbar paralysis. The immediate cause of death was respiratory failure. The diagnosis was established in both cases by isolation of the virus from the brains and was "confirmed in one instance by the presence of complement-fixing antibodies for LCM in serum drawn from the patient three days before his death" (no further details). It is to be regretted that the autopsy findings have not been published. Another fatality which may be said with some confidence to have been caused by the LCM virus was described by Scheid *et al.* (1956b). A 50-year-old man died with meningoencephalitis on the 33rd day after onset. The LCM virus was isolated in guinea-pigs from blood taken on the 30th day.

Of considerable interest is the report by Komrower *et al.* (1955) concerning a transplacental infection. A pregnant woman, resident in an area where human infections with LCM virus had previously occurred, fell ill with meningitis eight days before delivery. No virus isolation was attempted but the titer of complement-fixing antibody rose from 2 to 64. The newborn infant died at the age of 12 days. LCM virus was isolated from its liquor cerebrospinalis taken on the 11th day.

Viets and Warren (1937) based their diagnosis on the clinical picture only, and this was death from an acute abacterial meningitis; no laboratory confirmation was attempted. The agent isolated by Machella *et al.* (1939) in guinea-pigs from a fatal case of abacterial meningitis was not further characterized and its assumed identity with the LCM virus was not confirmed. No attempts were made by Silcott and Neubuerger (1940) to establish the etiology in three fatal cases which had been clinically diagnosed as acute lymphocytic choriomeningitis. Likewise of doubtful significance is the alleged LCM virus etiology of a chronic meningoencephalitis seen in a man by Skogland and Baker (1939) who died nine years after the onset (Baker, 1947). The mere demonstration of a "strong concentration of antibodies against the virus of lymphocytic choriomeningitis" six weeks and ten months after onset may not be accepted as establishing an etiologic connection in the light of what we know of nonspecific inhibitors in normal human sera (see Section V. H. 3).

The report on a "malignant lymphocytic choriomeningoencephalitis" with death described by Vedder (1948) has to be mentioned, even though the author himself discounts the LCM virus as the cause. Probably because of its title, the paper has occasionally been included in discussions on human infections with the LCM virus. The same is true of the report by Juba and Prievara (1948) on two fatal cases of abacterial meningitis; LCM was not mentioned by the authors.

With some anxiety I shall now turn to the three fatal cases documented by Howard (1940; 1940/41). They were described together with five additional patients who survived. Virus was recovered from all eight in guinea-pigs. It was never isolated in mice on direct inoculation, nor were these animals later immune to challenge. From guinea-pigs the disease could be transferred to mice, where it appeared to be a typical LCM. If this may seem unusual, then the isolation history from patient F. F. who had died of encephalitis appears even more bizarre. Cerebrospinal fluids had been repeatedly negative. First attempts with brain tissue had likewise failed. Renewed attempts at isolation with brain tissue, which had been stored in glycerin for 71 days (at room temperature?), in mice, three-day-old chickens, and one guinea-pig resulted in the death of the guinea-pig after 14 weeks and the death of one of six chickens ten weeks after inoculation. Material from these animals killed guinea-pigs but did not cause illness in mice. It was not before three guinea-pig passages had been performed that mice showed signs typical for LCM. Certainly, this report may not be accepted as being convincing and it becomes even less so when one reads that no neutralizing antibody appeared in either of the two patients where assays had been performed up to many weeks after infection.

In concluding this part of our discussion it may be said that since its discovery in 1934 this virus has been proved responsible for the death of not more than eight people (including the baby, and assuming an overlapping of Armstrong's and Smadel's reports).

Inasmuch as the syndromes for which the LCM virus may be responsible are also caused by a multitude of other agents, a diagnosis which is based on clinical considerations only or on insufficient virological evidence may not be accepted. Several such reports have already been discussed; others have yet to be mentioned. The two cases of acute benign lymphocytic meningitis described by Collis (1935) were not investigated virologically; the author himself does not discuss the possible etiology. None the less, they are often referred to as LCM virus infections. The three cases of acute abacterial meningitis, thought by Viets and Warren (1937) to have been caused by the LCM virus, were not substantiated by laboratory investigations. The same is to be said of the seven patients seen by Hammes (1938) of which three were described in some detail. One typical case of abacterial meningitis in a congenital syphilitic, thought by Howard (1939) to have been caused by the LCM virus, may not be accepted in spite of isolation of the virus. The neutralization tests with the patient's serum were highly irregular, being positive with a specimen from the 45th week but negative earlier and ten weeks later. In contrast, good protection was obtained with the control serum obtained from Rivers' case, "W.E". Findlay *et al.* (1940) isolated the LCM virus from the cerebrospinal fluid and the blood of a patient with an abacterial meningitis, but they failed to confirm their finding by serology. None of the eight cases described by Howard (1940; 1940/41), including the three fatal ones (see above), was unequivocally shown to have been caused by the LCM virus. Most probably, the virus came from the guinea-pigs used for isolation attempts. In two patients, the repeated search for neutralizing antibody remained unsuccessful for as long as 26 and 29 weeks, respectively, after onset. Nor may the case of a "recurrent lymphocytic choriomeningitis" described by Leichenger *et al.* (1940) be accepted. Though an LCM virus was isolated in guinea-pigs, this was not accomplished before the 13th week during the fifth meningeal attack. The clinical picture did not resemble an LCM meningitis; indeed, it was unlike any common virus disease. No antibody was demonstrable in the patient's serum 13 and 17 weeks after onset. The two cases of abacterial meningitis seen in the clinic of Dr. Merrit (Merrit, 1940) were insufficiently documented. The same must be said of the one case of Brown (1941) who did not confirm the infection by demonstrating antibody in the patient's serum.

No virology was done by AVERY (1945) who described the occurrence of a "benign lymphocytic choriomeningitis" in four patients. The agent isolated in mice by VAN HASSELT (1946) from the liquor cerebrospinalis of a patient with meningitis was serologically not identified. No virology accompanied the description by SREENIVASAN (1946) of lymphocytic choriomeningitis in eight patients living in the Singapore area. The same is true of the two cases of MURPHY (1947) where reduction of chlorides in the cerebrospinal fluids was the main result of laboratory tests. In Rumania, MESROBEANU and BADENSKI (1948) detected by guinea-pig inoculations filterable agents — which they believed to be strains of LCM virus — in the cerebrospinal fluids of two patients suffering from abacterial meningitis. In neither case was the identity of the isolates established, nor did the authors perform serological tests with the patients' sera. The same is to be said of the one case documented by SCHEID (1948). GRATER and RIDER (1949) reported successful treatment with aureomycin in two cases of lymphocytic choriomeningitis. In patient C. V. a doubtful diagnosis was based on the complement fixation test, which "was negative on admission but became positive six weeks later". No laboratory data substantiated the alleged etiology in patient J. T. An outbreak of "acute benign lymphocytic choriomeningitis" in Australia was not substantiated by laboratory data (PARRY, 1951). The same must be said of an epidemic in England, documented by SMITH and KINSELLA (1951). The etiology of a meningitis in a woman living in Budapest, ascribed by MOLNÁR (1953) to the LCM virus, is uncertain. An agent was isolated by mouse inoculation of the cerebrospinal fluid of the 18th day of illness which, presumably, was an LCM virus. Also, complement-fixing antibody increased from a titer of eight in the third to 32 in the tenth week and fell again to eight in the 35th week. However, no neutralization was obtained with the same sera, which should have become demonstrable in spite of the fact that they had been heat-inactivated. No virological observations supported the claim of JACOBIUS and GRANDI (1954) that a case of lymphocytic choriomeningitis was associated with a bilateral acute chorioiditis. Of the six alleged cases of lymphocytic choriomeningitis diagnosed in eastern Slovakia by MITTERMAYER *et al.* (1958), only one may be accepted to have been presumably caused by the LCM virus. The eight patients whose abacterial meningitis was blamed on the LCM virus by CÁRDENAS and YÉPEZ (1959) were not investigated in the laboratory. The LCM virus etiology of one case of meningitis which was characterized by a low sugar content of the cerebrospinal fluid (KINCAID, 1967) was insufficiently proved.

2. Pathology and Pathogenetic Mechanisms

From the above it is obvious that an analysis of the pathology in man rests essentially on two *post mortem* examinations. The findings in the cases reported by ARMSTRONG (1942) and SMADEL *et al.* (1942) and in the baby after transplacental infection (KOMROWER *et al.*, 1955) should not be expected to be characteristic of infections with this virus.

MITCHELL and KLOTZ (1942) found the brain to be swollen to such an extent that a cerebellar pressure cone resulted. The arachnoid was extremely thickened and infiltrated with large numbers of "chronic inflammatory cells", predominantly lymphocytes and macrophages. With the severely involved vessels the inflammation extended into the Virchow-Robin spaces. There was little infiltration of the nervous tissue itself but many ganglion cells in the cord — fewer in the brain — were swollen and the nuclei broken up into numerous minute, deeply stained globular masses which were concentrated at the cellular periphery. SCHEID *et al.* (1956b) described a hemorrhagic necrotizing meningoencephalitis which was less severe in the central portions of the brain where perivascular infiltrations and glial proliferations predominated. Capillary hemorrhages were found in the cerebellar cortex, in the nuclei of the pons, and in the nuclei of the cranial nerves with a pattern which was said to be reminiscent of an encephalitis due to *Rickettsia prowazeki*. The cases of ARMSTRONG (1942) and SMADEL *et al.* (1942) were unusual in that alterations of the central nervous system were all but absent. Indeed, in the first patient of Smadel, the immediate cause of death did not become apparent even at autopsy. The other two had widespread focal hemorrhages and, at least one of them, inconspicuous loose cuffs of lymphocytes about small vessels in several organs, most frequently present in the liver, meninges, and brain substance. The pathology in the 12-day-old baby who had died after transplacental infection was characterized by extensive subarachnoid hemorrhages and a hemorrhage in the occipital lobe. The leptomeninges were congested and the subarachnoid space — remote from the bleeding — was infiltrated with lymphocytes. Infiltrations were also found beneath the ependyma of the third, fourth, and lateral ventricles (KOMROWER *et al.*, 1955).

Little is known of the multiplication and the distribution of the virus. After the subcutaneous infection of man, Lépine and his collaborators found virus in the blood for two to three weeks. In the cerebrospinal fluid it became detectable only when a meningitis followed, being present a few days (hours?) before onset of meningeal signs (LÉPINE *et al.*, 1937b; LÉPINE, 1939). According to BLANC *et al.* (1951b), the blood was infectious from the 5th to the 20th (occasionally 25th) day and the liquor cerebrospinalis from the 15th to the 20th (occasionally the 25th) day. Virus appeared late in the urine (LÉPINE, 1939). In two patients, immunity was tested by challenge inoculation 375 and 577 days after primary infection and protection was found to be complete (LÉPINE, 1939).

As regards the mechanisms leading to LCM disease in man, no positive statement may be made with our present knowledge. However, there is nothing to indicate that disease and pathology are allergic phenomena similar to the ones in the mouse (see Section V. A. 4. b) apart from a possible immune component which is known to be involved in many diseases of viral origin (ALLISON, 1967; LEHMANN-GRUBE, Med. Klin., in press). BLANC *et al.* (1951b) elicited a marked skin reaction in humans by intradermal inoculation of the WE strain of LCM virus and a lesser reaction by inoculation of the Armstrong virus. This is a very interesting observation, but further details are needed before its significance can be evaluated.

3. Diagnosis

As with all virus diseases, the etiology may be established by either the isolation of the agent and/or the demonstration of an increase of specific antibody during convalescence. Ideally, corresponding results are obtained with both methods. Often, however, for technical or other reasons, the investigator has to be content with one or the other. Antibody carries more weight of evidence, but its demonstration usually takes longer and is also more laborious. Virus isolation, on the other hand, is as a rule more conveniently accomplished but is beset with risks of contamination either in the laboratory or from the host. In the case of LCM virus, the erroneous isolation from the assay host is a well recognized hazard, although I believe that its significance is often exaggerated. Spurious isolation due to insufficiently controlled laboratory conditions seems to occur much more frequently which, understandably, is not often mentioned when an isolation is appraised. For this reason, I firmly believe that a conclusive diagnosis should rest on serological evidence, in particular where the clinical course is unusual.

Two methods are generally available for the demonstration of LCM-specific antibody; the complement fixation test and the neutralization test. Technical considerations will be dealt with under Section XI. B. Here, their application to the diagnosis of human infections is to be evaluated. Complement-fixing antibody appears relatively early, *i.e.* one to three weeks after onset, sometimes even sooner, and reaches its maximum at five to eight weeks. In most cases it declines quickly and has disappeared within six months after onset (LÉPINE *et al.*, 1938a; 1938b; SMADEL and WALL, 1940; RASMUSSEN, 1947; SCHEID *et al.*, 1959). Therefore, its presence is of considerable diagnostic value (RASMUSSEN, 1947; LEVI *et al.*, 1951; SHVAREV, 1964a). There are, however, cases on record where the complement fixation tests gave positive results for years (MILZER and LEVINSON, 1942; SCHEID *et al.*, 1959; SHVAREV, 1964a).

According to SCHEID *et al.* (1959), false positive results have not to be feared when clean antigen preparations are used. However, ŽÁČKOVÁ *et al.* (1959) tested 162 presumably normal human sera with antigens prepared in three different ways and found them to be positive — though always in low titers — in 6.7, 8.6, and 15.4 per cent, respectively. Furthermore, it appears to be likely that many of the positive results obtained with the complement fixation test on sera from apparently healthy persons (see Section X. C) did not result from recent infections with the LCM virus but were rather due to technical inadequacies.

It is of importance to be aware that complement-fixing antibody does not always appear in cases where the infection is proved otherwise (SMADEL and WALL, 1940; RASMUSSEN, 1947; COHEN *et al.*, 1966). Why complement-fixing activity should be present in most cases but not in all is unknown. One could think of the appearance of blocking antibody which combines with the antigen but fails to fix complement, as has been shown to occur with a variety of virus antigens including that of LCM virus by SCHMIDT and HARDING (1956). Of course, technical faultiness can never be ruled out completely.

The unequivocal demonstration of a high concentration of LCM-specific complement-fixing antibody suggests, but does not prove, a recent infection with this virus; the same may not be said of neutralizing antibody (Fig. 14). This appears later and rises more slowly but remains at its maximum for years, possibly for life (SMADEL and WALL, 1940; MILZER and LEVINSON, 1942; SCHEID *et al.*, 1959; 1960). In earlier reports, it was often stated that even in proved cases neutralizing antibody not always appears. Thus, LÉPINE *et al.* (1938a) noted that it is "inconstante, tardive et souvent fugitive". Other authors arrived at similar conclusions. However, thanks mainly to the efforts of W. Scheid and his colleagues at Cologne, this assumption cannot be maintained any longer. If during an alleged

LCM virus infection neutralizing antibody remains undetected, it is the diagnosis that should be questioned and not the significance of the negative results.

It is conceivable that some such failures might have been due to heating of the serum. In contrast to most other viral antibodies, neutralizing antibody directed against the LCM virus is heat labile (Lehmann-Grube *et al.*, 1960; Scheid *et al.*, 1960). Ackermann *et al.* (1962) titrated eight human immune sera before and after inactivation for 20 minutes at 56° C and measured decreases of the neutralizing indices which ranged from 0.7 to 2.1 $\log_{10}$ with a mean of 1.51. This marked heat lability led Ackermann and his colleagues to study the effect of storage on neutralizing titers in human immune sera. Two weeks at 22° C or six weeks at 4° C slightly but definitely reduced the titers. If whole blood was kept at either temperature, no loss had become apparent after 14 days. The ability to neutralize the LCM virus

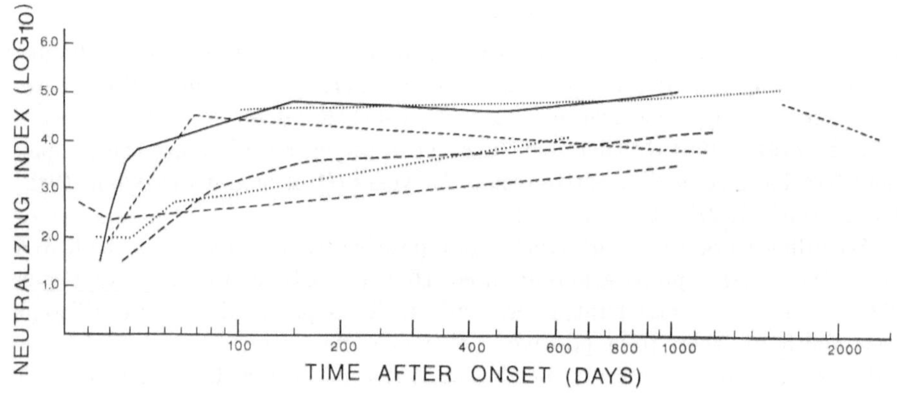

Fig. 14. LCM virus-specific neutralizing antibody in man after infection with the LCM virus. Curves represent antibody titers in sera of six patients taken repeatedly at intervals after onset of the LCM disease. Adapted from W. Scheid, R. Ackermann, K.-A. Jochheim, and F. Lehmann-Grube: Arch. ges. Virusforsch. 9, 295 (1960)

was well maintained for months at —30° C and results were even better after lyophylization. It is noteworthy, although unexplained, that the reduction in titer after heat inactivation was partly reversed by storage at 4° C or 22° C. Since, as we have seen, unheated sera lose some of their activity under these conditions, heat-inactivated and native aliquots of sera showed essentially the same neutralizing capacities when kept for some time at 4° C or 22° C. Storage was found not to affect complement-fixing activities in sera (Scheid *et al.*, 1959).

It has been stated that a single high titer of neutralizing antibody is of little diagnostic significance. This conclusion is based not only upon its prolonged persistence, but even more on the fact that most human sera contain natural inhibitors for the virus. When mixed with undiluted normal serum, the virus titer may be reduced up to 100-fold (Scheid *et al.*, 1960). We know little of these "nonspecific" substances. Just like "specific" antibody they are affected, but not eliminated, by heat inactivation. Again, loss due to heating is recovered on storage at 4° C or 22° C (Ackermann *et al.*, 1962). In fact, so far no difference has shown up between these two types of neutralizing activities apart from the concentrations they attain. Whereas neutralizing indices climb to $\log_{10}$ three or even five during the course of an LCM virus infection, the "natural" inhibitors remain low. Their upper limit has been set at an index of $\log_{10}$ two (SCHEID *et al.*, 1959), which appears to be justified from an analysis of the data (SCHEID *et al.*, 1960) on which this figure was based; the calculated mean from 36 determinations is 1.230 and the standard deviation of the single observation is 0.356. Thus, 95 per cent of all "natural" neutralizing indices may be expected to fall into the range of 0.52 to 1.94. As judged from their low titers, it may be assumed that the "neutralizing activity" in human sera, described by POLLIKOFF and SIGEL (1952; personal communication) to be heat labile, was actually such nonspecific inhibitors. These considerations make it obvious that antibody in a single human serum is of little diagnostic value. The only true serological proof of an infection with LCM virus in the immediate past lies in detecting the appearance or increase of antibody. However, as is the case with a few other viral infections, a tentative diagnosis may sometimes be based on a comparison of complement fixation and neutralization titers (SCHEID *et al.*, 1959; PANOV *et al.*, 1963).

The detection and titration of LCM-specific antibody by means of indirect immunofluorescence may turn out to be of value. Immune bodies detected by immunofluorescence were found to appear faster than those detected by either the complement fixation or neutralization tests and to remain demonstrable for at least three years with a slow decrease (TRIANDAPHILLI *et al.*, 1965; COHEN *et al.*, 1966). It is disconcerting, though, to read that in three of the twelve cases no neutralizing activities became apparent. Possibly, the sera were taken too early, namely "3 months or less after onset". It is to be hoped that more data will become available so as to permit an appraisal of this method's relative value (see also Section XI. B. 3).

There remains the question of optimal conditions for the isolation of the virus. Blood in the febrile stage and blood and cerebrospinal fluid in the stage of cerebral manifestations are reliable sources. Occasional reports on successful isolations from other materials (MACCALLUM and FINDLAY, 1939) should be regarded with suspicion, although, in at least one case, isolation from the throat has been reported from a patient whose infection was also proved by isolation of the virus from the blood and significant increases of complement-fixing, neutralizing, and immunofluorescing antibodies (COHEN *et al.*, 1966).

For isolation of the virus, of the available hosts the laboratory mouse is undoubtedly the animal of choice. Its susceptibility is high and clinical signs after the intracerebral inoculation may — for all practical purposes — be regarded as pathognomonic. I have not heard of any strain of virus which would not cause typical signs and death in mice with the possible exception of "E 53" which induced illness of two to three days duration but death only in a few animals (WIKTOR *et al.*, 1966). The high dose phenomenon (see Section V. A. 4. b) may safely be disregarded where isolation from clinical materials is concerned.

Although often recommended, the guinea-pig is less suitable for primary isolation. Most strains do not cause an overt disease in these animals and serology and protection tests have to follow. However, all but a few LCM virus strains multiply in these animals, and I have become aware of only three isolates which apparently did not infect guinea-pigs (ACKERMANN *et al.*, 1964; KÜPPER *et al.*, 1964/65; SCHEID *et al.*, 1966).

I. Immunization Procedures

1. Active Immunization with Vaccine

LCM virus vaccines were prepared repeatedly, either to provide a model for the study of virus vaccines in general or to serve certain experimental purposes. Traub (1938a) immunized guinea-pigs with two or three injections of a formalin-inactivated preparation derived from a variety of guinea-pig tissues after infection with a virulent strain. In most animals the protection was partial. Vaccines prepared from infected mouse tissues had no or little immunizing capacity, even though the original infectivity had been equally high. Also, the admixture of a formalin-treated normal mouse tissue suspension to a vaccine prepared from infected guinea-pig tissues reduced the immunizing capacity of the latter. The inhibitory effect was less marked when the foreign tissue vaccine was inoculated simultaneously on the opposite side of the body. Traub explained this phenomenon as immunologic competition. Vaccinated guinea-pigs developed neutralizing antibody faster than the unprepared controls when challenged with active virus. Occasionally, such animals had infectious virus and antibody together. A high degree of protection was produced in some guinea-pigs by prolonged treatment. These animals had neutralizing antibody before being challenged. Smadel and Wall (1940) did not succeed in inducing complement-fixing or neutralizing activities or specific protection in guinea-pigs by inoculation of noninfectious soluble antigen or partially purified, heat-inactivated virus. The repeated inoculation of a formalin vaccine induced complement-fixing antibody, specific protection, and neutralizing antibody, in this order. Alice and McNutt (1945) achieved partial resistance in guinea-pigs by treatment for many weeks with a vaccine prepared by incubating infected guinea-pig tissue suspensions with 0.15 per cent formalin for 24 to 36 hours at room temperature. Milzer and Levinson (1946; 1949) failed to immunize mice or monkeys by inoculation of virus which had been inactivated by heat or formalin. They had some success by treatment of the virus with ultraviolet light (see Section II. A). Mice inoculated at weekly intervals three times intraperitoneally with this vaccine resisted approximately 200 intracerebral LD_{50}, and rhesus monkeys, vaccinated in a similar manner, resisted ten subcutaneous LD_{50}. The extremely flat course of the curve relating virus doses and mortality in vaccinated mice is noteworthy. It indicates a great variation between these mice in their response to the infection as contrasted with the untreated control animals.

Great difficulties were encountered by Jochheim *et al.* (1957) who tried to render guinea-pigs resistant to challenge with the highly virulent WE strain by treatment with the virus after its inactivation by heat, ultraviolet light, or formalin. No protective immunity was achieved by Stock and Francis (1943) in mice inoculated with virus inactivated by ether or a fatty acid.

After having determined the optimal conditions for the formalin inactivation of the WE virus grown in monkey kidney cell cultures, Benda and Činátl (1964) compared the immunizing efficacy of this vaccine with that of a relatively non-pathogenic strain, "K". Prior infection with K protected guinea-pigs against large doses of WE aerosols. In contrast, the vaccine rendered only part of the animals resistant. When the guinea-pigs were challenged intraperitoneally, the average index of resistance (log_{10}) was 1.8 after treatment with WE vaccine but 4.0 to 5.0 after infection with active K virus. The low protection afforded by the vaccine as compared with infection was reflected by the pattern of virus multiplication after infection by inhalation with WE. While in the nonimmunized controls the infection spread rapidly, in the animals immunized with K the challenge virus was found only irregularly and in trace amounts. After immunization with WE vaccine and challenge with low inhalation doses of WE, the virus was similarly suppressed. With larger doses there was an initial delay, but by the second or third day the difference with the controls had vanished and both groups died at the same time. Monkeys could be protected to some extent against the lethal inhalation infection with WE by prior subcutaneous immunization with WE vaccine. Using an intracerebral mouse test, no neutralizing antibody was detected in sera from guinea-pigs or monkeys after vaccination with formalin-inactivated WE. This finding is of uncertain significance because no neutralizing activities were detected in the sera of guinea-pigs or monkeys after immunization with active virus K.

TRAUB (1964) inoculated mice six times with a formalized vaccine at four to seven days intervals. A moderate degree of protection was achieved against challenge virus, but neither neutralizing nor complement-fixing antibody became detectable.

2. Passive Immunization with Immune Serum

No experimental details were supplied by TRAUB (1939b) who stated that in mice the intravenous inoculation of hyperimmune guinea-pig serum three hours before intracerebral infection reduced lethality. MILZER and LEVINSON (1946; 1949) protected mice and guinea-pigs with monkey hyperimmune or human convalescent sera, respectively. Mice were spared if treated within 48 hours after infection. In guinea-pigs which received the serum two days after the virus the only effect was a prolongation of their life. TREUSCH *et al.* (1943) saw a beneficial effect of pooled human sera given in large quantities intravenously to a patient with "recurrent" encephalitis due to the LCM virus. According to NIKOLITSCH and FENJE (1959; NIKOLITSCH, 1959), treatment with immune serum reduced viremia and prolonged the lives of virus-infected guinea-pigs.

Treatment of mice intraperitoneally or subcutaneously with rabbit hyperimmune serum rendered them free from the general disease following foot pad inoculation. This protection was complete when the serum was given during the time period eight days before till five days after the virus inoculation. Even six days after infection, the mice could be partially protected. Significantly, the local reaction was not influenced by the antiserum. In such animals the virus had not spread throughout the body. No passive protection was possible of the general disease following the intracerebral or intraperitoneal inoculation of the virus (ROGER and ROGER, 1965b; 1966).

BENDA (1964) studied the effect of γ-globulin, prepared by precipitation from rabbit and sheep hyperimmune sera, on infection of guinea-pigs by inhalation of virus. The neutralizing indices of the 0.5 per cent solution ranged from log_{10} three to five. After the intramuscular injection of 0.1 g per kg body weight of γ-globulin peak neutralizing activities in the recipient sera ranging from log_{10} 1.5 to 2.0 were obtained after 48 hours. The protection afforded was slight; increases in survival were achieved only with minimal infectious doses and with large amounts of globulin administered before or immediately after the virus. When the treatment was delayed or when the infectious dose was increased some prolongation of survival time ensued. Passive immunization of guinea-pigs only slightly retarded the development of infectivity in various organs.

VI. Treatments Inhibiting Virus Multiplication or Abolishing Signs of Disease

In a previous chapter (see Section V. A. 4. b) the evidence has been summarized for our belief that the LCM disease of the mouse does not result from direct damage to the cells in consequence of the virus infection but rather from an allergic interaction between the host and some new antigen(s). Thus, treatment may be expected to succeed on two levels: (1) by suppression of virus multiplication and (2) by inhibition of the immunologic response of the host. Numerous examples have been cited which prove that mice may be saved by immunosuppression (see Table 5). In contrast, no evidence exists which would indicate that the disease in other species, and notably in man, likewise results from an immune conflict. Hence, immunosuppression may not be expected to result in a therapeutic success in species other than *M. musculus*.

1. Inhibition of Virus Multiplication

The extract of *Sambucus sieboldiana* inhibited the intracerebral multiplication of both encephalomyocarditis, strain Col. SK, and LCM viruses. Multiplication of the Col. SK virus was reduced throughout the observation period, but the concentration of the LCM virus was lower only during four days following the infection; on the seventh day it could not be distinguished from that of the controls (Furusawa *et al.*, 1968a). No further attempts to inhibit virus multiplication *in vivo* have come to my attention. Actinomycin D, halogen-deoxyuridines, 6-azauridine, and arabinosylcytosin were tested *in vitro*. The effects of these compounds have been discussed when dealing with the composition of the virus (see Section II. D). Pfau and Camyre (1968) observed inhibition of multiplication of LCM strains CA 1371, WCP, and Traub in HeLa cells by 2-(α-hydroxybenzyl)benzimidazole (HBB). The rate of inactivation of the virus was not influenced by the drug and adsorption onto the cells was not inhibited. No effect on virus multiplication was seen by guanidine-HCl at concentrations as high as 700 μM.

Further experiments *in vitro* with a variety of natural and synthetic substances were performed by Furusawa *et al.* (1964), Cutting *et al.* (1965), Furusawa and Cutting (1966), and Furusawa *et al.* (1967). These studies cannot be evaluated because the LCM identity of the used virus, which was the cell culture-adapted strain NY 621, is doubtful (see Section IX).

2. Abolition of Signs of the Disease

In the mouse a great number of measures have become known which reduce or even abolish the signs of the LCM disease. Most of them act by immunosuppression (see Section V. A. 4. b). With other treatments, the mode of action is less clear. ROSENTHAL *et al.* (1937) tested several sulfonamides and found prontosil to be effective. Though this may seem surprising, a synoptic analysis of the data from the six individual experiments reveals that, in all, 44 of 84 (=52.4 per cent) treated mice survived but only 12 of 94 (=12.8 per cent) controls, a difference which is highly significant at $p < 0.01$. Presumably, at the near toxic doses used, prontosil led to some immunosuppression, thus preventing clinical signs to develop. Of the experiments performed by TOOMEY and TAKACS (1944) with prontosil and neoprontosil, which seem to contradict Rosenthal's results, three are of no use because all controls died together with the virus-infected animals due to toxicity of the drugs. In three more experiments in which prontosil was tested in mice and neoprontosil in mice and guinea-pigs no therapeutic effects were demonstrated although toxic levels of the compounds were employed.

PANOV and REMEZOV (1960) protected mice by oxygen. Best results were obtained if, two days after intracerebral infection, the animals were kept for five to ten hours under pure oxygen with a pressure of one kg/cm^2. But treatment begun as late as five days after infection, *i.e.* immediately prior to the onset of illness, had some effect. In 3 of 37 mice thus protected, X-irradiation or cold water shock applied 30 days later induced typical disease during which virus was demonstrated. In the animals which did not respond to provocative measures no virus was found. Of 40 protected mice, 11 succumbed to intracerebral challenge 30 days later. Furthermore, it was said that in O_2-treated mice less virus was found (no data). No explanation was given towards the possible mechanism.

Interesting although unexplained is the observation of SIKORA *et al.* (1968) that mortality of mice was reduced by 50 per cent if the animals had been stressed by avoidance learning or hunger prior to the intracerebral infection with LCM virus. One would like to know whether the lymphatic system of these mice was affected such as is known to be the case following treatment with cortisone or severe stress (DOUGHERTY, 1952; ISHIDATE and METCALF, 1963).

Protection of mice from LCM death was reported by Furusawa and his colleagues to result from the subcutaneous inoculation of extracts from *Narcissus tazetta*, and *Magnolia kobus*, bulbs and buds, respectively, and propionin, a substance prepared from *Propionibacterium freudenreichii* (FURUSAWA and CUTTING, 1966; FURUSAWA *et al.*, 1967; 1968b). Partial purifications were accomplished by RAMANATHAN *et al.* (1965/66; 1966) and FURUSAWA *et al.* (1967). Although all three preparations markedly reduced the lethality of LCM virus-infected mice, none was found to inhibit the multiplication of the virus; titers in the brains of treated mice were equal and in the blood even higher than in controls. Nor were the protected mice depressed in their immunologic reactivity. On the contrary, higher titers of LCM-specific complement-fixing antibody developed in the treated animals. The development of hemagglutinins and hemolysins to sheep erythrocytes was temporarily depressed by *N. tazetta* extracts but not by the other preparations (FURUSAWA *et al.*, 1968b). Propionin B1, as used in these experiments, was further purified and characterized by RAMANATHAN *et al.* (1968) who showed the active principle — called 41B-I = fraction D — to have a molecular weight greater than 100,000 but smaller than 200,000. It contained *ca* 15 per cent protein and *ca* 50 per cent carbohydrates and was thought to be possibly a glycoprotein.

A further plant preparation, an extract from the bark of *Sambucus sieboldiana*, was also found to be active against LCM in mice. This drug retarded the multiplication of the virus in the mouse brain (Furusawa *et al.*, 1968a). Otherwise we have not a hint as to the possible mode of action of these natural products.

Reports dealing with the therapeutic efficacies in human cases of aureomycin (Grater and Rider, 1949) and sulfanilamide (Leichenger *et al.*, 1940) are not conclusive because the diagnoses were based on insufficient evidence (see Section V. H. 1).

VII. Interference Phenomena

An investigation into the question how the presence of one virus affects the host's ability to deal with another is one way to obtain a better understanding of the relationship between the agent and the infected organism. This is particulary true in the case of viruses, such as that of LCM, which by themselves are not pathogenic for the cell they have invaded. In evaluating experiments of this sort, a clear distinction must be maintained between homologous and heterologous interference, *i.e.* interference between identical or closely related and unrelated viruses, respectively.

A. Homologous Interference

1. Experiments Performed *in vivo*

A peculiar but highly significant aspect of the multiplication of LCM virus is that it is self-limited. When a newborn mouse is infected, the virus multiplies initially unchecked but, after having reached a certain maximum concentration, further propagation is limited such as to maintain an equilibrium between newly produced virus and virus lost due to excretion and inactivation (see Section V.A. 3). In these mice, closely related viruses are excluded from multiplication. One of my own unpublished experiments may be cited to illustrate this statement. The strain E-350 of Armstrong is of low pathogenicity for guinea-pigs, whereas strain WE of Rivers is invariably fatal in these animals. Two seven-month-old carriers, congenitally infected with E-350, were tested for viremia by mouse titration; per ml of blood, $10^{5.9}$ and $10^{6.1}$ ID_{50} were detected. They were then inoculated intraperitoneally on four consecutive days with WE virus, each one receiving altogether more than 10^{10} ID_{50}. Three weeks after the last WE injection, viremia was unaltered as determined by mouse titration, but the assay in guinea-pigs revealed that the blood of one mouse possibly contained a trace of WE, while the other animal was entirely free from it. A similar experiment with identical results had been performed by Traub (1961b) who employed strains with differing pathogenicities for newborn mice.

A striking example of homologous interference in adult mice was reported by Rowe (1954). When inoculated intraperitoneally, his "Armstrong" strain induced the production of pleural and ascitic fluids. In contrast, the "Institute" strain was virtually nonpathogenic when inoculated by the same route. After the simultaneous intraperitoneal inoculation of both strains in various proportions, significantly less fluids were produced, even if relatively little interfering virus had been admixed. If the "Institute" strain virus had been heat-inactivated, no interference became demonstrable.

Homologous interference may be inferred also from observations reported by MIMS and SUBRAHMANYAN (1966) using the fluorescing antibody technique. They failed to detect an increase of LCM virus antigen in the cells lining the cerebrospinal fluid spaces of the brain and the venous sinusoids of the liver (Kupffer's cells) in intracerebrally or intravenously superinfected carrier mice in spite of the fact that little antigen was present.

2. Experiments Performed *in vitro*

As in the mouse, the multiplication of the LCM virus in cultured cells is self-limited. Homologous interference is marked to the extent that the multiplication of a superinfecting identical or related virus is fully excluded (TRAUB and KESTING, 1964; MIMS and SUBRAHMANYAN, 1966; LEHMANN-GRUBE, 1967a; LEHMANN-GRUBE *et al.*, 1969).

Limitation of multiplication and homologous interference both *in vivo* and *in vitro* are probably closely related phenomena. The underlying mechanism is unknown. It is almost certainly not a matter of exhaustion of the infected cells, which are otherwise functionally intact (see Section III. A. C) and, furthermore, are fully able to support the multiplication of unrelated viruses (see Section VII. B. 2). It is probably also distinct from "immunity" in lysogenic bacteria (BERTANI, 1958); approximately five per cent of clones derived from an established carrier colony were free of virus but were readily infected, which excludes any inherent resistance (LEHMANN-GRUBE *et al.*, 1969). In cells infected *in vitro* with LCM virus, a small proportion always remained free of antigen as determined by immunofluorescence (SLENCZKA and LEHMANN-GRUBE, unpublished). With our present knowledge, the simplest interpretation of these phenomena seems to be a feedback mechanism, which is mediated either by a soluble substance or by incomplete forms of the virus produced and released together with the virions by the infected cells. TRAUB and KESTING (1964) searched for the presence of material able to inhibit virus multiplication in lymph node and mouse embryo cell cultures in media from infected lymph node cultures rendered free of infectivity by centrifugation and thermal inactivation at 36.5° C; none was found. Similar attempts of our own (unpublished) have likewise failed so far. BENSON (1962) claimed to have demonstrated the existence of an interfering substance in chronically infected L cells, the nature of which is unknown.

So far no evidence has come to light which would support the hypothesis advanced by MIMS and SUBRAHMANYAN (1966) that in a carrier mouse with its marked homologous interference all cells are infected "in the sense that they contain viral nucleic acid and may be capable of producing antigen".

B. Heterologous Interference

1. Experiments Performed *in vivo*

In a previous chapter the evidence was cited concerning the direct effects of the LCM virus on its host cells, and the conclusion was reached that the metabolism of the LCM virus-infected cell is not impaired to any measurable extent. If this is true, heterologous interference in LCM virus-infected cells should generally be absent although not necessarily in each combination.

SMADEL and WALL (1942) passaged LCM and St. Louis encephalitis viruses together intracerebrally in hamsters. After five transfers large amounts of both viruses were found in the brain. SINKOVICS (1955) reported that the multiplication of influenza A virus, strain PR8, in the mouse lung was not affected by simultaneous infection with LCM virus.

TRAUB and KESTING (1964) assayed vesicular stomatitis virus in normal and persistently LCM virus-infected mice and obtained the same final titers. They noticed, however, that the period between inoculation and appearance of the disease as well as the survival time were prolonged in the carriers. VOLKERT *et al.* (1964) failed to detect differences in susceptibility to the 17D yellow fever virus between normal AKR mice, AKR carriers, and AKR carriers adoptively immunized with immune syngeneic lymphoid cells. HOTCHIN and CINITS (1958) found LCM virus carrier mice to be susceptible to ectromelia virus. MIMS and SUBRAHMANYAN (1966) titrated ectromelia virus in normal and persistently infected mice with equal results. Superinfection did not change the pattern of immunofluorescing LCM virus antigen in sections from liver or brain. Also, mousepox immunofluorescence in these organs was not influenced by persistent LCM virus infection.

These observations indicate lack of heterologous interference, but this is not always true. A well-documented case is that of eastern equine encephalomyelitis (EEE) virus. TRAUB (1961b) titrated this virus and found carrier mice to be less susceptible than normal controls. WAGNER and SNYDER (1962) observed a moderate degree of resistance to EEE virus in mice previously inoculated intranasally with the WE strain of LCM virus. The resistance persisted for about eight days and disappeared *pari passu* with the LCM virus. Congenital and neonatal carriers were also slightly less susceptible to EEE virus inoculated intraperitoneally. Some further studies on this phenomenon were performed by TRAUB (1962a). He titrated the EEE virus intracerebrally in three groups of mice: (1) normal adults, (2) adults immunized with LCM virus by peripheral inoculation followed by cerebral challenge, and (3) LCM virus carriers. In all of six experiments the titers in the persistently infected animals were lower than in the controls with a mean of 0.6 $\log_{10}$ (four-fold). Surprisingly, the titers in the LCM-immune mice were decreased to the same extent, although the brains of parallel mice contained only traces of or no LCM virus infectivity at all at the time the titrations were done. The degree of resistance decreased as the interval between the intracerebral challenge with LCM virus and the intracerebral inoculation of EEE virus increased, but some resistance was found even when the mice had been inoculated with LCM virus by the subcutaneous route. Carrier mice were also significantly protected against western equine encephalomyelitis and St. Louis encephalitis viruses (HOTCHIN and CINITS, 1958; LEWIS and CLAYTON, 1969b).

DALLDORF *et al.* (1938b) reported on a sparing effect of canine distemper virus on poliomyelitis in rhesus monkeys. Later it was found that the distemper virus, which came from infected dog organs, contained LCM virus. Since LCM virus alone had the same effects as the mixture of both viruses, it was concluded that the clinical signs as well as the interference with poliomyelitis, recently ascribed to the distemper virus, had in fact been caused by the LCM virus (DALLDORF and DOUGLASS, 1938). More extensive experiments on the sparing effect of LCM virus infection on experimental poliomyelitis in monkeys were reported by DALLDORF (1939b). After various routes of inoculation, the LCM virus strain employed caused a disease which was distinct from poliomyelitis. In monkeys with established LCM disease no clinical signs developed after the intracerebral inoculation of the poliovirus. Moreover, in contrast to the controls, the cervical portions of the spinal cords were free of poliovirus, but they contained LCM virus. Also, few or no lesions typical of poliomyelitis developed. The same effects were obtained when poliovirus and LCM virus were given simultaneously but not when the poliovirus infection preceded the inoculation of the LCM virus. While the conclusion that the multiplication of poliovirus was suppressed by the LCM virus infection is convincing, the same cannot be said about the reverse. In fact, the data indicate that the multiplication of the LCM virus was not significantly affected by the concomitant poliovirus infection.

DALLDORF and WHITNEY (1943) observed that the paralysis caused in young hamsters by the intracerebral inoculation of MM, a member of the encephalomyocarditis group of viruses, could be prevented by the prior intracerebral injection of other "rodent paralyzing viruses" including LCM and polioviruses. RHODES and CHAPMAN (1949) were unable to detect a sparing effect of poliovirus on the paralysis due to MM. They did confirm, however, that the disease in hamsters following the intraperitoneal inoculation of MM was reduced if the animals had been inoculated intracerebrally at least four days previously with LCM virus. Also, inoculation of MM protected hamsters from the LCM disease, but the data supporting this conclusion are less convincing. Further experiments by RHODES and CHAPMAN (1950) revealed that some protection was afforded if MM was inoculated as late as 30 days after the LCM virus. In hamsters thus protected, MM multiplication in viscera, cord, and brain was reduced 100- to 1000-fold. In contrast, the multiplication of the LCM virus was not affected by the presence of MM virus in the tissues. Survivors from interference experiments resisted both LCM and MM virus inoculations 30 days later. Whether this resulted from active immunity or represented still existing interference could not be decided. RHODES and CHAPMAN (1950) concluded from their results that the LCM virus had altered a considerable number of the host cells, thus preventing multiplication of MM virus.

In the experiments just described, animals infected with the LCM virus were superinfected with viruses known to have direct destructive effects on the host cells. In another group of experiments the effects on viral neoplasias were evaluated. NADEL and HAAS (1955; 1956) studied the influence of LCM virus on the course of leukemia in guinea-pigs and mice. L2B leukemia of CONGDON and LORENZ (1954) was transplanted into inbred "Strain 2" guinea-pigs, which invariably resulted in the animals' death. Subcutaneous infection with a moderately pathogenic LCM virus during the period two days prior till seven days after transplantation prolonged the average survival time of the guinea-pigs from 18.3 to 32.5 days. Also, the onset of splenomegaly was slower and local tumor growth was retarded. Sequential injection of other viruses (St. Louis encephalitis, influenza, or yellow fever) did not afford a further benefit. No protection by LCM virus inoculation was seen in previously LCM virus-immunized animals, nor did heated virus affect leukemia. Thus, LCM virus multiplication was necessary for protection to develop. Similar experiments in mice with a mouse leukemia gave inconclusive results because of the (unprecedented) high pathogenicity of the LCM virus alone after subcutaneous inoculation.

I am not aware that attempts have been made to clear up the etiology of L2B leukemia. This has been done successfully, however, in the case of L2C, another transmissible lymphatic leukemia which originated at about the same time as L2B in the same strain of inbred guinea-pigs (Congdon and Lorenz, 1954). Jungeblut and Kodza (1963a) demonstrated that transmission was possible with various materials from leukemic animals after cellular disruption, high speed centrifugation, and filtration through bacteria-retaining filters. They also found that the agent was inactivated by heating for 30 minutes at 56° C, ultraviolet- and X-irradiation, and by treatment with ether or phenol, and it may safely be concluded that it is a virus. Interference experiments with L2C leukemia and an LCM virus strain, recently isolated from guinea-pigs, were performed by Jungeblut and Kodza (1963b); they confirmed and extended the reports by Nadel and Haas on L2B. If LCM virus was inoculated intraperitoneally concurrently or up to eight days after L2C, all guinea-pigs but one out of a total of 26 in 19 experiments had prolonged latent periods and three of them survived. Interference was found to be mutual; no LCM disease developed if L2C had also been inoculated. Five days after simultaneous inoculation, LCM virus but not L2C could be transmitted with the animals' blood; at 22 to 33 days the reverse was true. Apparently the two agents interfered with each other's multiplication. This is also indicated by the findings that all three survivors developed leukemia when challenged later and that in leukemia resistant guinea-pigs or mice the course of LCM was not influenced by L2C. (It should be mentioned that some of these experiments had been done with an L cell-adapted LCM virus, the true identity of which must be regarded as doubtful — see Section IX.)

Other experiments which belong in the same category are those performed with Rauscher leukemia in mice by Barski and Youn (1964; Youn and Barski, 1966). Inoculation of the Rauscher virus into adult BALB/c mice resulted in a more than 95 per cent incidence of leukemia. The intraperitoneal inoculation of the Armstrong strain of LCM virus prolonged the latent periods before first signs became apparent, prolonged the survival times, and reduced the overall incidence to approximately 75 per cent. The protective effect of the LCM virus was most marked when it was given one to two days before the Rauscher virus; protection was insignificant when given concurrently or one to three days later. In newborn mice, the protection afforded by infection with LCM virus was even more marked. At the same time the pathogenicity of the LCM virus seemed to be enhanced; more newborn mice receiving both viruses died with typical LCM signs. It is noteworthy that in Rauscher virus-infected controls which had escaped leukemia high levels of neutralizing antibody developed and none of eight responded with leukemia upon challenge. In contrast, in mice which had been protected by LCM virus no neutralizing activity to Rauscher virus could be detected, and in all of 13 which were challenged leukemia developed. Apparently, in these animals leukemia did not develop because of the exclusion from multiplication of the causative agent by the concurrent infection with the LCM virus, a conclusion which was also drawn in the LCM-L2C system described above. Attention must be drawn to the finding, however, that in one of two mice inoculated with both viruses as newborns and in one of two mice inoculated as adults, Rauscher virus was found 117 and 89 days, respectively, later. LCM virus was found after neonatal inoculation only.

A further case in point, which may or may not be related to the phenomena just described, is the sparing effect of persistent LCM virus infection upon tumor induction with polyoma virus (HOTCHIN, 1962a). Groups of newborn mice were inoculated either with LCM virus on day one followed by polyoma virus on day two of their life, or with polyoma virus only on day two. The tumor incidence after ten months in the group receiving both viruses (four per cent) was significantly lower than in the polyoma virus-only controls, where it was 35 per cent. This result is the more significant as the experiment was done with the UBC = WE strain of LCM virus (personal communication by Dr. J. Hotchin) which has been found by MIMS and WAINWRIGHT (1968) to cause immunosuppression in mice. Inasmuch as tumor formation due to neonatal infection with polyoma virus is increased by thymectomy (LAW and TING, 1965) or injection of antilymphocytic serum (ALLISON and LAW, 1968) one might have expected augmentation rather than reduction of tumor formation.

In this context, an observation reported by FINDLAY *et al.* (1938) may be mentioned. These authors isolated a "pleuropneumonia-like organism", strain "L_5", from LCM virus-infected mice. When injected by itself intracerebrally to mice no signs of illness became apparent, but when L_5 was inoculated together with other agents, *e.g.* LCM virus but also agar (!), "rolling disease" developed. In these mice no signs typical of LCM were seen. Since mice inoculated intracerebrally with the LCM virus alone fell ill as early as the fourth day, these findings are of uncertain significance.

2. Experiments Performed *in vitro*

According to HOTCHIN and CINITS (1958), cytopathic effects in chick embryo cells due to western equine encephalomyelitis virus were slightly retarded by prior infection with LCM virus, strain WE. LCM virus-infected HeLa cells were not protected against cellular destruction caused by poliovirus. By the same criterion, ACKERMANN (1961a) did not notice interference of LCM virus with Coxsackie B4, vesicular stomatitis (VS), and herpes viruses in mouse embryo cells or with poliovirus in FL cells. WAGNER and SNYDER (1962) found L cells, persistently infected with the WE strain virus, to exhibit a "moderately increased resistance" to superinfection with the VS virus. This was not confirmed by LEHMANN-GRUBE (1967a) in an essentially identical system. In a later study, VS and vaccinia viruses were found to multiply in L cells persistently infected with the E-350 strain of Armstrong just as well as they did in the control cells. When employed for a plaque assay, carrier cells were found to be slightly less susceptible to VS and ME viruses (LEHMANN-GRUBE *et al.*, 1969). It is doubtful whether this reduced susceptibility of the carrier cells to two RNA viruses was caused by the presence of LCM virus. At the time these titrations were performed, persistently infected and uninfected control cells had been passaged in parallel for approximately 17 months. During this time deviations between the two lines were bound to develop and the influence the LCM virus might have exerted is unknown.

Traub and Kesting (1964) titrated eastern equine encephalomyelitis and VS viruses in tube cultures of mouse lymph node cells infected either *in vivo* (derived from carrier mice) or *in vitro* with the LCM virus and found no differences to the controls. Mims and Subrahmanyan (1966) employed embryo fibroblast cultures from carrier and normal mice and found them to be equally susceptible to Semliki Forest and encephalomyocarditis viruses as determined by plaque titration. In contrast, cultivated macrophages from carrier as well as from normal mice infected *in vitro* exhibited slightly reduced susceptibility to the ectromelia virus as judged from the development of ectromelia-specific immunofluorescence, which was convincingly shown not to be due to the production of interferon by the LCM virus-infected cells. Wiktor *et al.* (1966) detected mutual interference of rabies and LCM viruses in BHK-21 cells, which might have been due to the cytopathic effect exerted by the latter.

When introducing the subject of heterologous interference, it was pointed out that the metabolic state of LCM virus-infected cells was such that the course of a superinfection with an unrelated virus should not be altered to any significant extent. As regards cells infected *in vitro*, this expectation was borne out by the experimental evidence. In the animal, however, a number of well-documented examples of heterologous interference are on record. No satisfactory explanation can be given at the present time which would account for these interference phenomena. LCM virus does not cross react immunologically with any of the viruses with which it interfered. Nor are true interferons produced by LCM virus-infected cells (see below). One could think of a competitive exclusion of certain superinfecting viruses, but not of others, from some metabolic pathways due to prior usurpation by the interfering agent.

Alternatively, in particular where tumor formation was affected, the LCM virus might have caused damage to the target cells leading to a reduction of their proliferative capacities as suggested by Nadel and Haas (1956) in the case of the retardation of leukemia in guinea-pigs. Finally, an interferon-like substance induced by the LCM virus *in vivo* and capable of inhibiting the multiplication of some of the superinfecting viruses (see below) could be responsible. A decision will most probably not come from animal experimentation alone. Studies *in vitro* must provide the ground on which further explorations of these complex phenomena may be based.

C. Interferon

Wagner and Snyder (1962) did not detect interferon by means of a plaque reduction assay employing vesicular stomatitis virus in tissues of mice infected as adults or newborns, nor was interferon demonstrated by Traub (1962a). Volkert *et al.* (1964) searched without success in organs of carrier mice adoptively immunized with syngeneic immune lymphoid cells. No interferon activity was detected by Mims and Subrahmanyan (1966) in the brain of a carrier mouse or in LCM virus-superinfected mouse embryo cells from carriers cultivated *in vitro*.

No resistance-promoting factors in the media of LCM virus-infected L cell cultures were detected by WAGNER and SNYDER (1962) and LEHMANN-GRUBE (1967a). TRAUB and KESTING (1964) failed to detect interferon activity in media from lymph node cell cultures from carriers or from normal mice infected *in vitro*. Thus, LCM virus-infected cultivated cells or animal tissues have never been shown to produce interferon. They are, however, quite capable of doing so and are susceptible to its action. After the intracerebral infection of an LCM virus carrier mouse with West Nile virus, large amounts of interferon were detected four days later. Cells from carrier mice cultivated *in vitro* resisted ectromelia virus infections like normal mouse cells when treated with stock interferon prepared from West Nile virus-infected mouse brain. Furthermore, normal mouse cells treated with interferon resisted LCM virus infection as efficiently as ectromelia virus infection (MIMS and SUBRAHMANYAN, 1966).

More recently, an interferon-like inhibitor was detected in brains and other organs of mice acutely infected with LCM virus, strain Armstrong. It affected cellular destruction *in vitro* due to Coxsackie A9, Coxsackie B1 through B6, ECHO 11, vesicular stomatitis, and influenza A viruses and reduced multiplication of poliovirus type 1. It did not inhibit cytopathic effects caused by vaccinia or Reo 1 viruses. The inhibitor required an induction period, was unaffected by LCM virus antiserum, was nonsedimentable, and showed a dose-response effect, all properties of a true interferon. However, it was acid labile, crossed species borders, and could be eliminated by a medium change at the time of addition of challenge virus. No similar activity was detected in tissues of WE strain-infected mice, nor was it present in infected cell culture fluids (VELTRI and KIRK, personal communication).

VIII. Enhancement Phenomena

The virologist is aware of innumerable examples of interference, involving practically all viruses. The opposite, namely enhancement, is rare. One example is known to occur with LCM virus. KOPROWSKI *et al.* (1966; WIKTOR *et al.*, 1966) infected WI 38 human diploid cells with rabies viruses. A maximum of between 2 and 12 per cent of the cells showed immunofluorescence when overlaid with conjugated rabies antiserum and the media contained less than 10^2 mouse LD_{50} per 0.03 ml. After superinfection with LCM virus, which had been obtained from inadvertently infected WI 38 cells, immunofluorescence rose to 80 to 100 per cent of the cells and infectivity in the media increased 20 to 100-fold. The most pronounced effect was obtained when LCM virus was given to the cells 24 hours prior to the rabies virus, but even in persistently rabies virus-infected cultures LCM virus led to enhancement. Unexpectedly, in such cells the stimulating effect was abolished by rabies-specific antiserum, although antiserum had no effect on persistent rabies virus infection by itself. Enhancement was also noted in rabbit endothelial cells. Ultraviolet irradiation of the LCM virus reduced the effect. Rabies virus infection was not stimulated by rubella, vesicular stomatitis, Newcastle disease, or SV40 viruses, nor was the propagation of rabies virus in mouse brain increased by LCM virus.

IX. Virus Variation

As a rule, viruses undergo alterations when transferred from one host to another and LCM virus is no exception. Traub (1937) passaged two strains, "A" and "B", isolated from an infected mouse stock, in mice and guinea-pigs. No change became apparent with A in mice or guinea-pigs, but B which had been highly pathogenic for guinea-pigs when isolated became markedly attenuated when passaged in mice. At the same time, its pathogenicity for this animal had increased. Essentially the same was seen by Howard (1939) with a fresh LCM virus isolate. The French strain of Lépine rapidly gained pathogenicity when passaged in guinea-pigs (Ronse, 1937). Lavillaureix and Minck (1955) compared the properties of seven human isolates before and after passages in mice and guinea-pigs. The ability of these strains to cause illness in either species was markedly increased. Different mice from an infected carrier colony were found by Traub (1938b) to harbor viruses with different pathogenicities for guinea-pigs.

Shwartzman (1946) tested the pathogenicity of strains WE, FA, and WWS which had been passaged serially 84 to 86, 23, and 33 to 34 times, respectively, intracerebrally in mice (mouse substrains) and 90, 38 to 39, and 28 times, respectively, intracerebrally or subcutaneously in guinea-pigs (guinea-pig substrains). In mice, all substrains caused close to 100 per cent lethality when inoculated intracerebrally. When inoculated intraperitoneally, the guinea-pig substrains were highly pathogenic but the mouse substrains were not. Guinea-pigs were invariably killed by strains WE and FA, independent of the previous history of these viruses. In contrast, differences were seen with the WWS substrains; after having been passaged in guinea-pigs, 19 of 19 animals of this species were killed, while only 4 of 20 succumbed to the inoculation of the mouse substrain. Apparently, the heightened pathogenicity for guinea-pigs, consequent on passages in this species, was associated with an increase of the virus' pathogenicity for the mouse when infection was done by the peripheral route. This increased pathogenicity was found to be reflected by the invasion of the organs of the infected mouse (see Section V. A. 4. a). No correlation, however, existed between the extent and the character of visceral histopathological lesions and the behavior of the substrains in the mouse after intracerebral or intraperitoneal inoculations. It should be stressed that in these studies a clear distinction between changes of the quality of the infectious particles towards higher or lower virulence and mere quantitative increases or decreases of their numbers was not always made.

Daneš *et al.* (1963) passaged the WE strain of LCM virus seven times in the lungs of cynomolgus monkeys and noted an increase of the virus' virulence; less virus was required to cause disease due to infection by inhalation. The clinical picture in the monkeys had not changed.

MacCallum and Findlay (1940) cultivated the original English strain of LCM virus in Maitland type tissue cultures of minced chick embryos. Around the 66th passage the properties of the carried virus changed abruptly. Test mice did not show signs typical for LCM. Rather, they became lethargic and flaccid paralyses of the hind legs developed, sometimes followed by similar signs in the forelegs. Passage in cell cultures or in mice did not alter the capacity of the virus to cause these new signs in the inoculated mouse, but transfer to guinea-pigs resulted either in fever and death with recovery of a typical LCM agent or in no clinical signs at all. Such animals did not resist challenge with the WE strain virus later, indicating a complete loss of the LCM antigenicity of the agent in addition to the profound changes of its pathogenicity. From what we know of virus variation in general and properties of the LCM virus in particular, this new agent was probably not a variant of LCM virus. Indeed, the whole pattern of conversion and reversion as described above could be explained by assuming that the tissue cultures had become contaminated with mousepox virus. At about the same time pseudolymphocytic choriomeningitis virus, later shown to be ectromelia virus, was discovered in the same laboratory.

An observation of a rather similar nature was reported by JUNGEBLUT and KODZA (1963b). From guinea-pigs, inoculated with a transmissible leukemia, a virus was isolated which turned out to be a strain of LCM virus (NY 621). A branch was maintained by passages in L cells where it increased in pathogenicity, finally bringing about complete cell destruction. At the same time it had lost more than 90 per cent of its original pathogenicity for mice and guinea-pigs. This "cell culture-adapted LCM strain" was extensively used by Furusawa and his colleagues (see Section VI) who noted that the pathogenicity for mice as well as the ability to induce immune protection to LCM virus was lost completely. Repeated attempts to obtain a similar variant by passages of the original isolate in KB cells failed (FURUSAWA, personal communication). Most probably this agent is not a true LCM virus strain. PFAU and CAMYRE (1968) reported that it had the properties of a picornavirus.

A more convincing example of LCM virus variation obtained *in vitro* was observed by LEHMANN-GRUBE *et al.* (1969). LCM virus, strain E-350 (= Armstrong), was carried together with L cells, which resulted in the establishment of a typical carrier culture. After prolonged cultivation, the carried virus was found to be functionally incomplete. Its ability to spread from cell to cell was greatly reduced; its ability to kill mice was abolished. The nature of this viral alteration, which has its precedent in Rustigian's finding that measles virus lost its infectivity when persistently infected HeLa cells were treated with specific antiserum (RUSTIGIAN, 1966), is not yet understood. A few facts, however, were established, and from these the following conclusions were drawn. The virus, as it was found after a certain number of passages in Armstrong virus-infected L cells, was immunologically indistinguishable from fully infectious Armstrong virus. It induced solid resistance to LCM virus infection in mice and reacted specifically with antibody as shown by immunofluorescence, complement fixation, and neutralization. Moreover, in the ultracentrifuge it sedimented similar to the original virus. The difference from the parent virus lay in its functional incompleteness. Though infectious in the sense that it multiplied within the host cell and was transmitted vertically to the cellular progeny, its infectiousness for other cells was greatly reduced. This loss of ability to spread did not appear to be absolute. Medium and cell extracts from Armstrong virus-infected cultures induced LCM-specific fluorescence in a few cells of heavily inoculated cultures. While this may simply indicate that antigen was taken up by a few predestined elements, other observations leave little doubt that horizontal transmission, if abortive, was still possible: (1) the immunizing capacity of carrier virus was neutralized by specific antibody; (2) in newborn mice some immunogenicity was found after four blind passages, although the estimated cumulative dilution by far exceeded the titer of the starting material; (3) carrier cultures were slowly cured when the culture medium contained virus-specific antibody. The question whether the functional incompleteness of the carrier virus was accompanied by structural defects, as it is known for a variety of other viruses, must remain unanswered at the present time.

X. Epizootiology

LCM virus strains have been isolated from a great variety of natural hosts as well as from laboratory products such as cell cultures and vaccines. The ultimate reservoir, however, seems to be the grey house mouse.

A. Sources of Isolation

1. *Mus musculus*

The suspicion of Armstrong and his associates that wild house mice were responsible for human infections was based largely on Traub's observation of a spontaneous LCM virus infection in a mouse colony in the U.S.A. which was followed by similar reports from England and France. Consequently, they investigated a number of *M. musculus* and were able to isolate the virus from animals that had been trapped in the homes of two persons suffering from abacterial meningitis (Armstrong and Sweet, 1939). The possibility that the mice had been infected by the patients rather than *vice versa* was discussed at length and refuted (Armstrong, 1941). Since then an ever increasing number of confirmative reports from many parts of the world leave no room for doubt that *M. musculus* is the principal reservoir of the virus in nature (Armstrong *et al.*, 1940; Farmer and Janeway, 1942; Howitt and van Herick, 1942; Alice, 1945a; 1945b; Dalldorf *et al.*, 1946a; 1946b; Jungeblut and Dalldorf, 1946; Havens, 1948; Green *et al.*, 1949; MacCallum, 1949; Koch *et al.*, 1950a; 1950b; Ivánovics and Koch, 1950; Duncan *et al.*, 1951; Levi *et al.*, 1951; Morris and Alexander, 1951; Smithard and Macrae, 1951; Bárdoš, 1957; Ackermann and Jansen, 1958; Gajdamovich, 1958; Ackermann, 1960; Traumann *et al.*, 1962; Grešíková and Casals, 1963; Ackermann *et al.*, 1964; Scheid *et al.*, 1964; Panov and Shvarev, 1966; Scheid *et al.*, 1966; Blumenthal *et al.*, 1968a; 1968b). It has been frequently stated that many colonies of experimental mice harbor the virus and, indeed, Maurer (1958) is of the opinion that this is the case with most of them. This, however, does not seem to be correct, and a variety of other viruses are much more commonly found in laboratory mice than that of LCM. In addition to the observation of Traub already mentioned, these are the reports of the presence of the LCM virus in albino mice: Lépine and Sautter (1936) detected the virus in one colony in France. Findlay *et al.* (1936) searched for it in England and found that "three strains of laboratory mice" were free from LCM virus; of 15 other colonies from as many different breeders the virus was present in one. In Japan, Kasahara *et al.* (1937a; 1937b; 1939; Yamada, 1940a; 1940b) isolated six strains of the virus, of which at least three probably had come from laboratory mice. During attempts to adapt poliovirus to rodents, WENNER (1948) encountered one strain; the source of the latter remained unknown but it most probably came from the mouse. BERGER and SCHOOP (1967) found that the BK strain of *Toxoplasma* was contaminated with LCM virus which had presumably come from mice used for its passage, and more recently SKINNER and KNIGHT (1969) detected LCM virus in a colony of albino mice at Pirbright, England. Although there are no more records available, it is of course possible that other such incidences, which sometimes entail embarrassing consequences, have remained unpublished. Furthermore, there may exist infected colonies, where the virus has never been suspected and thus never been searched for. However, many discussions with people intimately concerned with this problem have given no clue that infections with LCM virus of laboratory stock mice are frequent.

Most wild mice tested for LCM virus were killed which excluded the possibility of determining the category of infection to which they belonged. However, from laboratory experience and from a few longitudinal observations (TRAUB, 1960a) it seems safe to conclude that the great majority of infected *M. musculus* represented true carriers and were not undergoing a subclinical self-limited infection.

2. Vertebrates Other than *M. musculus*

In view of the number of house mice in which the virus can be detected, it is surprising that most other rodents have been found to be free of LCM virus, even those belonging to species closely related to *M. musculus.* In areas in West Germany where Scheid and his colleagues had found infected house mice, KÜPPER *et al.* (1964/65; SCHEID *et al.*, 1966) isolated LCM virus from one *Apodemus sylvaticus*; later, BLUMENTHAL *et al.* (1968a; 1968b) trapped one other infected member of that species. In Czechoslovakia BENDA *et al.* (1955) recovered the virus from one *A. flavicollis*. The agents isolated from two "field mice", identified as *Mus agrarius* (presumably *Apodemus agrarius*), by FENJE (1956; NIKOLITSCH and FENJE, 1957) were not identified serologically.

Besides *M. musculus,* man is no doubt the species from which the greatest number of strains has been isolated. This does not necessarily signify a higher proportion of infected humans as compared with animals but may simply be due to the fact that physicians usually employ more refined methods with their patients than do their veterinary colleagues. However, it may also reflect that man is one of the few species which react with illness to a natural infection with the virus.

Next to man, monkeys seem to be a source of some significance and Armstrong's original strain may possibly have originated in that species. Soon after the first isolation ARMSTRONG and WOOLEY (1935) recovered two additional strains, at least one of which came from a monkey. COGGESHALL (1939) has described an epidemic in a monkey colony which, although it exhibited some unusual aspects, appears to have been caused by LCM virus. MACCALLUM and FINDLAY (1939) detected virus in nasopharyngeal washings from a patient with a paralytic disease by intracerebral inoculation of a monkey, although the material used for isolation had been pretreated with ether. The human disease was probably not caused by LCM virus (see Section V. H. 1).

Dogs have been implicated several times. Thus, DALLDORF and DOUGLASS (1938; DALLDORF, 1939a) found LCM virus on two occasions associated with distemper virus obtained from dog spleens. Its origin remained unknown, but the dogs used for passaging the distemper virus were suspected. ARMSTRONG (1941) mentioned the recovery of LCM virus from a commercial distemper tissue vaccine presumably prepared from dog organs. The same author (ARMSTRONG, 1942) described three fatal infections with LCM virus, two of which occurred in persons engaged in the manufacture of distemper vaccine (see Section V. H. 1). FINDLAY *et al.* (1940) claimed the isolation of the virus from the spleen of an "apparently normal" dog. An agent supposedly responsible for an ascending paralysis in several dogs from a community in California (MEYER, 1939/40) has not been sufficiently characterized to consider that its identity has been established.

Several times the virus was discovered in Syrian hamsters *(Mesocricetus auratus)*. LEWIS *et al.* (1965) isolated LCM virus from a line of a spontaneous hamster fibrosarcoma. This virus not only infected hamsters with the tumor transplants but also spread to hamsters kept in the same and even distant rooms and infected animal attendants. A similar incidence was reported by D. ARMSTRONG *et al.* (1969); after having performed experimental surgery on hamsters, a man developed a typical LCM meningitis. Subsequently, the animals were shown to be infected with the LCM virus. During work with rabies virus, PETROVIĆ and TIMM (1968) found 24 of altogether 98 hamsters, which they had purchased from two different sources, to harbor the LCM virus. Mode of infection and origin remained unknown, but the authors suspected that house mice inhabiting the animal quarters might have spread the virus.

Some isolation histories suggest that the virus might have originated from guinea-pigs (TRAUB, 1936c; KASAHARA *et al.*, 1937a; 1937b; 1939; YAMADA, 1940a; MACCALLUM and FINDLAY, 1939; HOWARD, 1940/41; ALICE and MCNUTT, 1945; JUNGEBLUT and KODZA, 1963b). Nothing is known as to the circumstances under which they might have become infected, but carrier mice in the animal quarters are always a possibility.

In addition to the species already discussed, MAURER (1958; 1964) lists roaches (cockroaches?), chinchillas, cotton rats, and foxes as sources of LCM virus, but he gives no details.

The viruses obtained by CHASTEL (1965) from reptiles and amphibians are probably not LCM virus strains (see Section XII). Whether the nine agents isolated by REISS-GUTFREUND *et al.* (1962) in Ethiopia from sheep (five), goat (two), calf (one), and monkey (one) are true LCM virus strains is doubtful.

In concluding this chapter, it should be emphasized that there is no evidence, either from the laboratory or from the field, that persistent infections in animals other than *M. musculus* or its albino variety may exist. It appears more likely that all other animals are infected by carrier mice, thus representing side branches of the stem of vertical congenital infection perpetuated in mice. Secondary horizontal spread occurs (see Section X. C) but, no doubt, is rare.

3. Cell Cultures

CASALS-ARIET and WEBSTER (1940) encountered a typical strain of LCM virus contaminating a tissue culture used for the preparation of rabies vaccine, but its original source has remained unknown. WIKTOR *et al.* (1965; 1966) were confronted with the virus in various cell strains chronically infected with rabies virus. They found it impossible to separate the virus of LCM from that of rabies, either by inoculation of animals or by passage in other cell systems. In view of the usual absence of cytopathogenicity (see Section III. B. 4) and the ease with which cells may become persistently infected (see Section III. C), it is perhaps not surprising that chronic infections of cell cultures with LCM virus occur and remain undetected for possibly long times.

In the course of routine laboratory work, COUGHLIN and WHITNEY (1957) inoculated two human fecal specimens into various primate cell cultures and detected Coxsackie A9 virus. Unexpectedly, adult mice inoculated with material from the monkey kidney but not from human amnion cells used for the isolation became ill. This was found to be due to infection with LCM virus, but the source remained unknown. No LCM virus was found in the fecal specimens, nor could it be detected in cell cultures from 37 other rhesus or cynomolgus monkeys. The question remains, how did the virus contaminate the cells in the first place.

4. Other Sources

STEWART and HAAS (1956) searched 23 different transplantable mouse neoplasms and eight primary tumors for LCM virus. From four established and one primary neoplasms LCM virus was isolated. The source of the virus was not found and all stock mice were shown to be free of LCM virus.

Another example of an unexpected encounter with the virus was reported by BERGER and SCHOOP (1967) who had reason to suspect that the BK strain of *Toxoplasma gondii* was contaminated with LCM virus. It had been used by them and others for diagnostic work and research for many years. These investigators separated a virus from the *Protozoa*, and it was shown in Cologne (R. ACKERMANN, personal communication) and in our laboratory to be immunologically identical with LCM virus, although it differed in some other properties. Subsequently, the BK strain maintained for years in this institute was also found to be LCM virus-contaminated. Apparently, the virus had been transmitted from mouse to mouse by intraperitoneal passages for at least 12 years, which may not only invalidate some experimental work done with BK; this contaminant is probably responsible for at least one severe human illness, *i.e.* patient H.-L. W., documented by SCHEID *et al.* (1956a) (see Section V. H. 1). Another contamination of a *Toxoplasma* strain with a virus was reported by VERMEIL and MAURIN (1953) but in this instance the agent was not satisfactorily identified (see Section XII).

A few strains of virus isolated from arthropods (LEVI *et al.*, 1953; GLUSHCHENKO *et al.*, 1957; REISS-GUTFREUND *et al.*, 1962; CHASTEL, 1965) do not fulfill the criteria deemed necessary to classify them as LCM viruses.

B. Geographical Distribution

It is often said that the virus of LCM exists in all parts of the world. While this may be true, well-documented proof is available only for America and Europe. In other continents there is either no evidence at all (Australia) or else it does not stand up to a critical evaluation (Asia and Africa).

All three original isolations (see Section I. B) were made in the U.S.A. from places as widely separated as New Jersey and Missouri. Later, strains were recovered in many areas and it is probably safe to conclude that no part of the U.S A. is free of the virus. From Canada only one isolation seems to have been reported (MITCHELL and KLOTZ, 1942). In South America, the mice in Bahia (ALICE, 1945a; 1945b) were found to be infected with LCM virus. As noted, KASAHARA *et al.* (1937a; 1937b) in Japan isolated six strains.

In Europe, the evidence again indicates that the virus is present in most parts of the continent: in Belgium (NIHOUL and LECOMTE-RAMIOUL, 1953), Bulgaria (GREŠÍKOVÁ and CASALS, 1963), Czechoslovakia (BENDA *et al.*, 1955), England (FINDLAY *et al.*, 1936), France (LÉPINE and SAUTTER, 1936), Germany (SCHEID and JOCHHEIM, 1956b), Holland (VERLINDE, 1946; PRICK and VERLINDE, 1947), Hungaria (IVÁNOVICS *et al.*, 1948; KOCH *et al.*, 1950b), Portugal (PINTO and FERREIRA, 1954), Russia (CHUMAKOV, 1949).

The isolations reported from Rumania (MESROBEANU and BADENSKI, 1948) and Yugoslavia (FENJE, 1956) have not been sufficiently characterized to permit their inclusion in this list. The reports from China, Cambodia, Africa (CHANG *et al.*, 1954; CHASTEL, 1965; REISS-GUTFREUND *et al.*, 1961) are not conclusive.

Although it is probable that the virus is present in countries surrounded by neighbors in which it has been shown to exist, this is not necessarily so for other areas lying more in the periphery or for whole continents. It could be argued that this uneven distribution of the virus is apparent rather than real and that it is a function of the efforts which have been made to detect it. This may be true for some parts of the world, but it certainly is not generally applicable. In southern Sweden, AFZELIUS-ALM (1951) failed to demonstrate LCM virus on 37 occasions in pooled brains and spleens from *M. musculus* and in 210 spinal fluids and 60 blood specimens from patients with abacterial encephalomeningitis, or complement-fixing antibody in the sera of 147 such patients, although the methods of virus and antibody detection were suitable as evidenced by the diagnosis of a laboratory infection. In South Africa, BAYER and GEAR (1955) failed to isolate this virus from over 200 human cases of meningoencephalitis, although the methods employed should have been adequate. It seems unlikely that the virus would have been overlooked in Australia if it existed there which, apparently, is not the case (MILES, 1954). That the virus may be unequally distributed even in infested areas is shown by the extensive studies performed by Scheid and his colleagues (ACKERMANN *et al.*, 1964; SCHEID *et al.*, 1966). In 1960/61 and again in 1962, 1795 wild mice of the species *M. musculus* were caught in 376 trapping regions evenly distributed over the Federal Republic of Germany. Altogether 65 mice, caught in 44 regions in Nordrhein-Westfalen, Niedersachsen, Schleswig-Holstein, Baden-Württemberg, and Rheinland-Pfalz, were found to be positive; Hessen and Bayern were free (Fig. 15). This patchy occurrence of infection among mice has frequently been ascribed to the fact that they do not migrate, thus preventing spread of infection from one locality to another. This, however, applies only to members of established colonies (FREYE and FREYE, 1960).

M. musculus is said to have originated in two separated areas, one stretching between Japan and Marocco and the other in southern Russia. From these centers grey mice migrated to populate Asia and Africa and finally reached Europe where they met, *M. m. musculus* arriving from the east and *M. m. domesticus* from the west. The mouse populations of America and Australia were derived from animals introduced by man from the Old World (FREYE and FREYE, 1960). Although no house mouse from which the virus was isolated seems ever to have been identified as to its subspecies, the places of isolation make it clear that *domesticus* as well as *musculus* may be infected. This leaves us to conclude that the common ancestor

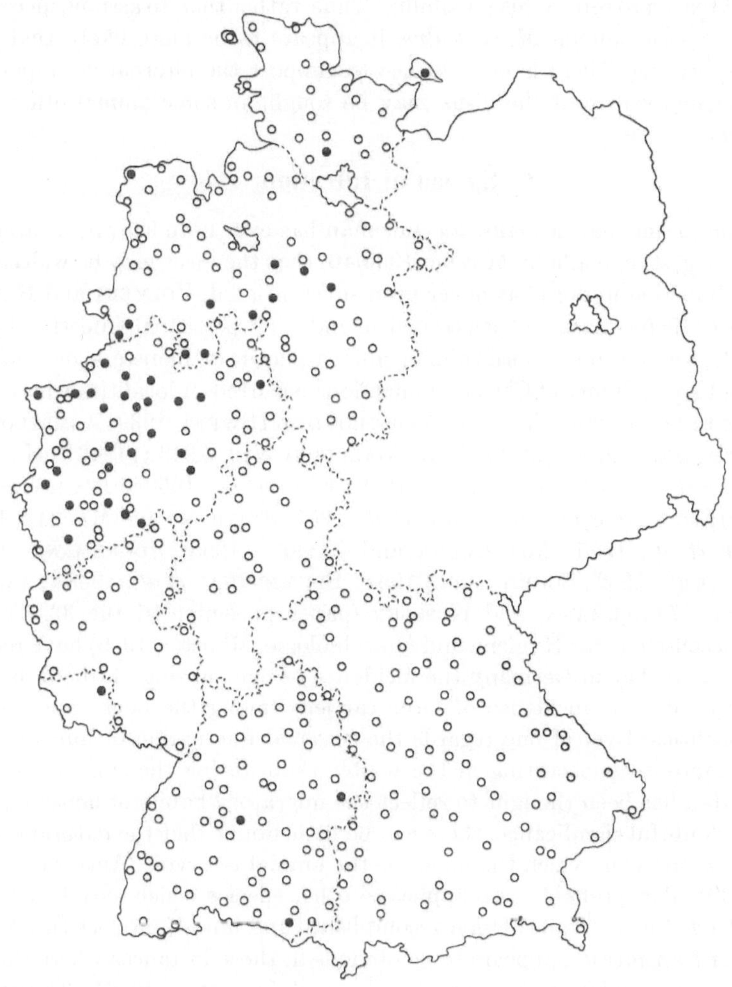

● TRAPPING AREAS WITH VIRUS-INFECTED MICE
○ AREAS WITHOUT VIRUS-INFECTED MICE

Fig. 15. Occurrence of LCM virus-carrying house mice in the Federal Republic of Germany. Each circle represents a trapping area; each closed circle represents a trapping area in which mice harboring the LCM virus were caught. From R. ACKERMANN, H. BLOEDHORN, B. KÜPPER, I. WINKENS, and W. SCHEID: Zbl. Bakt., I. Abt. Orig. 194, 407 (1964). (With permission of the authors and of Gustav Fischer Verlag, Stuttgart.)

believed to have lived in Persia-Turkistan (H.-A. FREYE, personal communication) carried LCM virus, and hence one would expect virus carriers to be evenly distributed among the mice of the world. As we have seen, this is not the case. The most plausible explanation would be that an occasional mouse loses the virus and, due to biological advantages, outgrows the carriers. There is sufficient evidence to support the latter part of this hypothesis (see Section V. A. 3). However, that mice may occasionally get rid of the virus is known only where the chronic infection was induced artificially shortly after birth (LEHMANN-GRUBE, 1964b). Whether this may occur also in congenital carriers is unknown, but there is no cogent reason to refute this possibility. Thus, rather than to assume increasing spread of the virus among *M. musculus*, it appears to be more likely that it is slowly disappearing. There is no evidence to support the alternative hypothesis that the original source of the virus may be sought in some animal other than *M. musculus*.

C. Spread of Infection

No animal other than *M. musculus* nor man has ever been shown to carry the virus. The suggestion made by MEYER (1939/40) that the virus may be widespread as a latent infection in dogs has never been substantiated. VOLKERT and HANNOVER LARSEN (1965a) have not succeeded in inducing persistent infection by inoculating the virus into newborn rabbits, guinea-pigs, rats, hamsters, or chickens.

Time and again, human LCM virus infections occurred in localities where mice were shown to be carrying the virus (ARMSTRONG and SWEET, 1939; ARMSTRONG *et al.*, 1940; FARMER and JANEWAY, 1942; DALLDORF *et al.*, 1946a; 1946b; HAVENS, 1948; GREEN *et al.*, 1949; MACCALLUM, 1949; KOCH *et al.*, 1950a; IVÁNOVICS and KOCH, 1950; DUNCAN *et al.*, 1951; LEVI *et al.*, 1951; SMITHARD and MACRAE, 1951; KOMROWER *et al.*, 1955; ACKERMANN and JANSEN, 1958; ACKERMANN, 1960; TRAUMANN *et al.*, 1962; SCHEID *et al.*, 1964; BLUMENTHAL *et al.*, 1968a; 1968b). BLUMENTHAL, ACKERMANN, and KESSLER (paper presented at the 32. Tagung Deutsche Gesellschaft für Hygiene und Mikrobiologie, Münster, 1969) have recently demonstrated that in Germany the incidence of neutralizing antibody in man is correlated with the incidence of virus carriers among the house mice in the relevant localities. Even if one regards the seasonal fluctuation of human infections with more cases occurring in the winter than during the summer months — which often has been thought to reflect the migratory habits of house mice — as being of doubtful significance, there can be little doubt that the natural disease in man is a zoonosis in which the mouse is the animal reservoir (ARMSTRONG and SWEET, 1939). This probably also applies to other species which may be infected in nature. How, then, is transmission accomplished and how often does this occur? The mode of transmission appears to be obvious in those instances where the disease has followed the bite of a mouse (SCHEID and JOCHHEIM, 1956b; TRAUMANN *et al.*, 1962; SCHEID *et al.*, 1964) but in most cases it is obscure. Carrier mice are highly contagious for other mice on close contact (TRAUB, 1936c; 1938b; 1939b; HAAS, 1941; SKINNER and KNIGHT, 1969), and nasal secretions and saliva were incriminated by Traub and Haas. According to TRAUB (1960a), the milk from carrier females is also infectious. PANOV and SHVAREV (1966) mentioned three possible modes of spread from mice to other animals: (1) by means of dust containing excreta from infected mice; (2) with food contaminated by mice; (3) through a vector. Possibly, the virus is transmitted by inhalation of virus-contaminated materials, and the ease with which other species may be infected experimentally by aerosols is remarkable. Working with *M. cynomolgus* and *M. rhesus* and the

WE strain of virus, DANEŠ *et al.* (1963) found that less than 200 and about ten mouse LD_{50}, respectively, initiated infection. Guinea-pigs were even more susceptible, and again with the WE strain it was found that the 50 per cent lethal inhalation dose was equal to 0.2 to 1.0 mouse LD_{50}. When the exhalation was taken into account, the susceptibility of these animals to inhalation was estimated to be greater than to intranasal inoculation and about as high as to intracerebral or subcutaneous infection (BENDA *et al.*, 1964).

Another way by which this virus may enter the prospective host seems to be through the skin. Surprising as this may be, SHAUGHNESSY and ZICHIS (1939; 1940) have presented unrefutable evidence that the virus may penetrate the intact skin of the guinea-pig. The precautions taken by these authors to forestall criticism are impressive. They concede "that minute abrasions, not visible with a hand lens, may have been present", but one has to follow their conclusion that this would be a "factor encountered in any normal skin". It may be mentioned that KELLER (1958) observed passage of *Bacillus megatherium* phage through the unprepared and apparently intact skin of the mouse by either immersion of the tail into the phage-containing suspension or by gentle spreading of the phage preparation on the abdominal skin. After inunction with LCM virus of the shaven but apparently undamaged skin of monkeys a disease developed which was less severe than the one following other routes of infection (DALLDORF, 1939b). FINDLAY and STERN (1936) transmitted the virus to mice and monkeys by applying it "on the lightly scarified skin". SHAUGHNESSY and MILZER (1939) infected guinea-pigs by rubbing the WE virus into the skin which had been lightly scarified so as not to draw blood.

The role of the alimentary tract for infections with this virus is difficult to assess. Infectivity is unlikely to pass beyond the barrier set up by the stomach. Penetration of the mucosa of the upper digestive parts must be considered a possibility. Experiments indicate that infection by feeding may succeed although with a low probability (FINDLAY and STERN, 1936; TRAUB, 1936c; 1939b; SHAUGHNESSY and ZICHIS, 1940; JOCHHEIM *et al.*, 1957; TYUSHNYAKOVA, 1962; GLADKIJ, 1965).

It may be concluded that LCM virus is easily transmitted by aerosols. It is also proposed that infection may occur *via* the skin. Both ways are likely to account for laboratory infections but hardly explain how the virus normally spreads from mice. The assumption that this occurs by means of dust containing feces, urine, and saliva from persistently infected mice, or by food stuff contaminated with such excretions is not a likely one because the virus is extraordinarily labile and would not be expected to remain infective under such unfavorable conditions. Work done by HAAS (1941) underlines this statement. In one typical experiment he transferred ten normal mice to a glass jar which had not been cleaned after carriers had lived in it for 22 days; during 16 days none of the new occupants became infected. The same carriers had transmitted the virus to 18 normal mice kept together with them in the same cage. In similar experiments performed by TRAUB (1936c) infection was not transmitted to mice which had been placed into cages "heavily contaminated" with virus-containing urine. In years of work with carrier mice I have not experienced one human laboratory infection which could be traced to them. Nor are vectors known which could be incriminated (see

Section X. D). It should be mentioned, however, that occasionally, under certain experimental conditions, LCM virus was found to be relatively stable. For instance, MILZER (1942) succeeded in infecting four of four guinea-pigs with dried feces from bed bugs, 3, 9, 14, and 85 days, respectively, after they had had infectious meals. It is not impossible, however, that the virus had multiplied in the arthropods (see Section X. D).

Although early in his work TRAUB (1936c) had drawn the conclusion that the virus may be readily transmitted from acutely infected mice to untreated cage mates, it later turned out that, in contrast to carriers, mice undergoing clinical or subclinical infection when infected as adults almost never spread the virus, even on close contact (RIVERS and SCOTT, 1936a; TRAUB, 1939b; HAAS, 1941; LEHMANN-GRUBE, 1969b). Evidence presented by PANOV and SHVAREV (1966) and thought by them to prove the contrary does not convince. Infections from species other than mice have not been documented to have taken place under natural conditions.

It may be accepted as a general rule that man is the last link in an infectious chain. The same may be said about infections in other species but a few exceptions must be mentioned. TRAUB (1936c) observed spread of infection from diseased guinea-pigs to healthy cage mates in a few instances. COGGESHALL (1939) reported on an epidemic of LCM in a colony of monkeys and FINDLAY *et al.* (1940) traced the spontaneous disease in two rhesus monkeys in the laboratory to hay and sawdust which had been in contact with infected guinea-pigs (no details). ARMSTRONG (1942) mentioned three laboratory infections in monkeys during work with an isolate from fatal human cases. DALLDORF (1939a; 1943) infected dogs with the virus and observed neutralizing antibody to appear in control cage mates. Spread of the virus between hamsters and from these to persons was reported by LEWIS *et al.* (1965), BAUM *et al.* (1966), and D. ARMSTRONG *et al.* (1969).

The example given by FARMER and JANEWAY (1942) which was thought to illustrate a possible spread from a sick dog to its owner is open to question. The evidence for an LCM virus etiology of an encephalitis epidemic in a convalescent home (VERLINDE *et al.*, 1948a; 1948b) may not be regarded as conclusive. The suggestion made by ARMSTRONG and WOOLEY (1937) that a veneral transmission in man may play a role is hardly more than a historical curiosity.

The conditions under which the virus is transmitted may be rather complex, and the question may be raised as to the probability of species other than the mouse becoming infected with this virus. The answer to this cannot be given on a global basis. Whole continents have to be left out because we know next to nothing about the frequency of infections with LCM virus there. Other large areas, *e.g.* Australia or Scandinavia, seem to be free of the virus and we must therefore restrict the discussion to Europe and the U.S.A., and even there our knowledge is limited.

WOOLEY *et al.* (1937) tested sera from 1248 persons residing in various parts of the U.S.A. by means of a semiquantitative neutralization test. Unfortunately, the data which seemed to indicate a rather high incidence of previous exposure to the virus cannot be accepted today, for no provision was made to exclude the "neutralization" by spontaneously occurring virus inhibitors (see Section V. H. 3). It seems reasonable to assume that the so-called "moderate protection" found in 73 sera belonged in this category. If the assumption is made that the test virus contained $10^{7.5}$ mouse LD_{50} per g of brain tissue and if it is accepted that the neutralization of 100 LD_{50} or more of virus by serum diluted two-fold may be considered proof for the existence of true antibody (see Section V. H. 3), then sera which exhibited "strong protection" may be regarded as having come from persons with LCM virus infections in their past. Of 1248 sera, 65 (five per cent) were found in this group. Applying similar considerations to a follow-up study by WOOLEY *et al.* (1939), 56 of 680 individuals (eight per cent) might have had an infection, but the details in this latter publication make the analysis uncertain.

No such additional evaluation is possible with the results of neutralization tests done with sera from 166 persons by ARMSTRONG and WOOLEY (1935). Nor does it seem that the negative results obtained by HEYL *et al.* (1948) with (two ?) preparations of human γ-globulin from plasma pools of up to 5500 individual donors are of real value.

In Europe, studies on small numbers of people were reported from various places. Of 21 persons living in Bohemia where LCM virus is known to occur, one had antibody neutralizing more than 100 mouse LD_{50} (BENDA *et al.*, 1955). ACKERMANN (1960) found no complement-fixing but neutralizing activities with indices of $\log_{10}$ 3.7, 3.7, and 3.9, respectively, in the sera of 3 of 14 healthy persons who lived near Bremen in Germany in the immediate neighborhood of patients known to have had infections with the LCM virus, and in the same area trapped house mice carried the virus. Of 42 persons who lived farther away, six had indices of higher than $\log_{10}$ 2.0; none exhibited complement-fixing activity.

Of great value is the investigation conducted by Blumenthal and his colleagues (BLUMENTHAL, 1968; paper presented at the 32. Tagung Deutsche Gesellschaft für Hygiene und Mikrobiologie, Münster, 1969). Sera from 2013 persons living in rural areas of West Germany were tested for LCM virus neutralizing antibody. Of these, 68 (=3.4 per cent) neutralized more than 100 mouse LD_{50} in a constant serum-variable virus test which may be taken as evidence of recent contact with the virus. While no differences were found between groups classified according to employment, the proportion of positive results increased with the age of the donors. What is more important, a significant correlation was found to exist between incidence of LCM antibody and LCM virus infection of house mice in the district. Of 560 persons living in areas where ACKERMANN *et al.* (1964) had demonstrated many mice to be infected, 51 (=9.1 per cent) were positive, while in those parts of Germany which had been found to be free of carrier mice only 17 of 1453 people (1.2 per cent) had LCM virus antibody in their sera.

The overall occurrence of neutralizing antibody in 3.4 per cent of a population consisting of people with and without potential contact with LCM virus-infected mice is not far from the figure (five per cent) concluded from the data of WOOLEY *et al.* (1937) (see above). Thus, human infections with LCM virus appear to be rare, and figures of up to 20 per cent among unselected people which are sometimes quoted seem to highly overestimate the true incidence.

As far as screening employing the complement fixation test is concerned, it was found by BLUMENTHAL (1968) that of 73 sera which had exerted doubtful protection in a mouse neutralization test only two showed a low degree of fixation. In France, LÉPINE *et al.* (1938a; 1938b) tested for control purposes the sera from

64 persons; none was found to fix complement in the presence of LCM-specific antigen. Balek *et al.* (1954) found complement-fixing antibody in the sera of 14 of 460 unselected normal people residing in Slovakia. In a group in France consisting of 209 persons not suspected to suffer or to have recently suffered from LCM virus infections, Sohier and Buissière (1954) detected complement-fixing antibody with low titers, *i.e.* eight, in two of them. Chastel and Le Noc (1968), also working in France, searched for complement-fixing antibody in 281 sera and found only one positive with a titer of 16. Of uncertain significance are the results of the complement fixation tests obtained by Bauzá *et al.* (1965). In 13 of 268 sera collected from children living in Montevideo they found titers varying from 5 to 20; 20 occurred in two instances. It is not clear from the report whether these children had been ill; nor was anything said concerning their previous history. It has been pointed out before (see Section V. H. 3) and should be stressed again that positive results obtained by means of the complement fixation test with single sera from apparently healthy individuals must be evaluated with caution.

We may now ask the question, what is the frequency of infections with the LCM virus among patients with diseases, such as acute abacterial meningitis or acute encephalitis, which it is known to cause. The negative results obtained by Brodie (1937) who tested sera from 24 cases of "nonparalytic poliomyelitis" for LCM virus-neutralizing antibody are open to criticism because of technical problems. Baird and Rivers (1938) investigated 34 cases of "acute aseptic meningitis" and proved that an LCM virus infection had occurred in one of them by demonstrating an increase of neutralizing antibody. In seven "presumptive" cases of this group the diagnosis was based on neutralizing antibody in convalescence only, which cannot be accepted because of the possible presence in the sera of nonspecific virus-neutralizing substances. As judged from the strongly positive complement fixation reactions, 13 of 18 patients suspected clinically by Lépine *et al.* (1938a; 1938b) were shown to have had recent LCM virus infections. The reason for this unusually high number is not clear. Smadel (1942b) investigated 165 cases of abacterial meningitis and proved by virus isolation and by the demonstration of complement-fixing or neutralizing antibody in convalescence that 25 (= 15.2 per cent) of them had been caused by LCM virus.

Of 75 patients with sporadic diseases, mainly of the central nervous system, which occurred in the Chicago area, LCM virus was held responsible in nine (Milzer, 1943). Of these the case "J. P.", related previously by Leichenger *et al.* (1940) is doubtful for the reasons already discussed (see Section V. H. 1). Thus, eight of the 75 cases (= 10.7 per cent) were presumably true LCM virus infections. (Besides "J. P.", two more cases had been documented more fully elsewhere: "A. M." by Milzer and Levinson, 1942, and "B. D." by Treusch *et al.*, 1943.) Of a total of 102 persons with acute abacterial meningitis, MacCallum (1949) obtained 24 specimens of cerebrospinal fluid, 36 paired sera and 66 single sera taken during convalescence. In two patients the LCM virus was isolated and the etiology confirmed by the appearance of antibody; in one patient, the diagnosis was based on the development of neutralizing and complement-fixing antibodies, and in two more it was tentative as shown by the presence of complement-fixing antibody in convalescence only, no early sera having been available. In 115 patients with abacterial meningitis residing in various parts of Holland, Verlinde and van Tongeren (1949) proved the LCM virus etiology in 5 of 30 by virus isolation plus antibody development, in 10 of 38 by antibody development alone, and in 1 of 47 by virus isolation only. Disregarding the latter, the LCM virus was shown to have caused meningitis in 15 of 115 (13 per cent) cases. Goldberg (1950) found infectious agents in 2 of 22 patients with abacterial meningitis by inoculating blood plus cerebrospinal fluid or the latter only into mice and guinea-pigs. The author assumed that they were strains of LCM virus, but they were not identified. In Hungaria, Koch *et al.* (1950a; Ivánovics and Koch, 1950) inoculated cerebrospinal fluids from 19 patients with meningitis and two more with encephalitis into mice and recovered strains from three of them; two of these patients also developed significant concentrations of neutralizing antibody. Thus, in at least two of the 21 patients with affections of the central nervous system was the LCM virus etiology established. (Ten cases were later shown to have been caused by mumps virus, *Mycobacterium tuberculosis, etc.*) In the Ukraine, Levi *et al.* (1951) performed complement fixation tests on sera from 204 patients. In 20 the titers were equal to or higher than four, which was considered proof of a recent infection with LCM virus. In 15 of these, the neutralizing indices were also determined. They were equal to or greater than 100 in seven and greater than 1000 in two. In ten additional cases which had been found free of complement-fixing activities, neutralization tests revealed indices of greater than 100 in two and greater than 1000 in one. Although these high titers leave no doubt that the patients had had infections with LCM virus in the past, it is questionable whether it had been responsible for all the diseases under consideration. In the three patients, for instance, with indices of more than 1000, the diagnoses were "myelitis", "keratitis with scarification", and "grippe with hypertension", none of which may be regarded as being characteristic of an infection with LCM virus. The positive serology in 4 of 25 cases of meningitis or encephalitis reported by Bieling and Koch (1952) was insufficiently documented. In a study on the etiology of acute abacterial infections of the central nervous system in France, Sohier *et al.* (1953; Sohier and Buissière, 1954) investigated 242 patients with meningitis or meningoencephalitis. In 8 of 186 persons from whom adequate materials were available, infections with LCM virus were established by complement fixation tests. Of these, five had meningitis and three meningoencephalitis.

Out of an unknown number of cases, Balek *et al.* (1954) proved the LCM virus etiology by increases of complement-fixing titers 16 times; on three occasions isolation of the virus was achieved. The diagnoses ranged from acute lymphocytic meningitis, meningoencephalitis, encephalitis, and subarachnoid bleeding in connection with meningitis to "grippe" and neuritis nervi vestibuli. The virological part in this study was not exhaustive enough to permit a critical appraisal. The same is to be said of the attempts by Laigret and Lavillaureix (1954; Lavillaureix, 1954) and by Lavillaureix and Reeb (1957) to clarify the role the LCM virus might have played in diseases of the central nervous system which occurred in Alsace. Haussmann (1955) tried to establish serologically the etiology of various central nervous system diseases in 490 patients who lived in North, West, or South Germany or in the eastern part of Switzerland. LCM virus was not incriminated, which may cast doubts on the reliability of the methods employed. Bárdoš (1957) in Czechoslovakia established the LCM virus etiology in 1 of

34 cases of abacterial meningitis or meningoencephalitis. Of doubtful value is the LCM diagnosis made by Tyushnyakova and Zagromova (1960) in 20 patients living in the Tomsk region of Siberia, for the virological part of the study was not convincingly executed. No details concerning the virological techniques were included in a report from Yugoslavia by Todorović *et al.* (1961) on 222 patients with lymphocytic meningoencephalitis of whom four were said to have been caused by the LCM virus. Reiss-Gutfreund *et al.* (1961) isolated eight agents in mice and guinea-pigs from people living in Ethiopia with a variety of diseases, including meningitis and encephalitis. LCM virus might have been present, but the virological part of the report is not detailed enough. The same must be said of a study conducted by Shvarev (1964b) during eight years on patients from hospitals in Leningrad. From an unspecified number of cases with infections (of the central nervous system?) the LCM virus etiology was established 54 times. The diagnoses were variable and included acute meningitis and meningoencephalitis, paraplegia, arachnitis, and polyradiculitis as well as acute and chronic hydrocephalus. Likewise of uncertain significance is a report from southern India. By means of the complement fixation test, Carey *et al.* (1969) investigated 66 pairs of sera from patients with diseases of the central nervous system residing in the Vellore area; none gave a positive reaction with LCM virus antigen.

In all these studies, the results were derived from small or insufficiently defined numbers of patients, which does not permit conclusions to be drawn as to the relative frequency of LCM virus infections among patients with diseases of the central nervous system. Furthermore, it does not appear permissible to pool the data. Neither the techniques employed nor the criteria according to which the patients had been selected were uniform. For the answer to our question, we may rely on the longitudinal study begun in 1941 by Rasmussen (1947), continued from 1947 by Adair *et al.* (1953), and concluded between 1953 and 1958 by Meyer *et al.* (1960). This extensive work is valuable, not only because it provides us with an unusual large number of patients classified according to similar clinical signs, *i.e.* "acute infectious disease with CNS manifestations of apparent viral etiology" (Meyer *et al.*, 1960); it furthermore represents a model investigation into the relative role this virus plays in such syndromes and should satisfy the most critical reader. Of altogether 1568 patients, 126 or eight per cent were considered proved LCM virus infections. This is perhaps to some a surprisingly low estimate but again stresses that lymphocytic choriomeningitis is a rare disease under natural conditions.

After having presented a survey of the numerous reports dealing with the frequency with which the LCM virus may infect — with or without manifestation of illness — people, we shall now turn to answering the question: how often is this virus transmitted to animals other than *M. musculus*?

Frequent attempts have been made to detect the virus in species closely related to *M. musculus*. In California, Howitt and van Herick (1942) tested 101 wild rodents which, besides *M. musculus*, included *Peromyscus maniculatus, Reithrodontomys megalotis, Perognathus californicus, Citellus beecheyi, Ammospermophilus nelsoni*, and two rat species, by inoculating organ homogenates intracerebrally into white mice. LCM virus was detected in two house mice only. In areas in West Germany where Scheid and his collaborators had found infected house mice, EMMERICH (1962) examined 132 *Microtus agrestis*, 109 *M. arvalis*, 5 *M. oeconomus*, 114 *Clethrionomys glareolus*, 109 *Apodemus sylvaticus*, 23 *A. flavicollis*, 10 *A. agrarius*, 2 *Rattus norvegicus*, and 6 *Sorex araneus*. Of 23 isolates from these animals, which were pathogenic for mice, not one was identified as LCM virus. Later, KÜPPER *et al.* (1964/65; SCHEID *et al.*, 1966) searched for this virus in the same general area. They examined 460 wild mice other than *M. musculus* of the following species: *Microtus arvalis* (311), *M. agrestis* (30), *Apodemus sylvaticus* (94), *Pitymus subterraneus* (5), *Clethrionomys glareolus* (4), *Micromys minutus* (3), and *Arvicola terrestris* (1). LCM virus was isolated from one *A. sylvaticus* only. BLUMENTHAL *et al.* (1968a; 1968b) looked for the virus in small mammals which they had trapped in the immediate neighborhood of the residence of a man with proved LCM encephalitis in a village east of Aachen, Germany. They found that 139 of 356 *M. musculus* and 1 of 5 *Apodemus sylvaticus* harbored the virus. None of 65 *Soricidae* nor a litter with eight rats were infected. BÁRDOŠ (1957) investigated 757 small rodents trapped in the Danube area of Czechoslovakia. One isolation of LCM virus was made in 1 of 30 *M. musculus*, but 122 *Apodemus flavicollis*, 33 *A. sylvaticus*, 1 *A. microps*, 323 *Clethrionomys glareolus*, 1 *Crocidura leucodon*, 2 *C. suaveolens*, 44 *Microtus arvalis*, 1 *Mus musculus spicilegus*, 196 *Sorex araneus*, 3 *S. minutus*, 1 *S. minimus* (?) were found to be free of LCM virus, although other viruses were isolated. In the north-east of Bohemia, BENDA *et al.* (1955) found 1 *A. flavicollis* to be infected among 17 "small mammals". In 5 of 40 other animals in the same area (19 *A. flavicollis*, 9 *A. sylvaticus*, 3 *Clethrionomys glareolus*, 9 *Sorex araneus*) significant complement-fixing antibody titers were found, which was interpreted as indicating recent infections with LCM virus. JUNGEBLUT and DALLDORF (1946) isolated no LCM virus in 11 *Rattus norvegicus* trapped in New York, while during the same period in the same area they secured 11 isolations from 290 house mice. BALEK *et al.* (1954) trapped 528 small mammals in Slovakia and found complement-fixing antibody to LCM virus in 42. The animals with positive sera were 5 of 34 *Clethrionomys glareolus*, 12 of 145 *Apodemus flavicollis*, 5 of 64 *A. sylvaticus*, 3 of 26 *A. microps*, 7 of 175 *Microtus arvalis*, 1 of 14 *Sorex araneus*, 4 of 19 *Crocidura suaveolens* and *leucodon*, and 5 of 51 *Mus musculus*.

BLANC *et al.* (1960) in Morocco isolated infectious agents from a variety of wild small mammals, which they considered to be strains of LCM virus on the basis of their pyrogenicity in guinea-pigs, their relative stability at 4° C when suspended in water, and the presence of numerous granules in the neutrophiles of spleens of infected animals. None of these criteria, however, may be accepted to suffice for identification.

As already mentioned, the first LCM virus to be recovered was isolated in but not necessarily from a monkey. Its origin has remained obscure. No immune animals were found in the monkey colony at that time (ARMSTRONG and LILLIE, 1934), but later two further strains of virus seem to have come from this colony (ARMSTRONG and WOOLEY, 1935). The significance of "moderate to strong neutralizing properties" found by these authors in the sera of 5 of 44 monkeys is doubtful on grounds which have been presented above (see Section V. H. 3). The "strong" neutralization by sera from 2 of 35 monkeys found later by WOOLEY *et al.* (1937) may indicate previous exposure to the virus. In the brains and cords of a great number of monkeys KOLMER (1936) did not encounter LCM virus. Natural dissemination of virus to monkeys apparently is a rare event. There is no reason, however, to deny the possibility, and monkeys, particularly those kept in captivity, may be expected to be infected, presumably by carrier mice, much in the same way as humans are, although the mode of spread is essentially unknown.

Infections of dogs seem to be likewise rare. DALLDORF (1943) found no complement-fixing activities in 331 healthy adult dogs and no LCM virus in brains and/or spleens of 17 dogs which had died from diseases characterized by neurological signs. The significance of the occasional "presence of immune bodies" detected by FINDLAY *et al.* (1940) in pooled sera from English dogs cannot be assessed, because no quantitative data were supplied. The same must be said of the complement-fixing antibody to "benign lymphocytic meningitis" (presumably choriomeningitis) found in two Alsatian dogs by SMITH and KINSELLA (1951).

D. Quest for a Vector

The natural host, if not the ultimate source, of the LCM virus is the common house mouse. But we have seen that other species become infected and hence it may be asked, how is the virus transmitted from mice to other animals and man. It has been pointed out that virus-contaminated dust or food stuff are unlikely vehicles (see Section X. C). Thus, the possibility has to be entertained that a vector is requisite, perhaps in the same way as with the arboviruses. Employing the isolate from an epidemic among laboratory monkeys, COGGESHALL (1939) proved *Aedes aegypti* to be infectious after having had a meal on infected guinea-pigs. Transmission was accomplished for up to two passages by transfer of the mosquitoes as early as the fourth and as late as the 15th day after feeding. Using the WE strain, SHAUGHNESSY and MILZER (1939) found larvae, nymphs, and adults of the Rocky Mountain wood tick, *Dermacentor andersoni*, to have taken up the virus from viremic guinea-pigs. Stage to stage persistence from larvae to nymphs, from nymphs to adults, and even from adults to eggs and larvae occurred. It was not possible, however, to demonstrate transmission by adult ticks which had fed on infected guinea-pigs in one of the previous stages of their life cycle, although such experiments with nymphs which had fed as larvae were said to have succeeded. Guinea-pigs could be infected by applying crushed infectious ticks or feces from ticks which had engorged in the previous stage on infected animals to the scarified skin. No data were presented by SHAUGHNESSY and MILZER (1939) to support their claim that ticks which had engorged as nymphs on an infected animal became infectious only after having fed on a normal guinea-pig.

FINDLAY *et al.* (1940) found that human lice *(Pediculus humanus)* had taken up the LCM virus from infected monkeys. ARMSTRONG (1941; 1942) reported that in two instances, "out of several trials", the virus was transmitted between monkeys by lice but not by bed bugs, rat and mouse fleas, and blood-sucking mites.

An extensive study was conducted by MILZER (1942) who employed a variety of arthropods and the J. P. strain of LEICHENGER *et al.* (1940). With *Aedes aegypti*, successful transmission depended on the temperature under which the insects were maintained. At the optimum of 28°—32° C transmission between guinea-pigs was achieved up to 38 days after the infectious meal. Trials with *A. albopictus* or *Culex pipiens* were negative, but both had been kept at room temperature. Of 18 attempted transmissions with bed bugs *(Cimex lectularius)* 11 were successful with intervals between the two meals of from ten minutes to 85 days. Since guinea-pigs could be infected by rubbing feces from infected bed bugs into their scarified skin, it was thought that transmission might occur when the parasite's feces contaminated the bitten area. In one experiment bed bug larvae remained infectious through one stage of molting but not to further ones. In one of three experiments virus was found to be transmitted from adult bugs to the eggs and further to the larvae. Bed bugs could be shown to spread infection between guinea-pigs kept together under conditions simulating those in nature. No transmission was achieved in one experiment between rhesus monkeys by lice *(Eupedicinus longiceps)* or between mice by mites *(Atricholaelaps glasgowi)* in four experiments. Panov and Shvarev (1966) reported that the LCM virus was transmitted from infected mice to cage mates by *Bdellonyssus (Liponyssus) bacoti*, but the experimental details are insufficient to permit evaluation.

Blanc and Ascione (1960) fed nymphs and larvae of an African tick *(Amblyomma variegatum)* on rabbits which had been made viremic by the intravenous inoculation of infectious guinea-pig blood and organ suspensions. After having engorged, which took six to seven days, the ticks were emulsified and tested for virus by the inoculation of guinea-pigs; both larvae and nymphs were infectious. Furthermore, nymphs originating from infected larvae after incubation at 30° C not only had retained their infectivity but were capable of transmitting by feeding virus to a normal rabbit which subsequently became viremic. Adults which developed from infectious nymphs likewise contained virus, as did excreta from infectious ticks. (It is to be regretted that the virus strain which was used in these interesting experiments was not specified.)

There can be little doubt that experimentally the LCM virus may be transmitted by arthropods. It is another matter whether this occurs under natural conditions. Claims by Russian workers (Levi *et al.*, 1953; Glushchenko *et al.*, 1957) to have proved this by repeated isolation of the virus from a variety of arthropods trapped in areas where the virus was also found in small rodents have to be regarded with caution; in none of the reports which have come to my attention was the identity of the isolates unequivocally established. The same has to be said of a survey made in Morocco by Blanc *et al.* (1960). It would seem that the above reports no more than hint at the possibility that LCM virus may infect arthropods and multiply in them. It is noteworthy, however, that of 22 different viruses tested, only those belonging to the arbovirus group and LCM virus multiplied in cells from *Hyalomma dromedarii* ticks cultivated *in vitro* (Řeháček, 1965).

Syverton and his colleagues investigated the possibility that *Trichinella spiralis* may act as a vehicle for the transport of the LCM virus (Syverton *et al.*, 1947). Guinea-pigs were infected orally with *T. spiralis* larvae and 15 to 18 days later by subcutaneous route with the WE strain of LCM virus. When the animals died, the carcasses were digested with pepsin and the larvae of *T. spiralis* were recovered. These were treated with acid to remove superficial virus and tested for infectivity in guinea-pigs either by feeding live larvae or after trituration by subcutaneous inoculation. Although not all experiments were successful, the results showed that trichinae not only take up infectious virus but also may acquire the ability to transmit it to new hosts. It should be added, however, that neither Syverton's experiments nor later evidence has established that *T. spiralis* ever functions as a vector for the LCM virus in nature.

XI. Technical Procedures

It is one of the basic characteristics of the LCM virus not to cause the disintegration of the cell in which it multiplies (see Section III. B. 4), thus barring the use of simple assay procedures based on cytopathic effects.

For the diagnosis of human and animal infections and the identification of isolates both the neutralization and the complement fixation tests have been employed.

A. Virus Titration

1. Quantal Procedures

A quantal assay is one in which every assay unit gives a nongraded yes-or-no response. Since its discovery, the LCM virus has been most commonly titrated by means of dilution assays performed intracerebrally in mice, where the animal's death is taken as the positive response. The usual estimate is the LD_{50} being that virus dose which kills 50 per cent. It is to be stressed that this method is highly unsatisfactory. Most strains of LCM virus exhibit a marked zone phenomenon with fewer mice dying in the high dosage region than would be expected (see Section V. A. 4. b). Thus, the basic prerequisite for a quantal assay, the — at least approximate — symmetry of the response curve, is not fulfilled, thereby grossly exaggerating the low precision which is inherent in every quantal virus assay (Meynell, 1957). It is difficult to understand why this method is still in wide use. It has been known for 30 years that this source of error can be excluded by the challenge of the surviving mice, thus deriving the ID_{50}, based on the animals which had died from the first inoculum plus those which survived the challenge (Scott and Elford, 1939). Indeed, if the second infection is performed with a strain and a dose known to produce 100 per cent mortality in nonimmune animals, this simple expedient not only causes the dose-response curve to be symmetrical (Fig. 10) but also provides the highest possible accuracy in an assay of this kind (Lehmann-Grube, 1969b). The danger that infected mice may spread the virus to cage mates thus invalidating the results of challenge may be dismissed. It has been shown again and again that, in contrast to carriers which are highly contagious, adult mice undergoing clinical or subclinical infection have a low probability of transmitting the virus even if in close contact (see Section X. C). Challenge of mice reveals another phenomenon which deserves our attention. The ID_{50} values are not only more accurate but also higher than the LD_{50} values, which is not so much due to the high zone survivors but rather reflects the fact that at high dilutions a certain number of mice, though infected, escape death. From 15 titrations of the WE strain — taken at random from our records — all performed with infected mouse brain homogenates employing five mice per decimal dilution step, the mean of the titer differences — LD_{50} *versus* ID_{50} — and the single standard error of the mean were found to be $\log_{10} 0.443 \pm 0.079$; the corresponding figures for the Armstrong strain are 0.351 ± 0.067. These data make it difficult to understand why ROGER and ROGER (1964c) failed to detect a difference between LD_{50} and ID_{50} of the WE strain, and even stated that challenge of mice after intracerebral inoculation was absolutely useless ("totalement inutile").

From experiments done by CAIRNS (1950) and MIMS (1960) it is known that upon inoculation of liquid material into the mouse brain the larger part immediately spills into the blood stream, thus turning the intended intracerebral injection into a combined cerebral and intravenous one. Around the end point, where single infectious units count, these may be deposited in the periphery rather than in the brain, initiating a peripheral subclinical instead of a cerebral fatal infection. If this is true, then peripheral and intracerebral inoculations should in terms of immunity lead to the same titers. This is indeed the case. ROWE (1954) titrated two strains intraperitoneally and intracerebrally and found the ID_{50} values to be indistinguishable. HAAS (1960) reported a similar result. In my own experiments, four virus strains (WE, E-350, Traub, and CA 1371) were tested. Each was diluted serially ten-fold and each dilution was inoculated intracerebrally, intraperitoneally, or subcutaneously into five mice. After 21 days the survivors were challenged intracerebrally with 1000 LD_{50} of Armstrong's virus E-350, a strain known to produce 100 per cent mortality. The results of two such trials conform to our expectation, *i.e.* titers obtained with different initial inoculation routes did not differ significantly (LEHMANN-GRUBE, unpublished). HOTCHIN and BENSON (1963) obtained similar results. They did, however, see much greater differences between LD_{50} and ID_{50} values after the intracerebral inoculation of the liver-passaged UBC (=WE) strain. Presumably, the calculations were based on the whole dose range, thereby including all the high dose survivors. Thus, even after intracerebral inoculations, the ID_{50} is a measure of peripheral infection, and the only reason to prefer a primary infection *via* the brain is the high death rate which follows, thereby considerably increasing the economy of the method.

From the available data yet other conclusions may be drawn. CAIRNS (1950) estimated that only two to eight per cent of the material remained in the brain and the meninges of a mouse after intracerebral inoculation. From this, the difference between LD_{50} and ID_{50} in mice should be more than ten-fold. As we have seen, it is only two- to three-fold which indicates that the average sensitivity of the tissues within the skull is approximately five times higher than the average sensitivity of the rest of the body. It also indicates that the mouse titration underestimates the number of potentially infectious units by a factor of at least five.

Recently, OLDSTONE and DIXON (1968a; 1968b) claimed that certain inbred mouse strains, notably C3H, are significantly less susceptible to the CA 1371 (=NIH 7022) strain than are ordinary albino mice. Since this observation had been based on deaths only, the question remained whether the survivors had been infected at all, and if so whether they were actively immune or carriers. In my own experiments (LEHMANN-GRUBE, 1969d) it was found that the differences in susceptibility based on deaths as well as on infections between a variety of inbred strains were slight and not significant, even with mice from the same source and the same virus strain as had been used by OLDSTONE and DIXON (1969d). HANNOVER LARSEN (1969d) did not observe differences between mouse strains either. His criticism of the work of Oldstone and Dixon on which their conclusion was based appears to be fully justified. However, since MIMS and TOSOLINI (1969) reported from Canberra that C57BL mice were refractory to the WE virus, which is contrary to the results in Marburg, true differences between laboratories seem to exist for which no explanation is available.

As has already been discussed (see Section V. A. 2), the inoculation of the LCM virus into the foot pad of the mouse is followed by a local inflammatory reaction. This foot pad reaction has been recommended as the criterion for a quantal response. Its advantage lies in the fact that the final reading may be made much sooner than after intracerebral inoculation followed by challenge. However, the method still rests on the use of mice, and since only one foot per animal is employed, the same number is required as for the intracerebral test. Furthermore, the individual inoculation is slower and the daily inspection more time-consuming so that it appears questionable whether the overall economy of the test is improved. (There is *a priori* no reason why all four feet of a mouse should not be utilized as independent assay units. This possibility should be explored experimentally and may make the quantal titration in mice much more economical.) Use of loss of weight of the individual mouse as a criterion of infection (HOTCHIN and BENSON, 1962; 1963) does not appear to be of advantage.

In order to overcome the difficulties which are associated with the use of animals, we have worked out an *in vitro* method which utilizes the production and the release into the medium of complement-fixing antigen by culture cells infected with LCM virus (LEHMANN-GRUBE and HESSE, 1967). In brief, L cell tube cultures are inoculated with virus diluted serially and are incubated in a stationary position at 37° C for six or seven days depending on the virus strain under study. Each tube is then individually tested for complement-fixing antigen and the ID_{50} is estimated according to one of the known procedures. It should be mentioned that the amount of antigen released by the cells is considerable. In repeated experiments 16 to 128 units were found in the medium of E-350 or WE-infected L tube cultures, as determined in conventional complement fixation tests against five times 10^7 sensitized sheep red cells employing two full units of complement. The final amount of released antigen varied little and was always independent of the initial inoculum.

This method which has been used in our laboratory for more than four years is easy to perform, relatively fast, and much more economical than any assay based on mouse inoculations. The dose-response relationship conforms with the most simple hypothesis, namely that one and only one unit initiates infection, which is mathematically expressed by the zero term of the Poisson distribution. For this reason, the test recommends itself to be used for the estimation of the most probable number which, on theoretical grounds, is preferable to the ID_{50} (LEHMANN-GRUBE, 1969b; 1969c).

Based on the cytopathic effect in chick embryo fibroblasts, BENSON and HOTCHIN (1960) performed virus titrations in tube cultures. For the same type of assay, DEIBEL *et al.* (1965) found adaptation of the virus to the cells to be a prerequisite. As has been discussed (see Section III. B. 4), a reproducible cytopathic effect in these cells is difficult to obtain. A further quantal test has been recommended by OLDSTONE and DIXON (1968c). It is based on the development of immunofluorescence in infected tube cultures. Its interesting aspect is the fact that specific fluorescence was seen at virus dilutions as high as 10^{-10}. This is several orders of magnitude higher than the infectious titer to be expected in mouse titrations, indicating the presence in the stock virus (mouse brain suspension) of a great majority of viral units with reduced infectivity. It is to be regretted that the published information is not sufficiently detailed to permit the estimation of a minimal ratio of physical to infectious units, of which we know nothing as regards LCM virus.

2. Quantitative Procedures

Virus titrations based on quantal responses are of inherent low precision (MEYNELL, 1957). Given the same number of assay units, quantitative assays are much more accurate. Attempts to improve the titration of LCM virus by applying quantitative procedures have met with great difficulties. The time between inoculation of the mouse and its death — usually called the latent period or preferably the survival time — successfully employed with other viruses is not a useful measure of infectivity. Mice inoculated intracerebrally with LCM virus never show signs of illness or die before the fifth day, irrespective of the dose administered. Thereafter, they succumb within a relatively short time. Data from an Armstrong virus titration, which had been analyzed according to quantal criteria previously (LEHMANN-GRUBE, 1969b), have been re-evaluated quantitatively. The differences between survival times relative to the doses were too small to be of use for the quantitation of infectious units. They were, however, significant. The proportion of mice found dead on day five as opposed to those which died later differed significantly between dilutions. χ^2 was estimated to be 166.8 which, with five degrees of freedom, corresponds to $P<0.001$. A similar analysis with the WE strain was hampered by this virus' marked zone phenomenon (Fig. 10). However, taking only those mice into account which died in the high zone region (10^0 to 10^{-5}), the differences between dilutions were not significant, which confirms the finding of ROGER and ROGER (1964a) who, working with the same strain, observed no influence of the dose on the survival time. It is presumably for this reason that the "comparative index of virus activity" (HAAS, 1954) which, among other variables, is based on survival times has not found general acceptance in spite of its apparent advantages.

The possibility of using the foot pad response (see Section V. A. 2) for the quantitative assay of LCM virus was explored by ROGER and ROGER (1964d; 1964e). For reasons just pointed out in connection with the intracerebral inoculation, the latent period was not recommended. More promising results were reported with two other measurements: duration and extension of the local response.

BENSON and HOTCHIN (1960; BENSON, 1960) were the first to describe an *in vitro* method based on the focal destruction under agar of chick embryo fibroblasts caused by single infectious units of the WE strain of LCM virus. We have not succeeded in our efforts to employ this method, and other workers, including the original authors (HOTCHIN, personal communication), had great difficulties too.

Apparently, the assay conditions are very critical, and minor deviations may vitiate the results. The use of L cells (Benson, 1961 b) instead of chicken fibroblasts does not seem to have been pursued further.

Another test has been worked out by Ackermann (1961 a). He found that focal exclusion of neutral red developed in monolayers of tertiary mouse embryo cells maintained under agar after infection, even though cytopathic effects were absent. Probably because it has not become available in published form, this promising method has not attracted wider attention.

Hope of improvement was again raised by the report that the hemadsorption interference test, originally worked out for the rubella virus by Marcus and Carver (1965), was adaptable to the titration of LCM virus (Wainwright and Mims, 1967). Again, disappointment soon followed. In this laboratory my colleague, Dr. W. Slenczka, was not able to put the method on a solid footing, and further attempts were not made when Mims himself related (personal communication) that the results were not satisfactory for routine use.

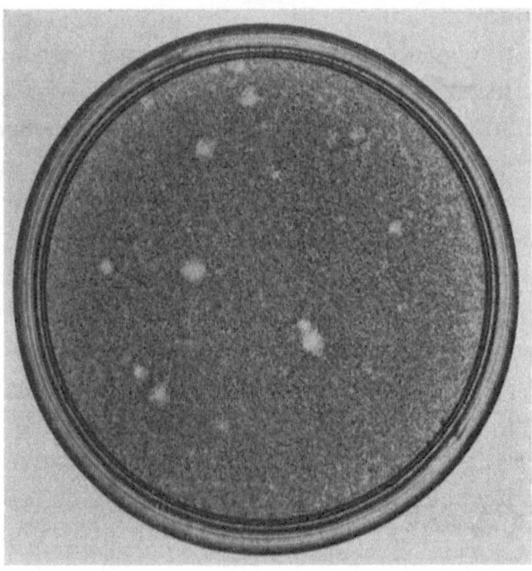

Fig. 16. Plaques of LCM virus on agar cell suspension culture of BHK-21/S 13 cells

So far, the last approach to this problem has been made by Sedwick and Wiktor (1967). Employing the agar cell suspension plaque assay of Cooper (1961), they found that various noncytopathogenic viruses, including that of LCM, caused focal exclusion of neutral red in BHK-21 clone S13 cells. We have modified the method which is now in use in this laboratory in the following way. Plastic Petri plates, six cm in diameter, receive a bottom layer which consists of minimal essential medium (Eagle, 1959) with two per cent fetal calf serum, solidified by 0.5 per cent agarose (Medium I). BHK-21/S 13 cells, grown in Roux bottles using Eagle's medium plus ten per cent tryptose phosphate broth (Difco) plus two per cent fetal calf serum (Medium II), are dispersed by the action of trypsin. They are resuspended in Medium II, counted, and diluted to a concentration of 10^7 cells per ml. Equal volumes of the cell suspension warmed to 37° C and Medium I warmed to 42° C are mixed and poured onto the bottom layers, one ml per plate. Virus is diluted with Medium II, and 0.1 ml portions are placed on the cells which are then incubated at 37° C in five per cent CO_2 for four days. Two ml of neutral red, 1: 5000 in 0.5 per cent agarose, are then layered on top of the cells and plaques are counted after four hours' further incubation. (We are grateful to Dr. T.J. Wiktor who supplied us with the cells and made valuable technical suggestions.) This method is satisfactory: the plaques are clearly defined and easy to count (Fig. 16); the efficiency has proved to be comparable to titrations in L cell tube cultures (see above); the relationship was found to be as expected; and virus clones are readily obtained (SCHOIERER and LEHMANN-GRUBE, unpublished) as could be expected from the report by ZGORNIAK-NOWOSIELSKA *et al.* (1967) who freed LCM virus preparations of contaminating mycoplasmas by plaque-picking procedures utilizing the just mentioned method.

Whether the seven isolates reported to cause cytopathic plaques on chick embryo fibroblasts under agar are true LCM viruses (CHASTEL, 1965) is doubtful (see Section XII).

B. Serology

1. Neutralization Test

In principle, the neutralization of infectivity may be assayed in two ways: (1) by keeping the serum constant and varying the virus, or (2) by keeping the virus constant and varying the serum. In the case of the LCM virus, with few exceptions the former method has been and still is being employed. In the early work guinea-pigs were often used as assay hosts, and TRAUB (1936b) reported that the subcutaneous inoculation of the serum virus mixture into the plantae of these animals revealed antibody with higher efficiency than inoculation into the brain. Later, the mouse was usually preferred; the details were worked out by LEHMANN-GRUBE *et al.* (1960) and SCHEID *et al.* (1960). With minor modifications based on more recent experience the test is performed as follows. Virus in the form of either infected tissue homogenate or infected cell culture fluid is diluted serially with buffered saline containing one per cent inactivated calf serum. Equal volumes of virus and undiluted, noninactivated test serum are mixed and held for two hours at 37° C. A control titration is run under similar conditions; but species-identical normal serum is not admixed for the following reason: most human sera, and possibly some animal sera as well (but not calf sera), contain nonspecific virus-inactivating substances (see Section V. H. 3) which may confound the estimation of the neutralizing activity. Besides, the virus is perfectly stable for two hours at 37° C in the presence of one per cent bovine serum. Mice are inoculated intracerebrally. If Armstrong's strain E-350 is employed, the estimation of the titer may be based on mortality between the 5th and the 14th day (LD_{50}). With other strains, challenge on the 21st day and estimation of the ID_{50} is considered necessary for obtaining optimal accuracy (see Section XI. A. 1). The neutralizing activity of a serum is expressed as the neutralizing index, which is the quotient of the virus titers determined without and with antiserum. There can be no doubt that human sera lose specific neutralizing potency upon heating at 56° C (see Section V. H. 3). Whether this applies to animal sera as well seems to be unknown. I found the neutralizing potency of mouse antisera to be reduced by heating, but TRAUB (1961a) noticed augmentation under similar conditions.

The constant serum-variable virus technique was criticized by Fazekas de St. Groth (1962) who considered it "uninformative, wasteful of material, and prone to nonspecific inhibition". Certainly the latter two accusations apply to our previously recommended procedure. Indeed, there is no good reason not to employ the much more widely used constant virus-variable serum technique. Using a recently developed *in vitro* virus assay (see Section XI. A. 1), a quantal neutralization test is now worked out in this laboratory in much the same way as it is done with many other viruses, the neutralizing titer of a serum being the reciprocal of that dilution which reduces 100 ID_{50} down to one ID_{50}.

The foot pad of the mouse has repeatedly been recommended for assaying the neutralizing capacities of antisera. Titers were found to be higher when based on the foot pad reaction rather than on mortality following intracerebral inoculation (Roger and Hotchin, 1962; Hotchin, 1962b; Traub, 1964; Wilsnack and Rowe, 1964; Roger and Roger, 1964 f.; 1965a; Hotchin *et al.*, 1969). The question whether this phenomenon is due to different dilution and dissociation effects after intracerebral or foot pad inoculation or whether it reflects differences of the host cells' ability to compete successfully with antibody for the virus cannot be answered from the available data. It is noteworthy that the virus may be partially neutralized to the extent that a general infection is prevented and immunity to intracerebral challenge does not develop, although local immunity may be present as demonstrated by failure of the foot to respond to reinoculation (Hotchin, 1962b).

According to Barlow and Wieland (1960), confirmed by Hotchin *et al.* (1969), use of a diluent for virus and antiserum consisting of 0.05 to 0.1 per cent bovine serum albumin in water and incubation for 18 to 24 hours at 2° to 12° C raise the titer 100-fold or more.

The preparation of antiserum poses no problem. Almost any animal will react to the inoculation of the virus with the production of usually low to moderate concentrations of specific inhibiting substances. In mice, high neutralizing serum titers may be induced by adoptive immunization of carriers (see Section V. A. 4. b).

2. Complement Fixation Test

The complement fixation titer of a serum is defined as the reciprocal of that dilution which fixes all or a defined proportion of complement — which in turn is standardized against the number of sensitized erythrocytes present — with an excess of antigen. With this arrangement antiserum is the limiting component of the reaction. Occasionally another path is taken; the serum is kept constant and complement is varied (Kaup and Kretschmer, 1917). It goes without saying that both procedures may be adapted to the measurement of complement-fixing antigen. While in most laboratories LCM virus complement-fixing antibody or antigen is titrated by diluting one and keeping the specific partner constant in some excess, Scheid and his co-workers prefer the alternative method. The motivation given by Jochheim *et al.* (1957) does not convince. In fact, this method has *a priori* at least one major disadvantage; it does not accurately reflect the complement-fixing capacity of a given serum at a given dilution if the antigen becomes limiting. This, however, may occur. Eggers (1958) has shown experimentally that the linear relationship between the number of fixed complement units and the amount of serum present held only in the range of the lower antiserum concentrations.

With high titer sera, the antigen soon became limiting, as a consequence of which the curve flattened leading to a constant complement titer, irrespective of the amount of antibody present. Furthermore, Eggers could show that in the region of relative antigen excess less complement than expected was fixed, indicating a zone phenomenon. Finally, the slopes of the lines connecting amount of antiserum present with the amount of complement fixed varied considerably between antisera, thus making a conversion of the complement titers, given by Scheid and his colleagues in a number of papers, for a quantitative comparison with data from other laboratories difficult if not impossible.

Complement fixation antigen may be derived from various sources by a number of techniques. Howitt (1936/37; 1937) utilized homogenized and ether-extracted infected mouse brains. Lépine *et al.* (1938a; 1938b) employed hepatized portions from infected guinea-pig lungs made up to a one per cent homogenate and filtered through paper. Traub and Schäfer (1939) triturated livers or lungs from infected guinea-pigs or whole embryos from carrier mice and used the supernatant after slow centrifugation. Casals and Palacios (1941) prepared their antigen from infected mouse brains by five cycles of freezing and thawing followed by centrifugation. By a similar process, Whitney *et al.* (1952; 1953) obtained an antigen from chorioallantoic membranes and bodies of chick embryos infected *via* chorioallantoic membrane or yolk sac; the infectivity was inactivated by ultraviolet irradiation. Lewis *et al.* (1965) found an LCM virus-infected transplantable hamster tumor to be a good source of antigen. Ackermann (1961a) recommended use of cell-associated antigen from infected mouse embryo cells in culture. Schell *et al.* (1966) extracted antigen from LCM virus-infected African green monkey kidney cultures by three cycles of freezing and thawing followed by homogenization in a blendor. Brown and Kirk (1969) obtained their complement-fixing antigen from disrupted BHK-21 clone S13 cells after infection with either WE or Armstrong strains of LCM virus. In our laboratory, WE strain-infected sonicated L cells are often used.

Undoubtedly, the now most widely employed antigens are those of Smadel and his co-workers and Grešíková and Casals. Smadel's soluble antigen is prepared as follows (Smadel *et al.*, 1939a; 1939b). Spleens from WE strain-infected guinea-pigs are taken at the height of the disease and are homogenized with saline plus two per cent inactivated guinea-pig serum. The supernatant fluid after ultracentrifugation represents the antigen. Smadel *et al.* (1939b) had found less antigen in guinea-pig lungs and livers as compared with the spleens, but in our laboratory all three organs are homogenized together, which results in specific activity not inferior to the one found with spleens alone. According to Žáčková *et al.* (1959), ultracentrifugation may be omitted if the supernatant from low speed centrifugation is shaken with bentonite and thereafter centrifuged again. Grešíková and Casals (1963) adopted the sucrose acetone extraction method of Clarke and Casals (1958) for the preparation of LCM virus antigen. Seven days after the intracerebral infection of four-day-old mice a 20 per cent brain homogenate is prepared with 8.5 per cent sucrose in water. This is extracted three times with acetone, dried, resuspended in saline, and centrifuged at 10,000 r.p.m. The specific activity of the supernatant fluid is said to be very high. A similar approach was chosen by Chastel and Le Noc (1968). They infected three- to five-day-old mice intracerebrally. Five days later, the brains were homogenized and treated four days at 4° C with trichlorotrifluoroethane. The aqueous phase was centrifuged and the supernate served as antigen.

While the provision of complement-fixing antigen causes no serious difficulties, obtaining complement-fixing antisera may be more laborious. In this laboratory, rabbit antisera are routinely produced by intravenous inoculation of cell culture-grown WE strain virus on days zero, one, two, and five. On days 10, 13, 16, 19, 22, 25, and 28 the rabbit is bled and the sera are assayed for complement-fixing antibody. Those with adequate titers are pooled and stored frozen. With rabbit sera, nonspecific and/or anticomplementary activities may be a great nuisance. They are, however, satisfactorily removed by heating for 20 minutes at 65° C rather than at the usual 56° C (Casals and Palacios, 1941; Jochheim *et al.*, 1957). Although approximately half the specific activity is lost, the net gain is considerable (Lehmann-Grube, unpublished). Some authors prefer guinea-pig sera which usually are less inhibitory. Smadel and Wall (1940) obtained sera with titers up to 512 by inoculating hyperimmune guinea-pigs with partially purified noninfectious s-antigen, "the simplest means so far available for regularly obtaining C-F serum of high titer". Others found the response in these animals to be unreliable; with some virus guinea-pig combinations no complement fixation activity at all developed (see Section V. B. 3).

Although the titers are not high and the amounts obtainable small, mouse sera are sometimes employed. Recently, their value as a source for antibody has risen considerably; Volkert *et al.* (1964) showed that adoptive immunization of carrier mice induced extraordinarily high titers. Indeed, specific fixation may still occur at serum dilutions as high as 1: 8000 (see Section V. A. 4. b). In our laboratory, sera from adoptively immunized LCM virus carriers have replaced other sera for most purposes. Using the microplate technique (Sever, 1962), no difficulty is encountered to make sufficient material available. The report that ascitic fluid from LCM virus-immunized mice exhibits adequate complement fixation activity (Barlow *et al.*, 1967) is likely to further stimulate use of the mouse as a source for LCM virus antibody. Sera from other species, notably man and monkey, are being employed occasionally.

3. Other Serological Methods

Detection of antibody by the indirect immunofluorescence method (Triandaphilli *et al.*, 1965; Cohen *et al.*, 1966; Benson and Hotchin, 1969; Lewis and Clayton, 1969a) promises to be of value. The necessary reagents may be prepared in advance to be used on demand. LCM virus-infected cells are spread on slides and, after fixation, are stored at —50° C. The fluorescein isothiocyanate-conjugated anti-γ-globulin is lyophylized and may then be kept at 4° C. In the test, the infected cells are exposed to serially diluted diagnostic serum and overlaid with conjugate. Typical immunofluorescence in at least three different fields is regarded positive. Apparently, this method poses some difficulties; Benda *et al.* (1965) employed it and found it to be insensitive and unsuitable. However, in a more recent report from the same laboratory, the usefulness of the immunofluorescence technique for the demonstration and titration of LCM-specific antibody was confirmed (Hronovský *et al.*, 1969).

A simple and quite reliable way to appraise qualitatively the serologic identity of an isolate is by cross immunization tests. Guinea-pigs and/or mice are immunized with a standard virus to be challenged with the unknown strain and *vice versa.* On occasion, passive protection of animals by means of immune sera has been explored experimentally (see Section V. I. 2). Finally, precipitation tests directly (Smadel *et al.*, 1940) or in agar (Barlow and Mustico, 1966) may be of value to answer certain questions.

XII. Virus Strains of Doubtful Association with LCM

Of the many agents reported over the years to represent strains of LCM virus many, but not all, were identified to everybody's satisfaction. Some of these agents have been excluded in the past, but many others are still awaiting further evaluation.

From the cerebrospinal fluids of two patients, MacCallum *et al.* (1939) isolated identical agents which were found to resemble LCM virus in some respects. They were named the virus of pseudo-lymphocytic choriomeningitis. This later turned out to be ectromelia virus (MacCallum *et al.*, 1957).

For years, swineherd's disease ("maladie des porchers") was thought to be caused by an agent related to LCM virus. Durand and his colleagues, on whose work this claim was mainly based, did not mention LCM (Durand *et al.*, 1936a; 1936b; 1936c). Indeed, their data revealed profound dissimilarities of the two agents. It is not possible, after so many years, to find the reason for this confusion. To make it short, swineherd's disease, as we know it today, is a leptospirosis (Gsell, 1944–46).

Durand (1940) isolated a virus "D" in guinea-pigs from his own blood during a febrile illness. Although the author himself found it to be different from other known agents, including that of LCM ("une autonomie complète"), it was sometimes associated with the latter, apparently without further experimental evidence.

An agent isolated by Cardoso (1941/42b) from the blood of a child with meningitis living in or near Lisbon, Portugal, was thought by the author to be a strain of LCM virus. The disease signs in mice, either as described or as illustrated by pictures, were not at all characteristic; nor was the agent identified by comparison with a prototype virus.

A virus was isolated by Humphreys *et al.* (1944) in guinea-pigs inoculated with *Dermacentor andersoni* ticks trapped in British Columbia which had previously fed on a normal guinea-pig. Although Humphreys and his colleagues did not make such claims, the new agent was later frequently thought to be at least related to LCM virus. No serologic studies have been reported, and the clinical signs as well as the pathology in experimental animals were different between the two agents (Humphreys *et al.*, 1944; Perrin and Steinhaus, 1944; Lillie and Armstrong, 1945). Thus, no reason exists to maintain that Humphreys' virus has anything to do with LCM.

Lépine *et al.* (1943) at the Pasteur Institute in Paris isolated a virus in guinea-pigs which had been inoculated with materials from a sick horse. From the pathology it caused in the experimental host it was named "virus de la pneumopathie des cobayes". Its true origin remained obscure; while it might have come from the horse, the authors considered the guinea-pigs the more likely origin. Some time later, BLANC *et al.* (1948; 1951a) received from the Institut Pasteur at Paris a guinea-pig which had been inoculated with material containing Q fever rickettsiae originating in Australia. From the animal's spleen they isolated an agent which caused a disease in guinea-pigs closely resembling "pneumopathie des cobayes". In initial studies, Blanc and his colleagues saw no apparent illness develop ("infection strictement inapparente") in a variety of mammalian species including man, except local reactions after inoculations into eye and skin (BLANC and BRUNEAU, 1948; BLANC *et al.*, 1948). Later, however, with man as the experimental host, BLANC *et al.* (1951a; 1951b) compared the new virus with prototype LCM strains and found that infection with the guinea-pig virus led to characteristic clinical signs which were indistinguishable from those following the inoculation of strains WE or Armstrong. Furthermore, infection with LCM virus induced immunity to the guinea-pig virus and *vice versa*. Finally, after infection with the new isolate, LCM complement-fixing antibody, and, after infection with LCM virus, antibody to the isolate appeared. The pathology in mice and guinea-pigs was said to be similar after infection with either virus. Thus, both in their pathogenetic potentials as well as serologically the agents under question seemed to be identical. However, there were differences, the most notable of which was the fact that the new agent killed mice as early as four days after infection, which true strains of LCM virus never do. Furthermore, the agent was found to be very heat stable which, again, contrasts with LCM virus. Nothing further has been reported of the relationship between Blanc's agent and Lépine's original "virus de la pneumopathie des cobayes"; the latter had been found by LÉPINE and SAUTTER (1945) to differ from true LCM strains. Thus, while the agent of Blanc and his colleagues may be a strain of LCM virus, this cannot be considered as having been unequivocally established. It is for this reason that the interesting experiments dealing with the transmission of the guinea-pig virus from inoculated pregnant guinea-pigs and rabbits to their embryos (BLANC and BRUNEAU 1951a; 1951b; BLANC *et al.*, 1951b; BLANC, 1952) will not be analyzed here.

With a yellow fever vaccine, prepared from infected mouse brains (batch No. 26), which had previously been shown to be innocuous, MOLLARET and FINDLAY (1936) inoculated four persons of whom three developed febrile illnesses and the fourth a meningoencephalitis. Two of six mice which had received intracerebrally blood from the patient with the disease of the central nervous system had spasms of the hind legs. Only one further passage in mice was successful. No antibody neutralizing LCM virus could be demonstrated in either the patient or in two monkeys inoculated with the vaccine. LAIGRET and DURAND (1936) demonstrated identical agents in the colony (from which the mice for the vaccine 26 had come?), in a patient, and in chicken embryos (!), used for the preparation of cell cultures. Serologic identification was not achieved. Although the authors themselves did not make such claim, these reports have frequently been taken to prove that the LCM virus may be a contaminant of yellow fever vaccines prepared from mice. While such an event must be considered a definite possibility, the published evidence does not permit the conclusion that this has ever happened.

A virus isolated by TAYLOR and MACDOWELL (1949) from a transplanted mouse leukemia was reported by LINDORFER and SYVERTON (1953/54) to be related, though not identical, to LCM virus. The accompanying data are insufficient. Furthermore, the signs in mice caused by the "MacD." virus were not characteristic of an LCM disease (TAYLOR and MACDOWELL, 1949). Essentially the same may be said of the M-P virus whose alleged relationship with LCM virus (MOLOMUT and PADNOS, 1965) was based on scanty serologic similarity; otherwise, there were marked differences.

Besides five strains of LCM virus, STEWART and HAAS (1956) isolated four more agents from mouse neoplasms whose identity as LCM virus they regarded as a "reasonable conjecture". The accompanying data are not sufficient to make a decision.

Some similarity was reported by CHUMAKOV (1949) (see also SHVAREV, 1966) to exist between the LCM virus and an agent which was said to have caused an epidemic, predominantly in children, of a subacute chorioencephalitis characterized by peculiar psychopathological alterations which had occurred in 1947/48 in Moscow. (I have not been able to obtain the original literature on the comparative study of these two viruses.)

An agent which had caused abacterial meningitis in at least 262 persons in a village near Heidelberg was thought by BINGEL (1951) to be a modified strain of LCM virus. The evidence is not convincing. SÉDALLIAN *et al.* (1954) isolated an agent from a human case of benign meningitis and considered it to be a variant of LCM virus in spite of marked biological as well as serological dissimilarities.

Other viruses whose identity is uncertain have already been mentioned. Neither the cell culture-adapted strain of JUNGEBLUT and KODZA (1963 b) nor the cell culture variant of MACCALLUM and FINDLAY (1940) may be accepted (see Section IX). The alleged LCM virus ("Tunis") isolated by VERMEIL and MAURIN (1953) from a toxoplasma strain, which — 295 intraperitoneal mouse passages previously — had been isolated in Holland from a patient, was serologically different from an LCM prototype virus.

During a search for arboviruses in Cambodia, CHASTEL (1965) isolated seven strains in suckling mice which he obtained from human serum (one), reptiles (four), amphibians (one), and a pool of *Culex fatigans* mosquitoes (one). Their identification was based on inhibition of plaques which they produced on monolayer cultures of chicken embryo fibroblasts by a reference antiserum. Otherwise they differed in many respects from true representatives of LCM virus. Neither the numerous isolates reported by BLANC *et al.* (1960) to have originated in small mammals trapped in Morocco, nor the ones Russian workers (LEVI *et al.*, 1953; GLUSHCHENKO *et al.*, 1957) found in small rodents, mosquitoes, and ticks have been sufficiently characterized as to allow their final identification. The same is to be said of the altogether 21 agents obtained by REISS-GUTFREUND *et al.* (1961; 1962; REISS-GUTFREUND, 1962) from a variety of mammals and arthropods in Ethiopia.

Acknowledgment

Work done in the author's laboratory was supported by a research grant from the Deutsche Forschungsgemeinschaft.

References[1]

ABELSON, H. T., G. H. SMITH, H. A. HOFFMAN, and W. P. ROWE: Use of enzyme-labeled antibody for electron microscope localization of lymphocytic choriomeningitis virus antigens in infected cell cultures. J. nat. Cancer Inst. **42**, 497—515 (1969).

ABERNATHY, R. S., G. M. BRADLEY, and W. W. SPINK: Increased susceptibility of mice with brucellosis to bacterial endotoxins. J. Immunol. **81**, 271—275 (1958).

ACKERMANN, R.: Serologische Untersuchungen auf latente Infektionen mit dem Virus der lymphozytären Choriomeningitis in einem Endemiegebiet Norddeutschlands. Zbl. Bakt., I. Abt. Orig. **179**, 298—307 (1960).

ACKERMANN, R.: Die Züchtung des Virus der Lymphozytären Choriomeningitis in der Gewebekultur. Habilitationsschrift. Köln. 1961 a.

ACKERMANN, R.: Über die Züchtung des Virus der lymphocytären Choriomeningitis in Mäuseembryo-Zellkulturen. Arch. ges. Virusforsch. **10**, 183—194 (1961 b).

ACKERMANN, R., H. BLOEDHORN, B. KÜPPER, I. WINKENS und W. SCHEID: Über die Verbreitung des Virus der Lymphocytären Choriomeningitis unter den Mäusen in Westdeutschland. I. Untersuchungen überwiegend an Hausmäusen (Mus musculus). Zbl. Bakt., I. Abt. Orig. **194**, 407—430 (1964).

ACKERMANN, R., und L. JANSEN: Zur Epidemiologie der Infektion mit dem Virus der lymphocytären Choriomeningitis. Z. klin. Med. **155**, 277—287 (1958).

ACKERMANN, R., W. SCHEID und K. A. JOCHHEIM: Der Einfluß der Lagerung auf die neutralisierenden Fähigkeiten von Seren gegenüber dem Virus der Lymphozytären Choriomeningitis. Zbl. Bakt., I. Abt. Orig. **185**, 343—354 (1962).

ADAIR, C. V.. R. L. GAULD, and J. E. SMADEL: Aseptic meningitis, a disease of diverse etiology: clinical and etiologic studies on 854 cases. Ann. intern. Med. **39**, 675—704 (1953).

AFZELIUS-ALM, L.: Aseptic (nonbacterial) encephalomeningitides in Gothenborg 1932 – 1950. Acta med. scand., Suppl. No. 263 (1951).

ALICE, F. J.: Ocurrência em camondongos cinzentos "Mus musculus" de um virus que se assemelha ao da coriomeningite linfocitária (nota prévia). Brasil-méd. **59**, 224 – 225 (1945 a).

ALICE, F. J.: Ocurrência do virus murino da coriomeningite linfocitária na Bahia. Brasil-méd. **59**, 339—350 (1945 b).

ALICE, F. J., and S. H. MCNUTT: A study of lymphocytic choriomeningitis virus. Amer. J. vet. Res. **6**, 54—60 (1945).

ALLISON, A. C.: Cell-mediated immune responses to virus infections and virus-induced tumours. Brit. med. Bull. **23**, 60—65 (1967).

ALLISON, A. C., and L. W. LAW: Effects of antilymphocyte serum on virus oncogenesis. Proc. Soc. exp. Biol. (N. Y.) **127**, 207—212 (1968).

ANDREWES, C. H.: Possible host-virus and cell-virus relationships. In: Symposium on Latency and Masking in Viral and Rickettsial Infections, Madison, Wis., 1957. Ed.: D. L. WALKER, R. P. HANSON, and A. S. EVANS. Minneapolis, Minn.: Burgess Publishing Co. 1958.

ANDREWES, C. H., and D. M. HORSTMANN: The susceptibility of viruses to ethyl ether. J. gen. Microbiol. **3**, 290—297 (1949).

ARMSTRONG, C.: Acute lymphocytic choriomeningitis: experimental considerations. Arch. Neurol. Psychiat. (Chic.) **36**, 1395 (only) (1936).

ARMSTRONG, C.: Studies on choriomeningitis and poliomyelitis. Harvey Lecture, October 31, 1940. Bull. N. Y. Acad. Med. **17**, 295—318 (1941).

ARMSTRONG, C.: Some recent research in the field of neurotropic viruses with especial reference to lymphocytic choriomeningitis and herpes simplex. Milit. Surg. **91**, 129—146 (1942).

ARMSTRONG, C., and P. E. DICKENS: Benign lymphocytic choriomeningitis (acute aseptic meningitis). A new disease entity. Publ. Hlth Rep. (Wash.) **50**, 831—842 (1935).

---

[1] The survey of the literature was concluded December 1969.

ARMSTRONG, C., and J. W. HORNIBROOK: Choriomeningitis virus infection without central nervous system manifestations. Report of a case. Publ. Hlth Rep. (Wash.) **56**, 907—909 (1941).

ARMSTRONG, C., and R. D. LILLIE: Experimental lymphocytic choriomeningitis of monkeys and mice produced by a virus encountered in studies of the 1933 St. Louis encephalitis epidemic. Publ. Hlth Rep. (Wash.) **49**, 1019—1027 (1934).

ARMSTRONG, C., and L. K. SWEET: Lymphocytic choriomeningitis. Report of two cases, with recovery of the virus from gray mice *(Mus musculus)* trapped in the two infected households. Publ. Hlth Rep. (Wash.) **54**, 673—684 (1939).

ARMSTRONG, C., J. J. WALLACE, and L. ROSS: Lymphocytic choriomeningitis. Gray mice, *Mus musculus*, a reservoir for the infection. Publ. Hlth Rep. (Wash.) **55**, 1222—1229 (1940).

ARMSTRONG, C., and J. G. WOOLEY: Studies on the origin of a newly discovered virus which causes lymphocytic choriomeningitis in experimental animals. Publ. Hlth Rep. (Wash.) **50**, 537—541 (1935).

ARMSTRONG, C., and J. G. WOOLEY: Benign lymphocytic choriomeningitis. Laboratory studies with the virus and their possible bearing on the infection in man. J. Amer. med. Ass. **109**, 410—412 (1937).

ARMSTRONG, C., J. G. WOOLEY, and R. H. ONSTOTT: Distribution of lymphocytic choriomeningitis virus in the organs of experimentally inoculated monkeys. Publ. Hlth Rep. (Wash.) **51**, 298—303 (1936).

ARMSTRONG, D., J. G. FORTNER, W. P. ROWE, and J. C. PARKER: Meningitis due to lymphocytic choriomeningitis virus endemic in a hamster colony. J. Amer. med. Ass. **209**, 265—267 (1969).

ASHERSON, G. L.: Antigen-mediated depression of delayed hypersensitivity. Brit. med. Bull. **23**, 24—29 (1967).

AVERY, L. W.: Benign lymphocytic choriomeningitis. Med. Clin. N. Amer. pp. 36—44, 1945.

AXELROD, A. E., and J. PRUZANSKY: The role of the vitamins in antibody production. Vitam. and Horm. **13**, 1—27 (1955).

BAIRD, R. D., and T. M. RIVERS: Relation of lymphocytic choriomeningitis to acute aseptic meningitis (Wallgren). Amer. J. publ. Hlth **28**, 47—53 (1938).

BAKER, A. B.: Chronic lymphocytic choriomeningitis. J. Neuropath. exp. Neurol. **6**, 253—264 (1947).

BAKER, F. D.: Changes in the level of tolerance in mice persistently infected with LCM virus. In: International Virology. I. Ed.: J. L. MELNICK. Proc. First Internat. Congr. Virology, Helsinki 1968. Basel: S. Karger 1969.

BAKER, F. D., and J. HOTCHIN: Slow virus kidney disease of mice. Science **158**, 502—504 (1967).

BALEK, F., H. LÍBIKOVÁ a M. ONDREJIČKA: Lymfocytárna choriomeningitída na Slovensku. I. Príspevok ku klinickej symptomatológii tzv. lymfocytárnej choriomeningitídy. II. Epidemiologicko virologický prieskum LCM. Bratisl. lek. Listy **34**, 1250—1269 (1954).

BÁNOS, Z., I. SZERI, P. ANDERLIK, and B. RADNAI: The course of lymphocytic choriomeningitis virus infection in mice treated by phytohaemagglutinin. Experientia (Basel) **25**, 1332—1333 (1969).

BARATAWIDJAJA, R. K., L. P. MORRISSEY, and N. A. LABZOFFSKY: Demonstration of vaccinia, lymphocytic choriomeningitis and rabies viruses in the leucocytes of experimentally infected animals. Arch. ges. Virusforsch. **17**, 273—279 (1965).

BÁRDOŠ, V.: Vírusové neuroinfekcie s prírodne ohniskovým výskytom v oblasti Dunaja. Čs. Epidem. **6**, 381—391 (1957).

BARKER, L. F., and F. R. FORD: Chronic arachnoiditis obliterating the spinal subarachnoid space. J. Amer. med. Ass. **109**, 785—786 (1937).

BARLOW, J. L.: The effect of alkylating agents on lymphocytic choriomeningitis infection in mice. A. R. for 1961, Div. Lab. Res., N. Y. St. Dep. Hlth (Albany) pp. 47—48, 1962.

Barlow, J. L., S. M. Cohen, and I. Triandaphilli: The effect of 5-halogen-2'-deoxyuridine derivatives on the synthesis of lymphocytic choriomeningitis virus. Fed. Proc. **24**, 319 (only) (1965).

Barlow, J. L., S. M. Cohen, I. Triandaphilli, and E. Keller: Identification of the nucleic acid of lymphocytic choriomeningitis virus. A. R. for 1965, Div. Lab. Res., N. Y. St. Dep. Hlth (Albany) pp. 59—60, 1966.

Barlow, J. L., and R. J. Fairley: Hyperreactivity to endotoxin in mice infected with lymphocytic choriomeningitis virus. A. R. for 1962, Div. Lab. Res., N. Y. St. Dep. Hlth (Albany) pp. 39—40, 1963.

Barlow, J. L., and J. Hotchin: The effect of certain drugs on lymphocytic choriomeningitis infection in mice. A. R. for 1960, Div. Lab. Res., N. Y. St. Dep. Hlth (Albany) pp. 22—23, 1961.

Barlow, J. L., and J. Hotchin: Induction of persistent tolerant infection with lymphocytic choriomeningitis virus in adult mice by amethopterin treatment. A. R. for 1962, Div. Lab. Res., N. Y. St. Dep. Hlth (Albany) p. 39, 1963.

Barlow, J. L., and E. Keller: Propagation of lymphocytic choriomeningitis virus in tissue cell cultures. A. R. for 1964, Div. Lab. Res., N. Y. St. Dep. Hlth (Albany) pp. 50—51, 1965 a.

Barlow, J. L., and E. Keller: Effect of 5-fluoro-2'-deoxyuridine on formation of lymphocytic choriomeningitis virus in continuous baby hamster kidney cells. A. R. for 1964, Div. Lab. Res., N. Y. St. Dep. Hlth (Albany) p. 51, 1965 b.

Barlow, J. L., and E. Keller: Studies of lymphocytic choriomeningitis virus in baby hamster kidney cells. A. R. for 1965, Div. Lab. Res., N. Y. St. Dep. Hlth (Albany) p. 61, 1966.

Barlow, J. L., T. E. Leibach, and W. J. Decher: Production of large quantities of viral antibodies in mouse ascites fluid. A. R. for 1966, Div. Lab. Res., N. Y. St. Dep. Hlth (Albany) pp. 70—71, 1967.

Barlow, J. L., and T. Mustico: Noninfectious antigens associated with lymphocytic choriomeningitis virus infection. A. R. for 1964, Div. Lab. Res., N. Y. St. Dep. Hlth (Albany) p. 52, 1965.

Barlow, J. L., and T. Mustico: Noninfectious antigens associated with lymphocytic choriomeningitis infection. A. R. for 1965, Div. Lab. Res., N. Y. St. Dep. Hlth (Albany) pp. 60—61, 1966.

Barlow, J., and M. H. Wieland: Effect of low salt concentration on neutralizing antibody reactions for lymphocytic choriomeningitis virus. A. R. for 1959, Div. Lab. Res., N. Y. St. Dep. Hlth (Albany) p. 23, 1960.

Barski, G., et J. K. Youn: Interférence entre la chorioméningite lymphocytaire et la leucémie de souris de Rauscher. C. R. Acad. Sci. (Paris) **259**, 4191—4194 (1964).

Battisto, J. R., and M. W. Chase: Induced unresponsiveness to simple allergenic chemicals. II. Independence of delayed-type hypersensitivity and formation of circulating antibody. J. exp. Med. **121**, 591—606 (1965).

Baum, S. G., A. M. Lewis, W. P. Rowe, and R. J. Huebner: Epidemic nonmeningitic lymphocytic-choriomeningitis-virus infection. An outbreak in a population of laboratory personnel. New Engl. J. Med. **274**, 934—936 (1966).

Bauzá, C. A., R. E. Somma, H. C. Tosi, E. F. Vallone, y R. M. Canto de Vallone: Encuesta seroepidemiologica de anticuerpos para el virus de la coriomeningitis linfocitica, en niños. Arch. Pediat. Urug. **36**, 705—708 (1965).

Bayer, P., and J. Gear: Virus meningo-encephalitis in South Africa. A study of the cases admitted to the Johannesburg Fever Hospital. S. Afr. J. Lab. clin. Med. **1**, 22—35 (1955).

Benda, R.: Passive immunoprophylaxis and immunotherapy of inhalation lymphocytic choriomeningitis in guinea-pigs. J. Hyg. Epidem. (Praha) **8**, 243—251 (1964).

Benda, R., and J. Činátl: Multiplication of lymphocytic choriomeningitis virus in bottle cell cultures. Experimental data for the preparation of highly infectious fluids. Acta virol. **6**, 159—164 (1962).

Benda, R., and J. Činátl: Active immunoprophylaxis of experimental inhalation lymphocytic choriomeningitis. J. Hyg. Epidem. (Praha) **8**, 252—261 (1964).

BENDA, R., L. DANEŠ, and M. FUCHSOVÁ: Experimental inhalation infection of guineapigs with the virus of lymphocytic choriomeningitis. J. Hyg. Epidem. (Praha) 8, 87—99 (1964).

BENDA, R., L. DANEŠ a R. RADVAN: Virus lymfocytární choriomeningitis. I. Isolace viru LCM z myši Apodemus flavicollis. Vojenská Lékařská Akademie Sborník Prací pp. 15—23, 1955.

BENDA, R., V. HRONOVSKÝ, L. ČERVA, and J. ČINÁTL: Demonstration of lymphocytic choriomeningitis virus in cell cultures and mouse brain by the fluorescent antibody technique. Acta virol. **9**, 347—351 (1965).

BENGTSON, I. A., and J. G. WOOLEY: Cultivation of the virus of lymphocytic choriomeningitis in the developing chick embryo. Publ. Hlth Rep. (Wash.) **51**, 29—41 (1936).

BENSON, L. M.: Tissue culture experiments and plaque assay with lymphocytic choriomeningitis virus. A. R. for 1959, Div. Lab. Res., N. Y. St. Dep. Hlth (Albany) pp. 22—23, 1960.

BENSON, L. M.: Suppression of lymphocytic choriomeningitis virus production in Maitland-type tissue culture by antibody. A. R. for 1960, Div. Lab. Res., N. Y. St. Dep. Hlth (Albany) p. 22, 1961 a.

BENSON, L. M.: The use of strain L mouse cells in an improved plaque assay of lymphocytic choriomeningitis virus. A. R. for 1960, Div. Lab. Res., N. Y. St. Dep. Hlth (Albany) pp. 23—24, 1961 b.

BENSON, L. M.: Autointerference due to lymphocytic choriomeningitis virus in tissue culture. A. R. for 1961, Div. Lab. Res., N. Y. St. Dep. Hlth (Albany) pp. 46—47, 1962.

BENSON, L.: The effect of x-ray on the foot-pad response of mice injected with lymphocytic choriomeningitis virus. A. R. for 1962, Div. Lab. Res., N. Y. St. Dep. Hlth (Albany) p. 41, 1963 a.

BENSON, L.: Effects of immune mouse lymphocytes on normal and virus infected mouse tissue culture. A. R. for 1962, Div. Lab. Res., N. Y. St. Dep. Hlth (Albany) pp. 41—42, 1963 b.

BENSON, L. M., and J. E. HOTCHIN: Cytopathogenicity and plaque formation with lymphocytic choriomeningitis virus. Proc. Soc. exp. Biol. (N. Y.) **103**, 623—625 (1960).

BENSON, L. M., and J. HOTCHIN: Tumor production in mice by strain L tissue culture cells carrying lymphocytic choriomeningitis virus. A. R. for 1961, Div. Lab. Res., N. Y. St. Dep. Hlth (Albany) pp. 44—46, 1962.

BENSON, L., and J. HOTCHIN: Antibody formation in persistent tolerant infection with lymphocytic choriomeningitis virus. Nature (Lond.) **222**, 1045—1047 (1969).

BENSON, L., A. MAGNUSON, and J. HOTCHIN: Long-term *in vitro* cultivation of lymphocytic choriomeningitis virus in tissue cultures. A. R. for 1960, Div. Lab. Res., N. Y. St. Dep. Hlth (Albany) pp. 21—22, 1961.

BENSON, L. M., H. WEIGAND, and J. E. HOTCHIN: Relationship between blood lymphocyte counts and susceptibility to lymphocytic choriomeningitis after x-irradiation. A. R. for 1959, Div. Lab. Res., N. Y. St. Dep. Hlth (Albany) pp. 21—22, 1960.

BERENBAUM, M. C.: Effect of cytotoxic agents on antibody production. Nature (Lond.) **185**, 167—168 (1960).

BERENBAUM, M. C.: Immunosuppressive agents and allogeneic transplantation. J. clin. Path. (Suppl.) **20**, 471—498 (1967).

BERGER, J., und G. SCHOOP: Über ein an den Toxoplasma-Stamm BK (Winsser, van Thiel, **1948**) gekoppeltes infektiöses Agens. Z. med. Mikrobiol. Immunol. **153**, 269 – 283 (1967).

BERTANI, G.: Lysogeny. Advanc. Virus Res. **5**, 151—193 (1958).

BIELING, R., und F. KOCH: Versuch einer klinischen Differentialdiagnose der abakteriellen Meningitis. Z. Kinderheilk. **72**, 85—112 (1953).

BILLINGHAM, R. E., and L. BRENT: A simple method for inducing tolerance of skin homografts in mice. Transplant. Bull. **4**, 67—71 (1957).

Billingham, R. E., and L. Brent: Quantitative studies on tissue transplantation immunity. IV. Induction of tolerance in newborn mice and studies on the phenomenon of runt disease. Phil. Trans. B **242**, 439—477 (1958—60).

Billingham, R. E., L. Brent, and P. B. Medawar: "Actively acquired tolerance" of foreign cells. Nature (Lond.) **172**, 603—606 (1953).

Billingham, R. E., L. Brent, and P. B. Medawar: Quantitative studies on tissue transplantation immunity. III. Actively acquired tolerance. Phil. Trans. B **239**, 357—414 (1955/56).

Bingel, K. F.: Ätiologische Untersuchung zu einer benignen epidemischen Meningitis. Z. Hyg. Infekt.-Kr. **132**, 173—201 (1951).

Blanc, G.: Pneumopathie du cobaye et chorioméningite lymphocytaire. Sem. Hôp. Paris **28**, 3805—3810 (1952).

Blanc, G., et L. Ascione: Rôle de certains arthropodes piqueurs dans la conservation et la transmission du virus de la chorioméningite lymphocytaire. Bull. Acad. nat. Méd. (Paris) **144**, 177—179 (1960).

Blanc, G., L. Ascione et M. Mailloux: Les petits mammifères sauvages peuvent-ils être porteurs du virus de la chorioméningite lymphocytaire? Enquête faite au Maroc. Bull. Acad. nat. Méd. (Paris) **144**, 645—649 (1960).

Blanc, G., et J. Bruneau: De l'infection inapparente à l'infection apparente avec le virus de la pneumopathie du cobaye. Ann. Inst. Pasteur **75**, 566—569 (1948).

Blanc, G., et J. Bruneau: Action du virus de la pneumopathie du cobaye sur la gestation ou cours de l'infection apparente et de l'infection inapparente. C. R. Acad. Sci. (Paris) **232**, 1716—1718 (1951a).

Blanc, G., et J. Bruneau: Comportement du virus de la chorioméningite chez la lapine en gestation. C. R. Acad. Sci. (Paris) **233**, 1704—1705 (1951b).

Blanc, G., J. Bruneau, B. Delage et R. Poitrot: Pneumopathie du cobaye et chorioméningite lymphocytaire. Bull. Acad. nat. Méd. (Paris) **135**, 255—262 (1951a).

Blanc, G., J. Bruneau, B. Delage et R. Poitrot: Etude comparative de virus de chorioméningite lymphocytaire d'origine humaine (W. E. Armstrong) et animale (pneumopathie du cobaye). Bull. Acad. nat. Méd. (Paris) **135**, 520—528 (1951 b).

Blanc, G., J. Bruneau et L.-A. Martin: La pneumopathie du cobaye est transmissible à l'homme et à certains animaux sous forme inapparente. C. R. Acad. Sci. (Paris) **227**, 787—788 (1948).

Blumenthal, W.: Spezifische Antikörper gegen das Virus der lymphozytären Choriomeningitis bei der Bevölkerung von Endemiegebieten in der Bundesrepublik Deutschland. Diss. Köln. 1968.

Blumenthal, W., R. Ackermann und W. Scheid: Durchseuchung mit dem Virus der Lymphozytären Choriomeningitis in einem Endemiegebiet. Dtsch. med. Wschr. **93**, 944—948 (1968 a).

Blumenthal, W., R. Ackermann, and W. Scheid: Distribution of lymphocytic choriomeningitis virus in an endemic area. German med. Mth. **13**, 587—590 (1968 b).

Bordet, P.: Contribution à l'étude de l'allergie. (Premier mémoire.) L'allergie non spécifique. Ann. Inst. Pasteur **56**, 325—352 (1936).

Borel, Y., M. Fauconnet, and P. A. Miescher: Selective suppression of delayed hypersensitivity by the induction of immunologic tolerance. J. exp. Med. **123**, 585 – 598 (1966).

Boyden, S.: Autoimmunity and inflammation. Nature (Lond.) **201**, 200—201 (1964).

Brent, L., and G. Gowland: Immunological competence of newborn mice. Transplantation **1**, 372—376 (1963).

Breyere, E. J., and L. B. Williams: Antigens associated with a tumor virus: rejection of isogenic skin grafts from leukemic mice. Science **146**, 1055—1056 (1964).

Brodie, M.: Tests of viruses of choriomeningitis and encephalitis (St. Louis) with serum from nonparalytic poliomyelitis (New York City, 1935). J. infect. Dis. **61**, 139—142 (1937).

Brooksaler, F., and S. E. Sulkin: Lymphocytic choriomeningitis. Clinical, epidemiologic, and laboratory aspects. Tex. St. J. Med. **44**, 364—367 (1948).

Brown, J. E.: Lymphocytic chorio-meningitis with isolation of the virus. Ohio St. med. J. **37**, 146—148 (1941).

Brown, P.: Evolution of lymphocytic choriomeningitis virus infection from neonatal inoculation through development of adult "late onset disease" and glomerulonephritis. An immunofluorescence study in mice. Arch. ges. Virusforsch. **24**, 220—230 (1968).

Brown, W. J., and B. E. Kirk: Complement-fixing antigen from BHK-21 cell cultures infected with lymphocytic choriomeningitis virus. Appl. Microbiol. **18**, 496—499 (1969).

Buck, L. L., and C. J. Pfau: Inhibition of lymphocytic choriomeningitis virus replication by actinomycin D and 6-azauridine. Virology **37**, 698—701 (1969).

Burgio, G. R., und F. Severi: Untersuchungen über Hämagglutinine der Blasenflüssigkeit. Proc. 10th Congr. Internat. Soc. Blood Transfus., Stockholm 1964. pp. 759 – 764, 1965.

Burnet, F. M.: Principles of Animal Virology. New York: Academic Press Inc. 1955.

Burnet, F. M., and F. Fenner: The Production of Antibodies. Second ed. Melbourne: Macmillan Co. 1949.

Cairns, H. J. F.: Intracerebral inoculation of mice: fate of the inoculum. Nature (Lond.) **166**, 910—911 (1950).

Campbell, J. B., R. F. Maes, T. J. Wiktor, and H. Koprowski: The inhibition of rabies virus by arabinosyl cytosine. Studies on the mechanism and specificity of action. Virology **34**, 701—708 (1968).

Camyre, K. P., and C. J. Pfau: Biophysical and biochemical characterization of lymphocytic choriomeningitis virus. IV. Strain differences. J. Virol. **2**, 161—166 (1968).

Cárdenas, G. E., y E. L. Yépez: Corio meningitis linfocitoria aguda. Arch. Crimin. Neuropsiq. **7**, 64—77 (1959).

Cardoso, A. M.: Coriomeningite linfocitária (Doença de Armstrong). Amat. lusit. **1**, 357—372 (1941/42 a).

Cardoso, A. M.: Tentativa de isolamento do vírus da coriomeningite linfocitária. Amat. lusit. **1**, 764—769 (1941/42 b).

Caren, L. D., and L. T. Rosenberg: Complement in skin grafting in mice. Immunology **9**, 359—364 (1965).

Carey, D. E., R. M. Myers, and J. K. G. Webb: Search for herpes simplex, mumps and lymphocytic choriomeningitis associated with central nervous system disease at Vellore, Southern India. Indian J. med. Res. **57**, 567—568 (1969).

Casals, J., and R. Palacios: The complement fixation test in the diagnosis of virus infections of the central nervous system. J. exp. Med. **74**, 409—426 (1941).

Casals-Ariet, J., and L. T. Webster: Characteristics of a strain of lymphocytic choriomeningitis virus encountered as a contaminant in tissue cultures of rabies virus. J. exp. Med. **71**, 147—154 (1940).

Ceglowski, W., and H. Friedman: Suppression of the primary antibody plaque response of mice following infection with Friend disease virus. Proc. Soc. exp. Biol. (N. Y.) **126**, 662—666 (1967).

Chang, H.-T., F.-H. Ch'iu, and H.-C. Wang: Lymphocytic choriomeningitis. Report of a chronic case. China med. J. **72**, 113—117 (1954).

Chase, M. W.: Immunologic tolerance. Ann. Rev. Microbiol. **13**, 349—376 (1959).

Chastel, C.: Technique des plages et de l'inhibition des plages en cultures cellulaires pour l'identification du virus de la chorioméningite lymphocytaire. Ann. Inst. Pasteur **109**, 874—886 (1965).

Chastel, C., et P. Le Noc: Antigène fixateur du complément de titre élevé et de préparation simple pour le virus de la chorioméningite lymphocytaire. Ann. Inst. Pasteur **114**, 698—704 (1968).

Chumakov, M. P.: Virusnyje nejroinfektsii. Klin. Med. (Mosk.) **27** (**6**), 3—10 (1949).

Clarke, D. H., and J. Casals: Techniques for hemagglutination and hemagglutination-inhibition with arthropod-borne viruses. Amer. J. trop. Med. Hyg. **7**, 561—573 (1958).

COGGESHALL, L. T.: The transmission of lymphocytic choriomeningitis by mosquitoes. Science **89**, 515—516 (1939).

COHEN, S. M., I. A. TRIANDAPHILLI, J. L. BARLOW, and J. HOTCHIN: Immunofluorescent detection of antibody to lymphocytic choriomeningitis virus in man. J. Immunol. **96**, 777—784 (1966).

COLLINS, D. N., H. WEIGAND, and J. HOTCHIN: The effects of pretreatment with x-rays on the pathogenesis of lymphocytic choriomeningitis in mice. II. The pathological histology. J. Immunol. **87**, 682—687 (1961).

COLLIS, W. R. F.: Acute benign lymphocytic meningitis. (Acute aseptic meningitis.) Brit. med. J. **II**, 1148—1150 (1935).

COLMORE, J. P.: Severe infections with the virus of lymphocytic choriomeningitis. J. Amer. med. Ass. **148**, 1199—1201 (1952).

CONGDON, C. C., and E. LORENZ: Leukemia in guinea-pigs. Amer. J. Path. **30**, 337—359 (1954).

COOPER, P. D.: An improved agar cell-suspension plaque assay for poliovirus: some factors affecting efficiency of plating. Virology **13**, 153—157 (1961).

COOPER, P. D.: The inhibition of poliovirus growth by actinomycin D and the prevention of the inhibition by pretreatment of the cells with serum or insulin. Virology **28**, 663—678 (1966).

COUGHLIN, J., and E. WHITNEY: Lymphocytic choriomeningitis virus latently infecting monkey kidney tissue cultures. A. R. for 1957, Div. Lab. Res., N. Y. St. Dep. Hlth (Albany) pp. 37—38, 1957.

CUTIE, T., and E. SIKORA: Effect of Evans blue on the foot pad reaction to lymphocytic choriomeningitis virus. A. R. for 1964, Div. Lab. Res., N. Y. St. Dep. Hlth (Albany) p. 52, 1965.

CUTTING, W., E. FURUSAWA, S. FURUSAWA, and Y. K. WOO: Antiviral activity of herbs on Columbia SK in mice, and LCM, vaccinia and adeno type 12 viruses *in vitro*. Proc. Soc. exp. Biol. (N. Y.) **120**, 330—333 (1965).

DALLDORF, G.: The simultaneous occurrence of the viruses of canine distemper and lymphocytic choriomeningitis. A correction of "Canine distemper in the rhesus monkey". J. exp. Med. **70**, 19—27 (1939 a).

DALLDORF, G.: Studies of the sparing effect of lymphocytic choriomeningitis on experimental poliomyelitis. I. Effect on the infectivity of monkey tissues. J. Immunol. **37**, 245—259 (1939 b).

DALLDORF, G.: Lymphocytic choriomeningitis of dogs. Cornell Vet. **33**, 347—350 (1943).

DALLDORF, G., and M. DOUGLASS: Simultaneous distemper and lymphocytic choriomeningitis in dog spleen and the sparing effect on poliomyelitis. Proc. Soc. exp. Biol. (N. Y.) **39**, 294—297 (1938).

DALLDORF, G., M. DOUGLASS, and H. E. ROBINSON: Canine distemper in the rhesus monkey *(Macaca mulatta)*. J. exp. Med. **67**, 323—332 (1938 a).

DALLDORF, G., M. DOUGLASS, and H. E. ROBINSON: The sparing effect of canine distemper on poliomyelitis in *Macaca mulatta*. J. exp. Med. **67**, 333—343 (1938 b).

DALLDORF, G., C. W. JUNGEBLUT und M. DOUGLASS UMPHLET: Multiple Fälle von Choriomeningitis in einer Wohnung, in welcher infizierte Mäuse festgestellt wurden. Wien. med. Wschr. **96**, 473—474 (1946 a).

DALLDORF, G., C. W. JUNGEBLUT, and M. DOUGLASS UMPHLET: Multiple cases of choriomeningitis in an apartment harboring infected mice. J. Amer. med. Ass. **131**, 25 (only) (1946 b).

DALLDORF, G., and E. WHITNEY: A further interference in experimental poliomyelitis. Science **98**, 477—478 (1943).

DALTON, A. J., W. P. ROWE, G. H. SMITH, R. E. WILSNACK, and W. E. PUGH: Morphological and cytochemical studies on lymphocytic choriomeningitis virus. J. Virol. **2**, 1465—1478 (1968).

DANEŠ, L., R. BENDA a M. FUCHSOVÁ: Experimentální inhalační nákaza opic druhů Macacus cynomolgus a Macacus rhesus virem lymfocitární choriomeningitidy (kmenem WE). Bratisl. lek. Listy **43**, 71—79 (1963).

DEIBEL, R., C. OSTERHOUT, and L. QUINLAN: Propagation of lymphocytic choriomeningitis virus in chick embryo fibroblast cells. A. R. for 1964, Div. Lab. Res., N. Y. St. Dep. Hlth (Albany) p. 50, 1965.

DENT, P. B., R. D. A. PETERSON, and R. A. GOOD: A defect in cellular immunity during the incubation period of passage A leukemia in C3H mice. Proc. Soc. exp. Biol. (N. Y.) **119**, 869—871 (1965).

DICKENS, P. F.: Benign lymphocytic choriomeningitis. Sth. med. J. (Bgham, Ala.) **30**, 728—730 (1937).

DINGLE, J. H.: Infectious diseases of mice. In: Biology of the Laboratory Mouse. Ed.: G. D. SNELL. Philadelphia: The Blakiston Company 1941.

DOMINICK, D.: Lymphocytic choriomeningitis. J. Amer. med. Ass. **109**, 247—250 (1937).

DOUGHERTY, T. F.: Effect of hormones on lymphatic tissue. Physiol. Rev. **32**, 379—401 (1952).

DRESSER, D. W., and N. A. MITCHISON: The mechanism of immunological paralysis. Advanc. Immunol. **8**, 129—181 (1968).

DUNCAN, P. R., A. E. THOMAS, and J. O'H. TOBIN: Lymphocytic choriomeningitis. Review of ten cases. Lancet **I**, 956—959 (1951).

DURAND, P.: Virus filtrant pathogène pour l'homme et les animaux de laboratoire, et à affinités méningée et pulmonaire (Premier mémoire). Arch. Inst. Pasteur Tunis **29**, 179—227 (1940).

DURAND, P., P. GIROUD, E. LARRIVÉ et A. MESTRALLET: Transmission expérimentale à l'homme de la maladie des porchers. C. R. Acad. Sci. (Paris) **203**, 830—832 (1936 a).

DURAND, P., P. GIROUD, E. LARRIVÉ et A. MESTRALLET: Réceptivité des animaux au virus de la maladie des porchers. C. R. Acad. Sci. (Paris) **203**, 957—959 (1936 b).

DURAND, P., P. GIROUD, E. LARRIVÉ et A. MESTRALLET: Virulence des humeurs dans la maladie des porchers. C. R. Acad. Sci. (Paris) **203**, 1032—1034 (1936 c).

EAGLE, H.: Amino acid metabolism in mammalian cell cultures. Science **130**, 432—437 (1959).

EAGLE, H., K. HABEL, W. P. ROWE, and R. J. HUEBNER: Viral susceptibility of a human carcinoma cell (strain KB). Proc. Soc. exp. Biol. (N. Y.) **91**, 361—364 (1956).

EAST, J., D. M. V. PARROTT, and J. SEAMER: The ability of mice thymectomized at birth to survive infection with lymphocytic choriomeningitis virus. Virology **22**, 160—162 (1964).

EGGERS, H. J.: Quantitative Untersuchungen zur Komplementbindungsreaktion bei der lymphozytären Choriomeningitis. Arch. ges. Virusforsch. **8**, 221—229 (1958).

ELSON, C. J., and D. M. WEIR: Development of anti-tissue antibodies in rats. Clin. exp. Immunol. **4**, 241—246 (1969).

ELSON, L. A.: A comparison of the effects of radiation and radiomimetic chemicals on the blood. Brit. J. Haemat. **1**, 104—116 (1955).

EMMERICH, R.: Untersuchungen über das Vorkommen des Virus der lymphocytären Choriomeningitis bei Wildmäusen in Deutschland. Diss. Köln. 1962.

FARMER, T. W., and C. A. JANEWAY: Infections with the virus of lymphocytic choriomeningitis. Medicine (Baltimore) **21**, 1—63 (1942).

FAZEKAS DE ST. GROTH, S.: The neutralization of viruses. Advanc. Virus Res. **9**, 1—125 (1962).

FENJE, P.: Virus limfocitnog koriomeningita izolovan iz mozga poljskog miša. Med. Pregl. **9**, 381—384 (1956).

FERNANDES, M. V., T. J. WIKTOR, and H. KOPROWSKI: Endosymbiotic relationship between animal viruses and host cells. A study of rabies virus in tissue culture. J. exp. Med. **120**, 1099—1116 (1964).

FINDLAY, G. M., N. S. ALCOCK, and R. O. STERN: The virus aetiology of one form of lymphocytic meningitis. Lancet **I**, 650—654 (1936).

FINDLAY, G. M., E. KLIENEBERGER, F. O. MACCALLUM, and R. D. MACKENZIE: Rolling disease. New syndrome in mice associated with a pleuropneumonia-like organism. Lancet **II**, 1511—1513 (1938).

FINDLAY, G. M., and R. O. STERN: Pathological changes due to infection with the virus of lymphocytic choriomeningitis. J. Path. Bact. **43**, 327—338 (1936).

FINDLAY, G. M., C. H. STUART-HARRIS, and F. O. MACCALLUM: Lymphocytic choriomeningitis with report of a case. J. roy. Army med. Cps **75**, 8—15 (1940).

FÖLDES, P., I. SZERI, Z. BÁNOS, P. ANDERLIK és M. BALÁZS: Újszülöttkorban thymusirtott egerek lymphocytás choriomeningitis vírusfertőzése. Orv. Hetil. **105**, 2122—2126 (1964).

FÖLDES, P., I. SZERI, Z. BÁNOS, P. ANDERLIK, and M. BALÁZS: LCM infection of mice thymectomized in newborn age. Acta microbiol. Acad. Sci. hung. **11**, 277—282 (1964/65).

FÖLDES, P., I. SZERI, Z. BÁNOS, P. ANDERLIK és M. BALÁZS: Adatok az újszülöttkori thymectomiát követő "wasting syndroma" pathogenesiséhez. Orv. Hetil. **108**, 1021—1025 (1967).

FREUND, J.: The effect of heterologous bacterial products upon tuberculous animals. J. Immunol. **30**, 241—253 (1936).

FREYE, H.-A., und H. FREYE: Die Hausmaus. Wittenberg Lutherstadt: A. Ziemsen Verlag 1960.

FRIEDMAN, H., and W. S. CEGLOWSKI: Cellular basis for the immunosuppressive properties of a leukaemogenic virus. Nature (Lond.) **218**, 1232—1234 (1968).

FURUSAWA, E., and W. CUTTING: Antiviral activity of higher plants on lymphocytic choriomeningitis infection *in vitro* and *in vivo*. Proc. Soc. exp. Biol. (N. Y.) **122**, 280—282 (1966).

FURUSAWA, E., W. CUTTING, and A. FURST: Inhibitory effect of antiviral compounds on Columbia SK, LCM, Vaccinia and adeno type 12 viruses in vitro. Chemotherapia (Basel) **8**, 95—105 (1964).

FURUSAWA, E., S. FURUSAWA, M. KROPOSKI, and W. CUTTING: Activity of *Sambucus sieboldiana* on Columbia SK and LCM virus infection in mice. Proc. Soc. exp. Biol. (N. Y.) **128**, 1196—1199 (1968 a).

FURUSAWA, E., S. FURUSAWA, S. RAMANATHAN, and W. CUTTING: Further studies of antiviral activity of natural products on lymphocytic choriomeningitis infection. Chemotherapy (Basel) **13**, 172—180 (1968 b).

FURUSAWA, E., S. RAMANATHAN, S. FURUSAWA, Y. K. WOO, and W. CUTTING: Antiviral activity of higher plants and propionin on lymphocytic choriomeningitis infection. Proc. Soc. exp. Biol. (N. Y.) **125**, 234—239 (1967).

GABRIELSEN, A. E., and R. A. GOOD: Chemical suppression of adaptive immunity. Advanc. Immunol. **6**, 91—229 (1967).

GAJDAMOVICH, S. YA.: Izuchenije zarazshennosti domovykh gryzunov nejrovirusami. Soobshchenije 1. Zarazshennost domovykh myshej virusom limfotsitarnovo choriomeningita. Vop. Virus. **3**, 171—172 (1958).

GLADKIJ, A. P.: Vivchennya shtamu virusu limfotsitarnovo choriomeningitu vidilenovo vid klishchiv Ix. ricinus zibranikh v zakhidnikh oblastyakh URSR. Mikrobiol. Zh. A. N. U. R. S. R. **27**, 10—15 (1965).

GLEDHILL, A. W.: Fatal effect of some bacterial toxins on mice pre-infected with mouse hepatitis virus (MHV 1). J. gen. Microbiol. **18**, p. XVII (1958).

GLEDHILL, A. W.: Protective effect of anti-lymphocytic serum on murine lymphocytic choriomeningitis. Nature (Lond.) **214**, 178—179 (1967).

GLEDHILL, A. W., D. L. J. BILBEY, and J. S. F. NIVEN: Effect of certain murine pathogens on phagocytic activity. Brit. J. exp. Path. **46**, 433—442 (1965).

GLEDHILL, A. W., G. W. A. DICK, and J. S. F. NIVEN: Mouse hepatitis virus and its pathogenic action. J. Path. Bact. **69**, 299—309 (1955).

GLEDHILL, A. W., and J. SEAMER: The effect of *Eperythrozoon coccoides* upon lymphocytic choriomeningitis in mice. A. R. for 1960. Div. Lab. Res., N. Y. St. Dep. Hlth (Albany) p. 21, 1961.

GLEDHILL, A. W., J. SEAMER, and J. HOTCHIN: The relationship between mouse hepatitis and lymphocytic choriomeningitis virus. A. R. for 1960, Div. Lab. Res., N. Y. St. Dep. Hlth (Albany) p. 24, 1961.

GLUSHCHENKO, P. A., A. V. GUTSEVICH i M. S. DUDKINA: Issledovanie komarov kak perenoschikov virusa limfotsitarnovo choriomeningita na zapade Ukrainy. Dokl. Akad. Nauk SSSR, Otd. Biol. **113**, 1181—1183 (1957).

Goldberg, B. Ts.: Limfotsitarnyj choriomeningit. Nevropat. i. Psichiat. **19**, 33—35 (1950).

Grabar, P.: The problem of auto-antibodies. An approach to a theory. Tex. Rep. Biol. Med. **15**, 1—16 (1957).

Grater, W. C., and J. A. Rider: Lymphocytic choriomeningitis. Treatment of two cases with aureomycin. Tex. St. J. Med. **45**, 568—570 (1949).

Green, W. R., L. K. Sweet, and R. W. Prichard: Acute lymphocytic choriomeningitis. A study of twenty-one cases. J. Pediat. **35**, 688—701 (1949).

Grešíková, M., and J. Casals: A simple method of preparing a complement-fixing antigen for lymphocytic choriomeningitis virus. Acta virol. **7**, 380 (only) (1963).

Gsell, O.: Aetiologie der Schweinehüterkrankheit. Bull. schweiz. Akad. med. Wiss. **1**, 67—78 (1944—46).

Haas, V. H.: Studies on the natural history of the virus of lymphocytic choriomeningitis in mice. Publ. Hlth Rep. (Wash.) **56**, 285—292 (1941).

Haas, V. H.: Some relationships between lymphocytic choriomeningitis (LCM) virus and mice. J. infect. Dis. **94**, 187—198 (1954).

Haas, V. H.: Serial passage of a lymphocytic tumor and choriomeningitis virus in immune mice. J. nat. Cancer Inst. **25**, 75—83 (1960).

Haas, V. H., G. M. Briggs, and S. E. Stewart: Inapparent lymphocytic choriomeningitis infection in folic acid-deficient mice. Science **126**, 405—406 (1957 a).

Haas, V. H., and S. E. Stewart: Sparing effect of a-methopterin and guanazolo in mice infected with virus of lymphocytic choriomeningitis. Virology **2**, 511—516 (1956).

Haas, V. H., S. E. Stewart, and G. M. Briggs: Folic acid deficiency and the sparing of mice infected with the virus of lymphocytic choriomeningitis. Virology **3**, 15—21 (1957 b).

Habel, H.: Virus-induced tumor antigens. Curr. Top. Microbiol. Immunol. **41**, 85—99 (1967).

Hackett, E., and A. Thompson: Anti-lens antibody in human sera. Lancet **II**, 663—666 (1964).

Hamacher, E.: Zur serologischen Diagnostik von Parotitis epidemica und lymphozytärer Choriomeningitis. Diss. Köln. 1956.

Hammes, E. M.: Acute lymphocytic meningitis. Minn. Med. **21**, 151—154 (1938).

Hanaoka, M., S. Suzuki, and J. Hotchin: Thymus-dependent lymphocytes: destruction by lymphocytic choriomeningitis virus. Science **163**, 1216—1219 (1969).

Hannover Larsen, J.: On the induction of immunological tolerance to LCM virus in the adult mouse. Acta path. microbiol. scand., Suppl. No. 187, pp. 60—61 (1967).

Hannover Larsen, J.: Den lymphocytaere choriomeningitis virusinfection hos musen. Undersøgelser over den immunologiske tolerance over for virus. Thesis. København. 1968 a.

Hannover Larsen, J.: Studies on immunological tolerance to LCM virus. 9. Induction of immunological tolerance to the virus in the adult mouse. Acta path. microbiol. scand. **73**, 106—114 (1968 b).

Hannover Larsen, J.: On the induction of immunological tolerance to a self-reproducing antigen. Immunology **16**, 15—23 (1969 a).

Hannover Larsen, J.: Development of humoral and cell-mediated immunity to lymphocytic choriomeningitis virus in the mouse. J. Immunol. **102**, 941—946 (1969 b).

Hannover Larsen, J.: The effect of immunosuppressive therapy on the murine lymphocytic choriomeningitis virus infection. Acta path. microbiol. scand. **77**, 433—**446** (1969 c).

Hannover Larsen, J.: Immunological tolerance and the significance of cell-mediated immunity in virus infections. Dan. med. Bull. **16**, 146—154 (1969 d).

Hannover Larsen, J., and M. Volkert: Studies on immunological tolerance to LCM virus. 7. Adoptive immunization of virus carrier mice by grafts of normal syngeneic lymphoid cells. Acta path. microbiol. scand. **70**, 95—106 (1967).

HASSELT, J. A. VAN: Meningitis lymphocytaria benigna idiopathica. Ned. T. Geneesk. **90, IV**, 1492—1494 (1946).

HAUSSMANN, H. G.: Welche Virus-Encephalitiden kommen in Europa vor? Schweiz. Z. allg. Path. **18**, 1046—1055 (1955).

HAVENS, W. P.: Lymphocytic choriomeningitis. Report of a case occurring in a granary harboring infected mice. J. Amer. med. Ass. **137**, 857—858 (1948).

HAVENS, W. P., D. W. WATSON, R. H. GREEN, G. I. LAVIN, and J. E. SMADEL: Complement fixation with the neurotropic viruses. J. exp. Med. **77**, 139—153 (1943).

HAYES, G. S., and T. L. HARTMAN: Lymphocytic choriomeningitis. Report of a laboratory infection. Bull. Johns Hopk. Hosp. **73**, 275—286 (1943).

HECHTEL, M., T. DISHON, and W. BRAUN: Hemolysin formation in newborn mice of different strains. Proc. Soc. exp. Biol. (N. Y.) **120**, 728—732 (1965).

HENLE, G., and W. HENLE: Studies on the toxicity of influenza viruses. I. The effect of intracerebral injection of influenza viruses. J. exp. Med. **84**, 623—637 (1946).

HERRIOTT, R. M.: Infectious nucleic acids, a new dimension in virology. Science **134**, 256—260 (1961).

HEYL, J. T., H. F. ALLEN, and F. S. CHEEVER: Quantitative assay of neutralizing antibody content of pools of gamma globulin from different sections of the United States against the viruses of herpes simplex, lymphocytic choriomeningitis and epidemic keratoconjunctivitis. J. Immunol. **60**, 37—45 (1948).

HILDEMANN, W. H., and R. L. WALFORD: Autoimmunity in relation to aging as measured by agar plaque technique. Proc. Soc. exp. Biol. (N. Y.) **123**, 417—421 (1966).

HIRSCH, M. S., and F. A. MURPHY: The effect of anti-lymphocyte serum on lymphocytic choriomeningitis (LCM) virus infection in mice. Fed. Proc. **26**, 481 (only) (1967).

HIRSCH, M. S., and F. A. MURPHY: Effects of anti-lymphoid sera on viral infections. Lancet **II**, 37—40 (1968).

HIRSCH, M. S., F. A. MURPHY, and M. D. HICKLIN: Immunopathology of lymphocytic choriomeningitis virus infection of newborn mice. Antithymocyte serum effects on glomerulonephritis and wasting disease. J. exp. Med. **127**, 757—766 (1968).

HIRSCH, M. S., F. A. MURPHY, H. P. RUSSE, and M. D. HICKLIN: Effects of anti-thymocyte serum on lymphocytic choriomeningitis (LCM) virus infection in mice. Proc. Soc. exp. Biol. (N. Y.) **125**, 980—983 (1967).

HOLTERMANN, O. A., and J. A. MAJDE: Rejection of skin grafts from mice chronically infected with lymphocytic choriomeningitis virus by non-infected syngeneic recipients. Nature (Lond.) **223**, 624 (only) (1969).

HOTCHIN, J. E.: Some aspects of induced latent infection of mice with the virus of lymphocytic choriomeningitis. In: Symposium on Latency and Masking in Viral and Rickettsial Infections, Madison, Wis., 1957. Ed.: D. L. WALKER, R. P. HANSON, and A. S. EVANS. Minneapolis, Minn.: Burgess Publishing Co. 1958.

HOTCHIN, J.: Discussion. In: "Allergic" Encephalomyelitis. Ed. M. W. KIES and E. C. ALVORD. Springfield: Charles C Thomas 1959.

HOTCHIN, J. E.: The role of immunological tolerance in neonatal infection of mice with lymphocytic choriomeningitis virus. Quart. Rev. Pediat. **16**, 97—101 (1961).

HOTCHIN, J.: The biology of lymphocytic choriomeningitis infection: virus-induced immune disease. In: Basic Mechanisms in Animal Virus Biology. Cold Spr. Harb. Symp. quant. Biol. **27**, 479—499 (1962 a).

HOTCHIN, J.: The foot pad reaction of mice to lymphocytic choriomeningitis virus. Virology **17**, 214—216 (1962 b).

HOTCHIN, J.: Chronic disease following lymphocytic choriomeningitis virus inoculation and possible mechanisms of slow virus pathogenesis. In: Slow, Latent, and Temperate Virus Infections. NINDB Monograph No. 2. Ed.: D. C. GAJDUSEK, C. J. GIBBS, and M. ALPERS. Washington: U. S. Department of Health, Education, and Welfare 1965.

HOTCHIN, J.: Immune and autoimmune reactions in the pathogenesis of slow virus disease. Curr. Top. Microbiol. Immunol. **40**, 33—43 (1967).

HOTCHIN, J.: Lymphocytic choriomeningitis as a model of a persistent virus infection. In: International Virology. I. Ed.: J. L. MELNICK. Proc. First Internat. Congr. Virology, Helsinki 1968. Basel: S. Karger 1969.

HOTCHIN, J., and L. M. BENSON: Mouse-weight measurements as an index of virus disease. A. R. for 1961, Div. Lab. Res., N. Y. St. Dep. Hlth (Albany) pp. 42—43, 1962.

HOTCHIN, J., and L. BENSON: The pathogenesis of lymphocytic choriomeningitis in mice: the effects of different inoculation routes and the foodpad response. J. Immunol. **91**, 460—468 (1963).

HOTCHIN, J., L. M. BENSON, and D. N. COLLINS: Late-onset kidney disease of mice with persistent tolerant infection with lymphocytic choriomeningitis virus. Fed. Proc. **22, No. 2 Part I**, 441 (only) (1963).

HOTCHIN, J., L. M. BENSON, and J. SEAMER: Factors affecting the induction of persistent tolerant infection of newborn mice with lymphocytic choriomeningitis. Virology **18**, 71—78 (1962).

HOTCHIN, J., L. BENSON, and E. SIKORA: The detection of neutralizing antibody to lymphocytic choriomeningitis virus in mice. J. Immunol. **102**, 1128—1135 (1969).

HOTCHIN, J. E., and M. CINITS: Lymphocytic choriomeningitis infection of mice as a model for the study of latent virus infection. Canad. J. Microbiol. **4**, 149—163 (1958).

HOTCHIN, J., and D. N. COLLINS: Glomerulonephritis and late onset disease of mice following neonatal virus infection. Nature (Lond.) **203**, 1357—1359 (1964).

HOTCHIN, J., and E. SIKORA: Protection against the lethal effect of lymphocytic choriomeningitis virus in mice by neonatal thymectomy. Nature (Lond.) **202**, 214—215 (1964).

HOTCHIN, J. E., and H. WEIGAND: Relationship between age at inoculation and outcome of infection of mice with lymphocytic choriomeningitis virus. A. R. for 1959, Div. Lab. Res., N. Y. St. Dep. Hlth (Albany) p. 21, 1960.

HOTCHIN, J., and H. WEIGAND: Studies of lymphocytic choriomeningitis in mice. I. The relationship between age at inoculation and outcome of infection. J. Immunol. **86**, 392—400 (1961 a).

HOTCHIN, J., and H. WEIGAND: The effects of pretreatment with X-rays on the pathogenesis of lymphocytic choriomeningitis in mice. I. Host survival, virus multiplication and leukocytosis. J. Immunol. **87**, 675—681 (1961 b).

HOWARD, J. G., and D. MICHIE: Induction of transplantation immunity in the newborn mouse. Plast. reconstr. Surg., Transplant. Bull. **29**, 91—96 (1962).

HOWARD, M. E.: Lymphocytic choriomeningitis. A discussion of its diagnosis in man. J. infect. Dis. **64**, 66—77 (1939).

HOWARD, M. E.: Virus of lymphocytic choriomeningitis in man. Arch. Path. (Chic.) **29**, 725 (only) (1940).

HOWARD, M. E.: Infection with the virus of choriomeningitis in man. Yale J. Biol. Med. **13**, 161—180 (1940/41).

HOWARD, R. J., A. L. NOTKINS, and S. E. MERGENHAGEN: Inhibition of cellular immune reactions in mice infected with lactic dehydrogenase virus. Nature (Lond.) **221**, 873—874 (1969).

HOWITT, B. F.: Complement fixation test differentiating 3 strains of equine encephalomyelitic virus and the virus of lymphocytic choriomeningitis. Proc. Soc. exp. Biol. (N. Y.) **35**, 526—528 (1936/37).

HOWITT, B. F.: The complement fixation reaction in experimental equine encephalomyelitis, lymphocytic choriomeningitis and the St. Louis type of encephalitis. J. Immunol. **33**, 235—250 (1937).

HOWITT, B. F., and W. VAN HERICK: Attempted adaptation of the virus of poliomyelitis to wild rodents. Proc. Soc. exp. Biol. (N. Y.) **46**, 431—435 (1941).

HOWITT, B. F., and W. VAN HERICK: Relationship of the St. Louis and the western equine encephalitic viruses to fowl and mammals in California. J. infect. Dis. **71**, 179—191 (1942).

HRABA, T.: Mechanism and Role of Immunological Tolerance. Monographs in Allergy. Vol. 3. Basel: S. Karger 1968.

HRONOVSKÝ, V., R. BENDA a O. PROCHÁZKA: Použití imunofluorescence k detekci protilátek a vizualizaci antigenu u lymfocytární choriomeningitidy. Čs. Epidem. **18**, 90—97 (1969).

HUMPHREYS, F. A., D. E. HELMER, and R. J. GIBBONS: Studies on a virus disease originating in a guinea pig injected with ticks (*Dermacentor andersoni* Stiles). J. infect. Dis. **74**, 109—120 (1944).

HUMPHREYS, S. R., J. P. GLYNN, and A. GOLDIN: Suppression of the homograft response by pretreatment with antitumor agents. Transplantation **1**, 65—69 (1963).

ISAKOVIĆ, K., S. B. SMITH, and B. H. WAKSMAN: Role of the thymus in tolerance. I. Tolerance to bovine gamma globulin in thymectomized, irradiated rats grafted with thymus from tolerant donors. J. exp. Med. **122**, 1103—1123 (1965).

ISHIDATE, M., and D. METCALF: The pattern of lymphopoiesis in the mouse thymus after cortisone administration or adrenalectomy. Aust. J. exp. Biol. med. Sci. **41**, 637—649 (1963).

IVÁNOVICS, G., und A. KOCH: Lymphozytäre Choriomeningitis Virus- (Armstrong) Erkrankungen in Ungarn. Acta physiol. Acad. Sci. hung. **1**, 91—99 (1950).

IVÁNOVICS, G., S. KOCH és G. TÖRÖK: Az első igazolt lymphocytás choriomeningitis virus (Armstrong) fertőzés hazánkban. Orv. Lapja pp. 1493—1498, 1948.

JACOBIUS, H. F., and J. GRANDI: Choroiditis with lymphocytic choriomeningitis. Amer. J. Ophthal. **38**, 231 (only) (1954).

JOCHHEIM, K.-A., W. SCHEID, G. LIEDTKE, I. HANSEN und G. STAUSBERG: Komplementbindende Antikörper gegen das Virus der lymphozytären Choriomeningitis im Serum von Versuchstieren und Beobachtungen zur Immunität. Arch. ges. Virusforsch. **7**, 143—162 (1957).

JUBA, A., und J. PRIEVARA: Die Histopathologie der atypischen lymphozytären Virus-Meningitis. Confin. neurol. (Basel) **9**, 381—391 (1948).

JUNGEBLUT, C. W., and G. DALLDORF: Epidemiological and experimental observations of poliomyelitis in New York City (1943—1944). Amer. J. Hyg. **43**, 49—64 (1946).

JUNGEBLUT, C. W., and H. KODZA: Studies of leukemia L_2C in guinea pigs. Arch. ges. Virusforsch. **12**, 537—551 (1963 a).

JUNGEBLUT, C. W., and H. KODZA: Interference between lymphocytic choriomeningitis virus and the leukemia-transmitting agent of leukemia L_2C in guinea pigs. Arch. ges. Virusforsch. **12**, 552—560 (1963 b).

KAJIMA, M., and M. POLLARD: Arterial lesions in gnotobiotic mice congenitally infected with LCM virus. Nature (Lond.) **224**, 188—190 (1969).

KASAHARA, S., R. HAMANO, and R. YAMADA: Choriomeningitis virus isolated in the course of experimental studies on epidemic encephalitis. Kitasato Arch. exp. Med. **16**, 24—35 (1939).

KASAHARA, S., R. HAMANO, R. YAMADA to S. TSUBAKI: Ryūkōseinōen no jikkenteki kenkyūchū, bunri seraretaru myakurakunōmakuen-byōdoku. Trans. Soc. path. Jap. **27**, 581—585 (1937 a).

KASAHARA, S., R. YAMADA, and R. HAMANO: Choriodal meningitis virus isolated during the study of experimental encephalitis. Kitasato Arch. exp. Med. **14**, Abstract Section pp. 7—8 (1937 b).

KAUP, J., und J. KRETSCHMER: Kritik der Methodik der Wassermannschen Reaktion und neue Vorschläge für die quantitative Messung der Komplementbindung. Münch. med. Wschr. **64**, 158—161 (1917).

KELIHER, T. F.: The encephalitic form of benign lymphocytic choriomeningitis. Report of a case. Med. Ann. D. C. **13**, 373—376 and 397 (1944).

KELLER, R.: Passage of bacteriophage particles through intact skin of mice. Science **128**, 718—719 (1958).

KERSTING, G., und H. LENNARTZ: Lymphozytäre Choriomeningitis und Gliaknötchenenzephalitis. Dtsch. med. Wschr. **80**, 629—630 and 639 (1955).

KIDD, J. G., and W. F. FRIEDEWALD: A natural antibody that reacts *in vitro* with a sedimentable constituent of normal tissue cells. I. Demonstration of the phenomenon. J. exp. Med. **76**, 543—556 (1942 a).

KIDD, J. G., and W. F. FRIEDEWALD: A natural antibody that reacts *in vitro* with a sedimentable constituent of normal tissue cells. II. Specificity of the phenomenon: general discussion. J. exp. Med. **76**, 557—578 (1942 b).

KINCAID, J. E.: Hypoglycorrhachia with viral meningitis, probably lymphocytic choriomeningitis. Michigan Med. **66**, 966—967 (1967).

KOCH, S., M. PINTÉR és G. IVÁNOVICS: A lymphocytás choriomeningitis virus kóroktani és járványtani jelentősége Magyarországon. Orv. Hetil. **91**, 865—871 (1950 a).

KOCH, S., M. PINTÉR és G. IVÁNOVICS: A hazai lymphocytás choriomeningitis virus törzsek tulajdonságai. Kísérl. Orvostud. pp. 337—343, 1950 b.

KOLMER, J. A.: Discussion. Arch. Neurol. Psychiat. (Chic.) **36**, 1397—1398 (1936).

KOLTAY, M., R. G. KINSKY, B. G. ARNASON, and J. B. SCHAFFNER: Immunoglobulins and antibody formation in mice during the graft versus host reaction. Immunology **9**, 581—590 (1965).

KOLTAY, M., B. RADNAI, Z. BÁNOS, I. SZERI, P. ANDERLIK, and I. VIRÁG: Interaction of graft-versus-host reaction and lymphocytic choriomeningitis infection in mice: histopathological changes. Experientia (Basel) **25**, 1081—1083 (1969).

KOLTAY, M., I. VIRÁG, Z. BÁNOS, P. ANDERLIK, and I. SZERI: Interaction of graft-versus-host reaction and lymphocytic choriomeningitis infection in mice. Experientia (Basel) **24**, 63—65 (1968).

KOMROWER, G. M., B. L. WILLIAMS, and P. B. STONES: Lymphocytic choriomeningitis in the newborn. Probable transplacental infection. Lancet **I**, 697—698 (1955).

KOPROWSKI, H., T. J. WIKTOR, and M. M. KAPLAN: Enhancement of rabies virus infection by lymphocytic choriomeningitis virus. Virology **28**, 754—756 (1966).

KRAFT, L. M., and I. GORDON: Propagation of lymphocytic choriomeningitis virus in embryonated hens' eggs. J. Bact. **54**, 275—276 (1947).

KREIS, B.: Chorio-méningite lymphocytaire (maladie d'Armstrong). In: C. LEVADITI et P. LÉPINE: Les Ultravirus des Maladies Humaines. Paris: Librairie Maloine 1938.

KREIS, B.: La maladie d'Armstrong (chorio-meningite lymphocytaire). Sem. Hôp. Paris **24**, 1018—1023 (1948).

KÜPPER, B., H. BLOEDHORN, R. ACKERMANN und W. SCHEID: Über die Verbreitung des Virus der Lymphozytären Choriomeningitis unter den Mäusen in Westdeutschland. II. Untersuchungen an Mäusen, ausgenommen Mus musculus. Zbl. Bakt. I. Abt. Orig. **195**, 1—11 (1964/65).

LACORTE, J. G.: A coriomeningite linfocitária. Hospital (Rio de J.) **43**, 153—163 (1953).

LACORTE, J. G.: Meningopatias provocadas por vírus. 2 - A coriomeningite linfocitária benigna: propriedades do vírus causador, imunidade, epidemiologia, diagnóstico e tratamento. Rev. bras. Med. **21**, 319—323 (1964).

LACORTE, J. G., E. MONTEIRO y J. C. LOURES: Ação do radium sôbre o vírus da coriomeningite linfocitária benigna. Mem. Inst. Osw. Cruz **66**, 181—195 (1968).

LAFFIN, R. J., W. A. BARDAWIL, W. N. PACHAS, and J. S. MCCARTHY: Immunofluorescent studies on the occurrence of antinuclear factor in normal human serum. Amer. J. Path. **45**, 465—479 (1964).

LAIGRET, J., et R. DURAND: Virus isolé des souris et retrouvé chez l'homme au cours de la vaccination contre la fièvre jaune. C. R. Acad. Sci. (Paris) **203**, 282—284 (1936).

LAIGRET, J., et J. LAVILLAUREIX: Méningites lymphocytaires en Alsace. Bull. Acad. nat. Méd. (Paris) **138**, 504—506 (1954).

LAVILLAUREIX, J.: Enquête préliminaire sur l'étiologie des syndromes méningés du type lymphocytaire rencontrés en Alsace. Strasbourg méd. **5**, 248—254 (1954).

LAVILLAUREIX, J., et R. MINCK: Etude expérimentale de sept souches de virus de chorio-méningite lymphocytaire du type Armstrong, isolées chez l'homme. C. R. Soc. Biol. (Paris) **149**, 582—584 (1955).

LAVILLAUREIX, J., et E. REEB: Résultats de 18 mois d'enquête sur les maladies à virus en Alsace. Strasbourg méd. **8**, 497—503 (1957).

LAW, L. W., and R. C. TING: Immunologic competence and induction of neoplasms by polyoma virus. Proc. Soc. exp. Biol. (N. Y.) **119**, 823—830 (1965).

LAWRENCE, J. S., J. T. SYVERTON, R. J. ACKART, W. S. ADAMS, D. M. ERVIN, A. L. HASKINS, R. H. SAUNDERS, M. B. STRINGFELLOW, and R. M. WETRICH: The virus of infectious feline agranulocytosis. II. Immunological relation to other viruses. J. exp. Med. **77**, 57—64 (1943).

LEHMANN-GRUBE, F.: Untersuchungen zur Wärmestabilität des Virus der lymphozytären Choriomeningitis. Arch. ges. Virusforsch. **9**, 56—63 (1960).

LEHMANN-GRUBE, F.: Lymphocytic Choriomeningitis in the mouse. I. Growth in the brain. Arch. ges. Virusforsch. **14**, 344—350 (1964 a).

LEHMANN-GRUBE, F.: Lymphocytic choriomeningitis in the mouse. II. Establishment of carrier colonies. Arch. ges. Virusforsch. **14**, 351—357 (1964 b).

LEHMANN-GRUBE, F.: A carrier state of lymphocytic choriomeningitis virus in L cell cultures. Nature (Lond.) **213**, 770—773 (1967 a).

LEHMANN-GRUBE, F.: Latente Infektionen. Zbl. Bakt., I. Abt. Orig. **205**, 136—139 (1967 b).

LEHMANN-GRUBE, F.: Untersuchungen über das Virus der lymphozytären Choriomeningitis. I. Stabilisierung des Virus. Arch. ges. Virusforsch. **23**, 202—217 (1968).

LEHMANN-GRUBE, F.: Infection of L cells with LCM virus. In: International Virology. I. Ed.: J. L. MELNICK. Proc. First Internat. Congr. Virology, Helsinki 1968. Basel: S. Karger 1969 a.

LEHMANN-GRUBE, F.: Dose-response relationships of lymphocytic choriomeningitis viruses in mice and L cell tube cultures. J. Hyg. (Lond.) **67**, 269—278 (1969 b).

LEHMANN-GRUBE, F.: Dosis-Wirkungsbeziehungen von LCM-Virusstämmen in Mäusen und Zellkulturen. Zbl. Bakt., I. Abt. Ref. **215**, 546 (only) (1969 c).

LEHMANN-GRUBE, F.: Lymphocytic choriomeningitis in the mouse. III. Comparative titrations of virus strains in inbred mice. Arch. ges. Virusforsch. **28**, 303—307 (1969 d).

LEHMANN-GRUBE, F., R. ACKERMANN, K.-A. JOCHHEIM, G. LIEDTKE und W. SCHEID: Über die Technik der Neutralisation des Virus der lymphozytären Choriomeningitis in der Maus. Arch. ges. Virusforsch. **9**, 64—72 (1960).

LEHMANN-GRUBE, F., and R. HESSE: A new method for the titration of lymphocytic choriomeningitis viruses. (Brief report.) Arch. ges. Virusforsch. **20**, 256—259 (1967).

LEHMANN-GRUBE, F., und W. SLENCZKA: Über die Vermehrung von LCM-Virus (Stamm WE_3) in Zellkulturen. Zbl. Bakt., I. Abt. Ref. **206**, 525 (only) (1967).

LEHMANN-GRUBE, F., W. SLENCZKA, and R. TEES: A persistent and inapparent infection of L cells with the virus of lymphocytic choriomeningitis. J. gen. Virol. **5**, 63—81 (1969).

LEICHENGER, H., A. MILZER, and H. LACK: Recurrent lymphocytic choriomeningitis treated with sulfanilamide. Isolation of virus. J. Amer. med. Ass. **115**, 436—440 (1940).

LÉPINE, P.: Experimental infection of man with lymphocytic choriomeningitis. Third Internat. Congress Microbiology, New York 1939. Abstracts of Communications. Baltimore: Waverly Press, Inc. 1939.

LÉPINE, P., B. KREIS et V. SAUTTER: Sensibilité de la souris, du cobaye et du rat au virus parisien de la chorio-méningite lymphocytaire. C. R. Soc. Biol. (Paris) **124**, 420—422 (1937 a).

LÉPINE, P., P. MOLLARET et B. KREIS: Réceptivité de l'homme au virus murin de la chorioméningite lymphocytaire. Reproduction expérimentale de la méningite lymphocytaire bénigne. C. R. Acad. Sci. (Paris) **204**, 1846—1848 (1937 b).

LÉPINE, P., P. MOLLARET et V. SAUTTER: Application de la déviation du complement, à l'étude de la méningite lymphocytaire. Ann. Inst. Pasteur **61**, 868—869 (1938 a).

LÉPINE, P., P. MOLLARET et V. SAUTTER: Déviation du complément dans l'infection par le virus de la chorioméningite lymphocytaire. C. R. Soc. Biol. (Paris) **129**, 925—927 (1938 b).

LÉPINE, P., et V. SAUTTER: Existence en France du virus murin de la chorio-méningite lymphocytaire. C. R. Acad. Sci. (Paris) **202**, 1624—1626 (1936).

LÉPINE, P., et V. SAUTTER: Contamination de laboratoire avec le virus de la chorioméningite lymphocytaire. Ann. Inst. Pasteur **61**, 519—526 (1938).

Lépine, P., et V. Sautter: Études sur la pneumopathie des cobayes. I. — La maladie des cobayes. Ann. Inst. Pasteur **71**, 102—120 (1945).

Lépine, P., V. Sautter et B. Kreis: Siège de la virulence dans la chorio-méningite lymphocytaire; caractères du virus. C. R. Soc. Biol. (Paris) **124**, 422—424 (1937c).

Lépine, P., V. Sautter et R. Lamy: Un nouvel ultravirus: le virus de la pneumopathie des cobayes. C. R. Soc. Biol. (Paris) **137**, 317—318 (1943).

Lerner, E. M., and V. H. Haas: Histopathology of lymphocytic choriomeningitis in mice spared by amethopterin. Proc. Soc. exp. Biol. (N. Y.) **98**, 395—399 (1958).

Levey, R. H., N. Trainin, L. W. Law, P. H. Black, and W. P. Rowe: Lymphocytic choriomeningitis infection in neonatally thymectomized mice bearing diffusion chambers containing thymus. Science **142**, 483—485 (1963).

Levi, M. I., N. N. Basova i P. V. Rutshtejn: Laboratornaya diagnostika limfotsitarnovo choriomeningita pri pomoshchi reaktsii svyazyvaniya komplementa. Nevropat. i Psichiat. **20 (2)**, 5—12 (1951).

Levi, M. I., V. M. Gusev, L. N. Kislyakova, G. I. Chueva i R. I. Kiselev: Prirodnaya ochagovost limfotsitarnovo choriomeningita. Zh. Mikrobiol. (Mosk.) **8**, 76—81 (1953).

Levy, H. B., and V. H. Haas: Alteration of the course of lymphocytic choriomeningitis in mice by certain antimetabolites. Virology **5**, 401—407 (1958).

Lewis, A. M., W. P. Rowe, H. C. Turner, and R. J. Huebner: Lymphocytic-choriomeningitis virus in hamster tumor: spread to hamsters and humans. Science **150**, 363—364 (1965).

Lewis, J. M., and J. P. Utz: Orchitis, parotitis and meningoencephalitis due to lymphocytic-choriomeningitis virus. New Engl. J. Med. **265**, 776—780 (1961).

Lewis, V., and D. Clayton: Detection of lymphocytic choriomeningitis virus antibody in murine sera by immunofluorescence. Appl. Microbiol. **18**, 289—290 (1969 a).

Lewis, V., and D. Clayton: Enhanced resistance to arboviruses of mice with persistent lymphocytic choriomeningitis virus infection. Canad. J. Microbiol. **15**, 1468—1469 (1969 b).

Lillie, R. D.: Histopathologic reaction to the virus of lymphocytic choriomeningitis in the chick embryo. Publ. Hlth Rep. (Wash.) **51**, 41—42 (1936 a).

Lillie, R. D.: Pathologic histology of lymphocytic choriomeningitis in monkeys. Publ. Hlth Rep. (Wash.) **51**, 303—310 (1936 b).

Lillie, R. D., and C. Armstrong: Pathologic reaction to the virus of lymphocytic choriomeningitis in guinea pigs. Publ. Hlth Rep. (Wash.) **59**, 1391—1405 (1944).

Lillie, R. D., and C. Armstrong: Pathology of lymphocytic choriomeningitis in mice. Arch. Path. **40**, 141—152 (1945).

Lindorfer, R. K., and J. T. Syverton: The characterization of an unidentified virus found in association with line I leukemia. Proc. Amer. Ass. Cancer Res. **1 (1)**, 33—34 (1953/54).

Lucchesi, P. F.: Nonparalytic poliomyelitis versus choriomeningitis. J. Amer. med. Ass. **108**, 1494—1496 (1937).

Lundstedt, C.: Interaction between antigenically different cells. Virus-induced cytotoxicity by immune lymphoid cells *in vitro*. Acta path. microbiol. scand. **75**, 139—152 (1969 a).

Lundstedt, C.: Effect of antilymphocyte serum on adoptive immunization of lymphocytic choriomeningitis virus carrier mice. Acta path. microbiol. scand. **77**, 518—526 (1969 b).

Lundstedt, C., and M. Volkert: Studies on immunological tolerance to LCM virus. 8. Induction of tolerance to the virus in adult mice treated with anti-lymphocytic serum. Acta path. microbiol. scand. **71**, 471—480 (1967).

Lyon, R. A.: Period of antibody development to lymphocytic choriomeningitis in mice. Publ. Hlth Rep. (Wash.) **55**, 2178—2180 (1940).

MacCallum, F. O.: The virus of lymphocytic choriomeningitis (L.C.M.) as a cause of benign aseptic meningitis. Laboratory diagnosis of five cases. Mth. Bull. Minist. Hlth Lab. Serv. **8**, 177—183 (1949).

MacCallum, F. O., and G. M. Findlay: Lymphocytic choriomeningitis. Isolation of the virus from the nasopharynx. Lancet I, 1370—1373 (1939).
MacCallum, F. O., and G. M. Findlay: The cultivation of lymphocytic choriomeningitis in tissue culture. Brit. J. exp. Path. **21**, 110—116 (1940).
MacCallum, F. O., G. M. Findlay, and T. M. Scott: Pseudo-lymphocytic choriomeningitis. Brit. J. exp. Path. **20**, 260—269 (1939).
MacCallum, F. O., T. F. M. Scott, G. Dalldorf, and R. Gifford: "Pseudo-lymphocytic choriomeningitis": a correction. Brit. J. exp. Path. **38**, 120—121 (1957).
Machella, T. E., L. M. Weinberger, and S. W. Lippincott: Lymphocytic choriomeningitis. Report of a fatal case with autopsy findings. Amer. J. med. Sci. **197**, 617—625 (1939).
Mahy, B. W. J., K. E. K. Rowson, and M. H. Salaman: Plasma enzyme levels in virus-infected mice. Virology **23**, 528—541 (1964).
Maksudova, N. F.: Vliyanie predvaritelnovo rentgenovskovo oblucheniya na techenie limfotsitarnovo choriomeningita u myshej linii BALB/c. Vop. Virus. **12**, 724—729 (1967).
Mannweiler, Kl., und S. Smerdel: Ultrastrukturelle Veränderungen an maserninfizierten HeLa-Zellen bei immunolytischen Reaktionen. Proc. Fourth European Regional Conference on Electron Microscopy, Rome 1968. Vol. II. Roma: Tipografia Poliglotta Vaticana 1968.
Marcus, P. I., and D. H. Carver: Hemadsorption-negative plaque test: new assay for rubella virus revealing a unique interference. Science **149**, 983—986 (1965).
Maurer, F. D.: Lymphocytic choriomeningitis. J. nat. Cancer Inst. **20**, 867—870 (1958).
Maurer, F. D.: Lymphocytic choriomeningitis. Lab. Anim. Care (Baltimore) **14**, 415—419 (1964).
Medawar, P. B.: Immunological tolerance. Science **133**, 303—306 (1961).
Medawar, P.: Immunosuppressive agents, with special reference to antilymphocytic serum. Proc. roy. Soc. B **174**, 155—172 (1969).
Mendoza, M. A.: Répartition du virus de la chorioméningite lymphocytaire et virulence comparée des différents organes dans l'infection expérimentale du cobaye. C. R. Soc. Biol. (Paris) **125**, 600—602 (1937).
Merrit, H. H. (Clinic of): Diseases of the brain and nervous system: differential diagnosis and treatment. Med. clin. N. Amer. pp. 1477—1487, 1940.
Mesrobeanu, I., et G. Badenski: Contribution à l'étude expérimentale de deux souches de virus choriomeningite lymphocytaire isolées à Bucarest. Arch. roum. Path. exp. Microbiol. **15**, 253—255 (1948).
Metcalf, D.: The Thymus. Its Role in Immune Responses, Leukaemia Development and Carcinogenesis. Berlin: Springer 1966.
Meyer, H. M., R. T. Johnson, I. P. Crawford, H. E. Dascomb, and N. G. Rogers: Central nervous system syndromes of "viral" etiology. A study of 713 cases. Amer. J. Med. **29**, 334—347 (1960).
Meyer, K. F.: The host-parasite relationship in the heterogenous infection chains. Harvey Lect. Series 35 pp. 91—134 (1939/40).
Meynell, G. G.: Inherently low precision of infectivity titrations using a quantal response. Biometrics **13**, 149—163 (1957).
Michelson, A. M., E. S. Russell, and P. J. Harman: *Dystrophia muscularis*: a hereditary primary myopathy in the house mouse. Proc. nat. Acad. Sci. (Wash.) **41**, 1079—1084 (1955).
Miles, J. A. R.: Benign lymphocytic meningitis. Med. J. Aust. **I**, 659—664 (1954).
Milgrom, F., G. Woźniczko, and Z. Dudziak: Physiological production of auto-antibodies. Schweiz. Z. Path. **20**, 373—381 (1957).
Miller, J. F. A. P., and D. Osoba: Current concepts of the immunological function of the thymus. Physiol. Rev. **47**, 437—520 (1967).
Milzer, A.: Studies on the transmission of lymphocytic choriomeningitis virus by arthropods. J. infect. Dis. **70**, 152—172 (1942).

MILZER, A.: Neurotropic virus infections in Chicago, 1939—1941. Nine cases of lymphocytic choriomeningitis. Proc. Soc. exp. Biol. (N. Y.) **54**, 279—282 (1943).

MILZER, A., and S. O. LEVINSON: Laboratory infection with the virus of lymphocytic choriomeningitis. A two year study of antibody response. J. Amer. med. Ass. **120**, 27—30 (1942).

MILZER, A., and S. O. LEVINSON: Production of potent inactivated vaccines with ultraviolet irradiation. V. Active and passive immunization with lymphocytic choriomeningitis vaccine. J. Bact. **51**, 622 (only) (1946).

MILZER, A., and S. O. LEVINSON: Active immunization of mice with ultraviolet-inactivated lymphocytic choriomeningitis virus vaccine and results of immune serum therapy. J. infect. Dis. **85**, 251—255 (1949).

MIMS, C. A.: Intracerebral injections and the growth of viruses in the mouse brain. Brit. J. exp. Path. **41**, 52—59 (1960).

MIMS, C. A.: Immunofluorescence study of the carrier state and mechanism of vertical transmission in lymphocytic choriomeningitis virus infection in mice. J. Path. Bact. **91**, 395—402 (1966).

MIMS, C. A.: Pathogenesis of viral infections of the fetus. Progr. med. Virol. **10**, 194—237 (1968).

MIMS, C. A.: Effect on the fetus of maternal infection with lymphocytic choriomeningitis (LCM) virus. J. infect. Dis. **120**, 582—597 (1969).

MIMS, C. A., and T. P. SUBRAHMANYAN: Immunofluorescence study of the mechanism of resistance to superinfection in mice carrying the lymphocytic choriomeningitis virus. J. Path. Bact. **91**, 403—415 (1966).

MIMS, C. A., and F. A. TOSOLINI: Pathogenesis of lesions in lymphoid tissue of mice infected with lymphocytic choriomeningitis (LCM) virus. Brit. J. exp. Path. **50**, 584—592 (1969).

MIMS, C. A., and S. WAINWRIGHT: The immunodepressive action of lymphocytic choriomeningitis virus in mice. J. Immunol. **101**, 717—724 (1968).

MITCHELL, C. A., and M. O. KLOTZ: Lymphocytic choriomeningitis. Canad. J. publ. Hlth **33**, 208—213 (1942).

MITCHELL, G. F., and J. F. A. P. MILLER: Cell to cell interaction in the immune response. II. The source of hemolysin-forming cells in irradiated mice given bone marrow and thymus or thoracic duct lymphocytes. J. exp. Med. **128**, 821—837 (1968).

MITCHISON, N. A.: Passive transfer of transplantation immunity. Nature (Lond.) **171**, 267—268 (1953).

MITCHISON, N. A.: Passive transfer of transplantation immunity. Proc. roy. Soc. B **142**, 72—87 (1954).

MITTERMAYER, T., V. POLJAK, V. BARDOŠ, A. ŠIMKOVA und E. ČUPKOVA: Lymphozytäre Choriomeningitis in der Ostslowakei. Wien. klin. Wschr. **70**, 649—654 (1958).

MÖLLER, G.: Regulation of cellular antibody synthesis. Cellular 7S production and longevity of 7S antigen-sensitive cells in the absence of antibody feedback. J. exp. Med. **127**, 291—306 (1968).

MOLLARET, P., et G. M. FINDLAY: Étude étiologique et microbiologique d'un cas de méningo-encéphalite au cours de la séro-vaccination anti-amarile. Bull. Soc. Path. exot. **29**, 176—185 (1936).

MOLLARET, P., P. LÉPINE et B. KREIS: Les modifications leucocytaires dans la choriomeningite expérimentale. C. R. Soc. Biol. (Paris) **131**, 1003—1005 (1939).

MOLNÁR, E.: Lymphocytás choriomeningitis virusizolálással igazolt esete Budapesten. Orv. Hetil. **94**, 208—211 (1953).

MOLOMUT, N., and M. PADNOS: Inhibition of transplantable and spontaneous murine tumours by the M-P virus. Nature (Lond.) **208**, 948—950 (1965).

MORI, R., K. NOMOTO, and K. TAKEYA: Effects of neonatal thymectomy on foot pad reaction caused by lymphocytic choriomeningitis virus inoculation. Proc. Jap. Acad. **40**, 772—775 (1964).

MORRIS, J. A., and A. D. ALEXANDER: Lymphocytic choriomeningitis virus from gray mice trapped in a rural area. Cornell Vet. **41**, 122—123 (1951).

MURPHY, B. W.: Benign lymphocytic meningitis. A report of two cases with reduction of chlorides in the cerebrospinal fluid. N. Z. med. J. **46**, 37—39 (1947).

MURPHY, F. A., P. A. WEBB, K. M. JOHNSON, and S. G. WHITFIELD: Morphological comparison of Machupo with lymphocytic choriomeningitis virus: basis for a new taxonomic group. J. Virol. **4**, 535—541 (1969).

NADEL, E., and V. HAAS: Inhibitory effect of virus of lymphocytic choriomeningitis on course of leukemia in guinea pigs. Fed. Proc. **14**, 414—415 (1955).

NADEL, E. M., and V. H. HAAS: Effect of the virus of lymphocytic choriomeningitis on the course of leukemia in guinea pigs and mice. J. nat. Cancer Inst. **17**, 221—231 (1956).

NAKANE, P. K., and G. B. PIERCE: Enzyme-labeled antibodies: preparation and application for the localization of antigens. J. Histochem. Cytochem. **14**, 929—931 (1966).

NAYAK, K. K., S. O. WALLER, and G. KUPPUSWAMY: Encephalitis syndrome of lymphocytic choriomeningitis virus infection. Brit. med. J. **I**, 162—164 (1964).

NIHOUL, E., et S. LECOMTE-RAMIOUL: Diagnostic sérologique de la chorioméningite lymphocytaire. Acta clin. belg. **8**, 482—483 (1953).

NIKOLITSCH, M.: Der Weg des neurotropen Virus, dargestellt in Modellversuchen an Tollwut und lymphozytärer Choriomeningitis. Zbl. Bakt., I. Abt. Orig. **175**, 1—10 (1959).

NIKOLITSCH, M., und P. FENJE: Viraemie und lymphocytäre Chorio-Meningitis. Arch. Hyg. (Berl.) **141**, 161—167 (1957).

NIKOLITSCH, M., und P. FENJE: Der Weg des von der Peripherie aus inokulierten lymphocytären Chorio-Meningitis-Virus. Arch. Hyg. (Berl.) **143**, 204—212 (1959).

NORINS, L. C., and M. C. HOLMES: Antinuclear factor in mice. J. Immunol. **93**, 148—154 (1964).

NOTKINS, A. L.: Lactic dehydrogenase virus. Bact. Rev. **29**, 143—160 (1965).

NOTKINS, A. L., S. E. MERGENHAGEN, A. A. RIZZO, C. SCHEELE, and T. A. WALDMANN: Elevated γ-globulin and increased antibody production in mice infected with lactic dehydrogenase virus. J. exp. Med. **123**, 347—364 (1966).

ODAKA, T., H. ISHII, K. YAMAURA, and T. YAMAMOTO: Inhibitory effect of Friend leukemia virus infection on the antibody formation to sheep erythrocytes in mice. Jap. J. exp. Med. **36**, 277—290 (1966).

OLDSTONE, M. B. A.: A neurologist looks at (to) the kidney. Trans. Amer. neurol. Ass. **94**, 42—43 (1969).

OLDSTONE, M. B. A., and F. J. DIXON: Lymphocytic choriomeningitis: production of antibody by "tolerant" infected mice. Science **158**, 1193—1195 (1967).

OLDSTONE, M. B. A., and F. J. DIXON: The immunological response of LCM viral carrier mice and associated pathologic changes. Fed. Proc. **27**, 261 (only) (1968 a).

OLDSTONE, M. B. A., and F. J. DIXON: Susceptibility of different mouse strains to lymphocytic choriomeningitis virus. J. Immunol. **100**, 355—357 (1968 b).

OLDSTONE, M. B. A., and F. J. DIXON: Direct immunofluorescent tissue culture assay for lymphocytic choriomeningitis virus. J. Immunol. **100**, 1135—1138 (1968 c).

OLDSTONE, M. B. A., and F. J. DIXON: Pathogenesis of chronic disease associated with persistent lymphocytic choriomeningitis viral infection. I. Relationship of antibody production to disease in neonatally infected mice. J. exp. Med. **129**, 483—505 (1969).

OLDSTONE, M. B. A., K. HABEL, and F. J. DIXON: The pathogenesis of cellular injury associated with persistent LCM viral infection. Fed. Proc. **28**, 429 (only) (1969).

OLSON, G. B., P. B. DENT, W. E. RAWLS, M. A. SOUTH, J. R. MONTGOMERY, J. L. MELNICK, and R. A. GOOD: Abnormalities of *in vitro* lymphocyte responses during rubella virus infections. J. exp. Med. **128**, 47—68 (1968).

OSBORN, J. E., A. A. BLAZKOVEC, and D. L. WALKER: Immunosuppression during acute murine cytomegalovirus infection. J. Immunol. **100**, 835—844 (1968).

OVERMAN, J. R., and W. F. FRIEDEWALD: Multiplication of certain neurotropic viruses in the rabbit eye following intraocular inoculation. J. exp. Med. **91**, 39—51 (1950).

OWEN, R. D.: Immunogenetic consequences of vascular anastomoses between bovine twins. Science **102**, 400—401 (1945).

PAUKALÉN, T.: On the development of non-specific hyperergy in experimental tuberculosis and its significance for the subsequent course of the infection. Acta path. microbiol. scand., Suppl. No. **91**, pp. 126—134 (1951).

PANOV, A. G., i P. I. REMEZOV: Vliyanije kisloroda pod davleniem na techenije nekotorykh eksperimentalnykh nejrovirusnykh infektsij u belykh myshej. Vop. Virus. **5**, 267—272 (1960).

PANOV, A. G., P. I. REMEZOV i A. I. SHVAREV: Diagnostika limfotsitarnovo choriomeningita. Zh. Nevropat. Psikhiat. **63**, 1441—1444 (1963).

PANOV, A. G., i A. I. SHVAREV: K epidemiologii limfotsitarnovo choriomeningita. Vo.-med. Zh. **6**, 53—55 (1966).

PARIKH, G. C.: Cytological changes by lymphocytic choriomeningitis virus in the human amnion cells. Jap. J. Microbiol. **5**, 129—132 (1961).

PARRY, J.: A small outbreak of acute benign lymphocytic choriomeningitis. Med. J. Aust. **I**, 745—749 (1951).

PEDERSEN, I. R.: Methanol precipitation of lymphocytic choriomeningitis virus. Acta path. microbiol. scand. **67**, 514—522 (1966).

PEDERSEN, I. R., and M. VOLKERT: Multiplication of lymphocytic choriomeningitis virus in suspension cultures of Earle's strain L cells. Acta path. microbiol. scand. **67**, 523—536 (1966).

PERRIN, T. L., and E. A. STEINHAUS: Pathologic reaction in guinea pigs to the Humphreys' virus strain. Publ. Hlth Rep. (Wash.) **59**, 1603—1609 (1944).

PETERSON, O. P., i N. F. MAKSUDOVA: Vozrastnaya chuvstvitelnost belykh myshej k virusu limfotsitarnovo choriomeningita. Vop. Virus. **14**, 42—48 (1969).

PETERSON, R. D. A., R. HENDRICKSON, and R. A. GOOD: Reduced antibody forming capacity during the incubation period of passage A leukemia in C_3H mice. Proc. Soc. exp. Biol. (N. Y.) **114**, 517—520 (1963).

PETROVIĆ, M., und H. TIMM: Latente Infektion des syrischen Goldhamsters (Mesocricetus auratus auratus) mit dem Virus der lymphocytären Choriomeningitis (LCM). Zbl. Bakt., I. Abt. Orig. **207**, 435—442 (1968).

PFAU, C. J.: Biophysical and biochemical characterization of lymphocytic choriomeningitis virus. 1. Density gradient studies. Acta path. microbiol. scand. **63**, 188—197 (1965 a).

PFAU, C. J.: Biophysical and biochemical characterization of lymphocytic choriomeningitis virus. 2. Partial purification by differential centrifugation and fluorocarbon techniques. Acta path. microbiol. scand. **63**, 198—205 (1965 b).

PFAU, C. J.: Purification of virus-like structures from cells infected with lymphocytic choriomeningitis virus. In: International Virology. I. Ed.: J. L. MELNICK. Proc. First Internat. Congr. Virology, Helsinki 1968. Basel: S. Karger 1969.

PFAU, C. J., and K. P. CAMYRE: Biophysical and biochemical characterization of lymphocytic choriomeningitis virus. III. Thermal and ultrasonic sensitivity. Arch. ges. Virusforsch. **20**, 430—437 (1967).

PFAU, C. J., and K. P. CAMYRE: Inhibition of lymphocytic choriomeningitis virus multiplication by 2-(α-hydroxybenzyl)benzimidazole. Virology **35**, 375—380 (1968).

PFAU, C. J., I. R. PEDERSEN, and M. VOLKERT: Inability of nucleic acid analogues to inhibit the synthesis of lymphocytic choriomeningitis virus. Acta path. microbiol. scand. **63**, 181—187 (1965).

PINHEIRO, F. P., R. E. SHOPE, A. H. PAES DE ANDRADE, G. BENSABATH, G. V. CACIOS, and J. CASALS: Amapari, a new virus of the Tacaribe group from rodents and mites of Amapa Territory, Brazil. Proc. Soc. exp. Biol. (N. Y.) **122**, 531—535 (1966).

PINTO, M. R., e C. F. FERREIRA: Un cas de chorioméningite lymphocytaire isolé à Lisbonne. Med. contemp. **72**, 417—418 (1954).

PIRQUET, C. VON: Allergie. Münch. med. Wschr. **53**, 1457—1458 (1906).

PIRQUET, C. VON: Klinische Studien über Vakzination und Vakzinale Allergie. Leipzig: Franz Deuticke 1907.

PLAYFAIR, J. H. L.: Strain differences in the immune response of mice. I. The neonatal response to sheep red cells. Immunology **15**, 35—50 (1968).

PLAYFAIR, J. H. L.: Specific tolerance to sheep erythrocytes in mouse bone marrow cells. Nature (Lond.) **222**, 882—883 (1969).

POLJAK, V., a V. BÁRDOŠ: Laboratorní nákaza virusem lymfocytární choriomeningitidy. Čas. Lék. čes. **97**, 1185—1191 (1958).

POLLARD, M., M. KAJIMA, and N. SHARON: LCM virus-induced immunopathology in congenitally infected gnotobiotic mice. In: Virus-Induced Immunopathology. Perspectives in Virology. VI. Ed.: M. POLLARD. Academic Press: New York 1968 a.

POLLARD, M., and N. SHARON: Immunoproliferative effects of lymphocytic choriomeningitis virus in germfree mice. Proc. Soc. exp. Biol. (N. Y.) **132**, 242—246 (1969).

POLLARD, M., N. SHARON, and B. A. TEAH: Congenital lymphocytic choriomeningitis virus infection in gnotobiotic mice. Proc. Soc. exp. Biol. (N. Y.) **127**, 755—761 (1968 b).

POLLIKOFF, R., and M. M. SIGEL: Factors influencing the neutralization of lymphocytic choriomeningitis virus. Bact. Proc. pp. 105—106, 1952.

POTTER, M., and V. H. HAAS: Relationships between lymphocytic choriomeningitis virus, amethopterin, and an amethopterin-resistant lymphocytic neoplasm in mice. J. nat. Cancer Inst. **22**, 801—809 (1959).

PRICK, J. J. G.: Virusmeningitis. I. Clinical part. Antonie v. Leeuwenhoek **11**, 177—180 (1946).

PRICK, J. J. G., en J. D. VERLINDE: Chorio-meningitis in Nederland. Ned. T. Geneesk. **91, II**, 1146—1157 (1947).

RABINOWITZ, Y.: Separation of lymphocytes, polymorphonuclear leukocytes and monocytes on glass columns, including tissue culture observations. Blood **23**, 811—828 (1964).

RAFF, M. C.: Theta isoantigen as a marker of thymus-derived lymphocytes in mice. Nature (Lond.) **224**, 378—379 (1969).

RAMANATHAN, S., E. FURUSAWA, and W. C. CUTTING: An anti-LCM agent from Propionibacteria. Chemotherapy (Basel) **13**, 271—275 (1968).

RAMANATHAN, S., E. FURUSAWA, G. READ, and W. CUTTING: Isolation and activity of propionin A, an antiviral polypeptide from Propionibacteria. Chemotherapia (Basel) **10**, 197—204 (1965/66).

RAMANATHAN, S., G. READ, and W. CUTTING: Purification of propionin, an antiviral agent from Propionibacteria. Proc. Soc. exp. Biol. (N. Y.) **123**, 271—273 (1966).

RASMUSSEN, A. F.: The laboratory diagnosis of lymphocytic choriomeningitis and mumps. Proceedings of the Rocky Mountain Conference on Infantile Paralysis, Denver, Col., 1946. Denver, 1947.

ŘEHÁČEK, J.: Cultivation of different viruses in tick tissue cultures. Acta virol. **9**, 332—337 (1965).

REIMANN, H. A.: Infectious diseases. Review of current literature. Arch. intern. Med. **60**, 337—384 (1937).

REISS-GUTFREUND, R. J.: Antagonisme entre un virus de chorioméningite lymphocytaire (C.M.L.) et *Rickettsia prowazeki*. Note préliminaire. Ann. Inst. Pasteur **102**, 227—231 (1962).

REISS-GUTFREUND, R. J., L. ANDRAL et C. SÉRIÉ: Étude d'un virus présentant les caractéristiques de la chorio-méningite lymphocytaire (C.M.L.) isolé en Éthiopie. Ann. Inst. Pasteur **102**, 36—43 (1962).

REISS-GUTFREUND, R. J., C. SÉRIÉ et L. ANDRAL: Étude de souches virales présentant les caractéristiques de chorioméningite lymphocytaire (C.M.L.) isolées en Éthiopie. Ann. Inst. Pasteur **101**, 427—442 (1961).

REMEZOV, P. I., i K. A. TOPLENINOVA: Obnaruzshenije virusa limfotsitarnovo choriomeningita s pomoshchyu nepryamovo metoda fluorestsiruyushchikh antitel. Vop. Psikhiat. Nevropat. (Leningrad) **7**, 113—120 (1961).

REMEZOV, P. I., i S. D. YAKOVLEVA: Izmeneniya urovnya properdina v syvorotkakh krovi obluchennykh i neobluchennykh belykh myshej pri eksperimentalnom limfotsitarnom choriomeningite. Vop. Virus. **5**, 431—435 (1960).

RHODES, A. J., and M. CHAPMAN: Some observations on interference between neurotropic viruses. Canad. J. Res., E **27**, 341—348 (1949).

RHODES, A. J., and M. CHAPMAN: Further observations on interference between lymphocytic choriomeningitis and MM viruses. Canad. J. Res., E **28**, 245—255 (1950).

RHODES, A. J., and C. E. VAN ROOYEN: Lymphocytic choriomeningitis. In: Textbook of Virology. Fifth ed. Baltimore: Williams and Wilkins Co. 1968.

RIVERS, T. M.: Lane Medical Lectures: Viruses and Virus Diseases. Stanford University Publications, University Series, Medical Sciences Vol. IV, number 1. Stanford, Calif.: Stanford University Press 1939.

RIVERS, T. M., and T. F. M. SCOTT: Meningitis in man caused by a filterable virus. Science **81**, 439—440 (1935).

RIVERS, T. M., and T. F. M. SCOTT: Meningitis in man caused by a filterable virus. II. Identification of the etiological agent. J. exp. Med. **63**, 415—432 (1936 a).

RIVERS, T. M., and T. F. M. SCOTT: Five cases of lymphocytic choriomeningitis in man. Trans. Amer. pediat. Soc. **48**, 41—42 (1936 b).

ROGER, F.: Étude sur le pouvoir pathogène du virus de la chorioméningite lymphocytaire. I. — Réactivité dermique chez le lapin. Ann. Inst. Pasteur **103**, 639—656 (1962).

ROGER, F.: Études sur le pouvoir pathogène expérimental du virus de la chorioméningite lymphocytaire. II. — Inoculation dans le derme du cobaye. Ann. Inst. Pasteur **104**, 274—283 (1963 a).

ROGER, F.: Études sur le pouvoir pathogène expérimental du virus de la chorioméningite lymphocytaire. III. — Une réaction inflammatoire directement visible chez la souris l'oedème viral du membre inférieur. Ann. Inst. Pasteur **104**, 347—360 (1963b).

ROGER, F., and J. HOTCHIN: Local reactivity to lymphocytic choriomeningitis virus in the mouse; its development as a new diagnostic test. A. R. for 1961, Div. Lab. Res., N. Y. St. Dep. Hlth (Albany) pp. 43—44, 1962.

ROGER, F., et A. ROGER: Études sur le pouvoir pathogène expérimental du virus de la chorioméningite lymphocytaire. IV. — Niveau de mortalité des souris après inoculation sous-cutanée plantaire. Ann. Inst. Pasteur **105**, 476—485 (1963 a).

ROGER, F., et A. ROGER: Études sur le pouvoir pathogène expérimental du virus de la chorioméningite lymphocytaire. V. — Distribution de la mortalité des souris au cours des réactions locales. Ann. Inst. Pasteur **105**, 612—623 (1963 b).

ROGER, F., et A. ROGER: Études sur le pouvoir pathogène expérimental du virus de la chorioméningite lymphocytaire. VI.— Mortalité des souris selon le mode d'inoculation et selon la dose. Ann. Inst. Pasteur **106**, 588—601 (1964 a).

ROGER, F., et A. ROGER: Études sur le pouvoir pathogène expérimental du virus de la chorioméningite lymphocytaire. VII. — L'allergie dans les réactions locales chez la souris et ses conditions de démonstration. Ann. Inst. Pasteur **107**, 354—365 (1964 b).

ROGER, F., et A. ROGER: Titrage local du virus de la chorioméningite lymphocytaire chez la souris. I. — Position du problème. Méthodes. Traitement "en tout ou rien". Ann. Inst. Pasteur **106**, 439—448 (1964 c).

ROGER, F., et A. ROGER: Titrage local du virus de la chorioméningite lymphocytaire chez la souris. II. — Étude quantitative par la méthode des courbes de latence. Ann. Inst. Pasteur **106**, 738—751 (1964 d).

ROGER, F., et A. ROGER: Titrage local du virus de la chorioméningite lymphocytaire chez la souris. III. — Liaison entre la durée ou l'étendue de la réaction locale et la concentration de virus inoculée. Implications théoriques et pratiques. Ann. Inst. Pasteur **106**, 878—893 (1964 e).

ROGER, F., et A. ROGER: Le "masquage immunologique" des virus. Influence des récepteurs sur le résultat apparent de la réaction antigène-anticorps en virologie. C. R. Acad. Sci. (Paris) **259**, 2571—2572 (1964 f).

ROGER, F., et A. ROGER: Effet des anticorps neutralisants, passivement transmis, sur les maladies à virus locales de type différé: le phénomène d'immunisation accélérée. C. R. Acad. Sci. (Paris) **259**, 4886—4888 (1964 g).

ROGER, F., et A. ROGER: Trois modalités d'action des anticorps en immunologie virale. I. — Le "masquage" des virus par les anticorps. Influence du récepteur sur les résultats apparents des réactions de séro-neutralisation. Ann. Inst. Pasteur **108**, 166—179 (1965 a).

Roger, F., et A. Roger: Immunité de diffusion et phénomènes de protection par les anticorps en virologie. C. R. Acad. Sci. (Paris) **261**, 2027—2029 (1965 b).

Roger, F., et A. Roger: Trois modalités d'action des anticorps en immunologie virale. II. — L'immunité de diffusion et les phénomènes de séro-protection. Ann. Inst. Pasteur **110**, 218—232 (1966).

Rogers, N. G.: The effect of Merthiolate on the infectivity of certain viruses. J. Lab. clin. Med. **38**, 483—485 (1951).

Ronse, M.: Le virus de la chorio-méningite de la souris. C. R. Soc. Biol. (Paris) **125**, 393—395 (1937).

Rooyen, C. E. van, and A. J. Rhodes: Acute lymphocytic choriomeningitis. In: Virus Diseases of Man. New York: Thomas Nelson and Sons 1948.

Rosenthal, S. M., J. G. Wooley, and H. Bauer: Studies in chemotherapy. VI. The chemotherapy of choriomeningitis virus infection in mice with sulfonamide compounds. Publ. Hlth Rep. (Wash.) **52**, 1211—1217 (1937).

Rowe, W. P.: Studies on pathogenesis and immunity in lymphocytic choriomeningitis infection of the mouse. Naval Medical Research Institute, Research Report: NM 005 048.14.01, 1954.

Rowe, W. P.: Protective effect of pre-irradiation on lymphocytic choriomeningitis infection in mice. Proc. Soc. exp. Biol. (N. Y.) **92**, 194—198 (1956).

Rowe, W. P., P. H. Black, and R. H. Levey: Protective effect of neonatal thymectomy on mouse LCM infection. Proc. Soc. exp. Biol. (N. Y.) **114**, 248—251 (1963).

Rowley, D. A., and F. W. Fitch: The mechanism of tolerance produced in rats to sheep erythrocytes. II. The plaque-forming cell and antibody response to multiple injections of antigen begun at birth. J. exp. Med. **121**, 683—695 (1965).

Rustigian, R.: Persistent infection of cells in culture by measles virus. II. Effect of measles antibody on persistently infected HeLa sublines and recovery of a HeLa clonal line persistently infected with incomplete virus. J. Bact. **92**, 1805—1811 (1966).

Salaman, M. H., and N. Wedderburn: The immunodepressive effect of Friend virus. Immunology **10**, 445—458 (1966).

Scheid, W.: Ueber akute idiopathische abakterielle Meningitiden. Dtsch. Z. Nervenheilk. **159**, 269—298 (1948).

Scheid, W.: Das Virus der lymphozytären Choriomeningitis und seine Bedeutung für die Neurologie. Fortschr. Neurol. Psychiat. **25**, 73—99 (1957).

Scheid, W.: Lymphozytäre Choriomeningitis. In: R. Haas und O. Vivell: Virus- und Rickettsieninfektionen des Menschen. München: J. F. Lehmanns Verlag 1965.

Scheid, W., a R. Ackermann: Postencefalitický Parkinsonov syndróm a otázka sporadickej encephalitis lethargica (v. Economo). Bratisl. lek. Listy **51**, 335—339 (1969).

Scheid, W., R. Ackermann, H. Bloedhorn und B. Küpper: Über die Verbreitung des Virus der Lymphozytären Choriomeningitis in Westdeutschland. Dtsch. med. Wschr. **89**, 325—328 (1964).

Scheid, W., R. Ackermann, H. Bloedhorn, B. Küpper und I. Winkens: Untersuchungen zur Epidemiologie des Virus der Lymphocytären Choriomeningitis (LCM) in Westdeutschland. Forschungsberichte des Landes Nordrhein-Westfalen Nr. 1633. Köln: Westdeutscher Verlag 1966.

Scheid, W., R. Ackermann und K. Felgenhauer: Lymphozytäre Choriomeningitis unter dem Bild der Encephalitis lethargica. Dtsch. med. Wschr. **93**, 940—943 (1968).

Scheid, W., R. Ackermann und K.-A. Jochheim: Die Bedeutung der komplementbindenden und der neutralisierenden Antikörper für die Diagnose der Infektionen mit dem Virus der lymphozytären Choriomeningitis. Dtsch. med. Wschr. **84**, 1293—1296 (1959).

Scheid, W., R. Ackermann, K.-A. Jochheim und F. Lehmann-Grube: Die neutralisierenden Serumantikörper des Menschen nach Infektionen mit dem Virus der lymphozytären Choriomeningitis und das Verhalten von Normalseren im Neutralisationsversuch. Arch. ges. Virusforsch. **9**, 295—309 (1960).

Scheid, W., und K.-A. Jochheim: Akute Encephalomyelitis und Virus der lymphocytären Choriomeningitis. Nervenarzt **27**, 385—388 (1956 a).

Scheid, W., und K.-A. Jochheim: Infektionen mit dem Virus der lymphozytären Choriomeningitis in Deutschland. Dtsch. med. Wschr. **81**, 700—703 (1956 b).

Scheid, W., K.-A. Jochheim und W. Mohr: Laboratoriumsinfektionen mit dem Virus der lymphocytären Choriomeningitis. Dtsch. Arch. klin. Med. **203**, 88—109 (1956a).

Scheid, W., K.-A. Jochheim und A. Stammler: Tödlicher Verlauf einer Infektion mit dem Virus der lymphocytären Choriomeningitis. Dtsch. Z. Nervenheilk. **174**, 123—139 (1956b).

Schell, K., R. J. Huebner, and H. C. Turner: Concentration of complement fixing viral antigens. Proc. Soc. exp. Biol. (N. Y.) **121**, 41—46 (1966).

Schleifstein, J., and D. N. Collins: The pathology of lymphocytic choriomeningitis in nonirradiated and radiated mice. A. R. for 1959, Div. Lab. Res., N. Y. St. Dep. Hlth (Albany) p. 22, 1960.

Schlesinger, M.: Spontaneous occurrence of autoantibodies cytotoxic to thymus cells in the sera of mice of the 129 strain. Nature (Lond.) **207**, 429—430 (1965).

Schmidt, N. J., and H. B. Harding: The demonstration of substances in human sera which inhibit complement fixation in antigen-antibody systems of lymphogranuloma venereum, psittacosis, mumps, Q fever, and lymphocytic choriomeningitis. J. Bact. **71**, 217—222 (1956).

Scott, T. F. M., and W. J. Elford: The size of the virus of lymphocytic choriomeningitis as determined by ultrafiltration and ultracentrifugation. Brit. J. exp. Path. **20**, 182—188 (1939).

Scott, T. F. M., and T. M. Rivers: Meningitis in man caused by a filterable virus. I. Two cases and the method of obtaining a virus from their spinal fluids. J. exp. Med. **63**, 397—414 (1936).

Seamer, J.: The growth, reproduction and mortality of mice made immunologically tolerant to lymphocytic choriomeningitis virus by congenital infection. Arch. ges. Virusforsch. **15**, 169—177 (1965 a).

Seamer, J.: Mouse macrophages as host cells for murine viruses. Arch. ges. Virusforsch. **17**, 654—663 (1965 b).

Seamer, J., J. L. Barlow, A. W. Gledhill, and J. Hotchin: Increased sucseptibility of mice to lymphocytic choriomeningitis virus after peripheral inoculation. Virology **21**, 309—316 (1963).

Seamer, J., and A. W. Gledhill: Role of the central nervous system in fatal murine lymphocytic choriomeningitis. Arch. ges. Virusforsch. **17**, 664—668 (1965).

Seamer, J., A. W. Gledhill, J. L. Barlow, and J. Hotchin: Effect of *Eperythrozoon coccoides* upon lymphocytic choriomeningitis in mice. J. Immunol. **86**, 512—515 (1961).

Seamer, J., and J. Hotchin: The effect of subcutaneous inoculation upon subsequent intracerebral challenge with lymphocytic choriomeningitis virus. A. R. for 1960, Div. Lab. Res., N. Y. St. Dep. Hlth (Albany) p. 20, 1961.

Sédallian, P., A. Bertoye, P. Détolle, G. Limet-Piloz et J.-P. Garin: Sur un virus d'origine méningitique, apparenté au virus d'Armstrong, mais anormal par sa résistance, ses dimensions et sa répartition dans l'organisme. Ann. Inst. Pasteur **86**, 785—787 (1954).

Sedwick, W. D., and T. J. Wiktor: Reproducible plaquing system for rabies, lymphocytic choriomeningitis, and other ribonucleic acid viruses in BHK-21/13S agarose suspensions. J. Virol. **1**, 1224—1226 (1967).

Sever, J. L.: Application of a microtechnique to viral serological investigations. J. Immunol. **88**, 320—329 (1962).

Shaughnessy, H. J., and A. Milzer: Experimental infection of *Dermacentor andersoni* Stiles with the virus of lymphocytic choriomeningitis. Amer. J. publ. Hlth **29**, 1103—1108 (1939).

Shaughnessy, H. J., and J. Zichis: Infection of guinea pigs by application of virus of lymphocytic choriomeningitis to their normal skins. Proc. Soc. exp. Biol. (N. Y.) **42**, 755—757 (1939).

SHAUGHNESSY, H. J., and J. ZICHIS: Infection of guinea pigs by application of virus of lymphocytic choriomeningitis to their normal skins. J. exp. Med. **72**, 331—343 (1940).

SHVAREV, A. I.: Limfotsitarnyj choriomeningit (sovremennoe sostoyanie problemy). Vop. Psikhiat. Nevropat. (Leningrad) **10**, 19—43 (1964 a).

SHVAREV, A. I.: Spinalnye i koreshkovye formy limfotsitarnovo choriomeningita. Zh. Nevropat. Psikhiat. **64**, 1290—1294 (1964 b).

SHVAREV, A. I.: Chorioentsefalit i choriomeningit. Vop. Psikhiat. Nevropat. (Leningrad) **12**, 159—165 (1966).

SHWARTZMAN, G.: Association of the virus of lymphocytic choriomeningitis with erythrocytes of infected animals. J. Bact. **46**, 482—483 (1943).

SHWARTZMAN, G.: Recovery of the virus of lymphocytic choriomeningitis from the erythrocytes of infected animals. J. Immunol. **48**, 111—127 (1944).

SHWARTZMAN, G.: Alterations in pathogenesis of experimental lymphocytic choriomeningitis caused by prepassage of the virus through heterologous host. J. Immunol. **54**, 293—304 (1946).

SIDWELL, R. W., G. ARNETT, and G. J. DIXON: In vitro studies on the antiviral activity of 1,3-bis(2-chloroethyl)-1-nitrosourea. Appl. Microbiol. **14**, 405—416 (1966).

SIDWELL, R. W., G. J. DIXON, S. M. SELLERS, and F. M. SCHABEL: In vivo antiviral activity of 1,3-bis(2-chloroethyl)-1-nitrosourea. Appl. Microbiol. **13**, 579—589 (1965).

SIEGEL, B. V., and J. I. MORTON: Depressed antibody response in the mouse infected with Rauscher leukaemia virus. Immunology **10**, 559—562 (1966 a).

SIEGEL, B. V., and J. I. MORTON: Serum agglutinin levels to sheep red blood cells in mice infected with Rauscher virus. Proc. Soc. exp. Biol. (N. Y.) **123**, 467—470 (1966 b).

SIKORA, E.: Protective effect of neonatal thymectomy on lymphocytic choriomeningitis virus disease in mice. A. R. for 1963, Div. Lab. Res., N. Y. St. Dep. Hlth (Albany) pp. 43—44, 1964.

SIKORA, E., and J. HOTCHIN: Effect of amethopterin on the foot-pad response of mice to lymphocytic choriomeningitis virus. A. R. for 1962, Div. Lab. Res., N. Y. St. Dep. Hlth (Albany) pp. 40—41, 1963.

SIKORA, E., J. HOTCHIN, and L. BENSON: Mutual interaction between behavior and animal virus infections. Bact. Proc. p. 166, 1968.

SILCOTT, W. L., and K. NEUBUERGER: Acute lymphocytic choriomeningitis. Report of three cases with histopathologic findings. Amer. J. med. Sci. **200**, 253—259 (1940).

SINKOVICS, J.: Virus neutralisation experiments with lymphoid cell- and lymph node-extracts. Acta microbiol. Acad. Sci. hung. **2**, 385—400 (1955).

SINKOVICS, J., és E. MOLNÁR: Az ellenanyagképzés specifikus bénulása lymphocytás choriomeningitis-virussal fertőzött egerekben. Kísérl. Orvostud. pp. 647—653, 1955.

SKINNER, H. H., and E. H. KNIGHT: Studies on murine lymphocytic choriomeningitis within a partially infected colony. Lab. Anim. **3**, 175—184 (1969).

SKOGLAND, J. E., and A. B. BAKER: An unusual form of lymphocytic choriomeningitis. Arch. Neurol. Psychiat. (Chic.) **42**, 507—512 (1939).

SLENCZKA, W., und F. LEHMANN-GRUBE: Über den Einfluß von Actinomycin auf die Vermehrung des LCM-Virus in L-Zellen. Zbl. Bakt., I. Abt. Ref. **206**, 526 (only) (1967).

SMADEL, J. E.: Common neurotropic virus diseases of man. Their diagnosis and mode of spread. U. S. nav. med. Bull. **40**, 1020—1036 (1942 a).

SMADEL, J. E.: Aseptic meningitis of known and unknown etiology. J. clin. Invest. **21**, 646 (only) (1942 b).

SMADEL, J. E., R. D. BAIRD, and M. J. WALL: Complement-fixation in infections with the virus of lymphocytic choriomeningitis. Proc. Soc. exp. Biol. (N. Y.) **40**, 71—73 (1939 a).

SMADEL, J. E., R. D. BAIRD, and M. J. WALL: A soluble antigen of lymphocytic choriomeningitis. I. Separation of soluble antigen from virus. J. exp. Med. **70**, 53—66 (1939 b).

SMADEL, J. E., R. H. GREEN, R. M. PALTAUF, and T. A. GONZALES: Lymphocytic choriomeningitis: two human fatalities following an unusual febrile illness. Proc. Soc. exp. Biol. (N. Y.) **49**, 683—686 (1942).

SMADEL, J. E., and T. M. RIVERS: Complement-fixing antigen in lymphocytic choriomeningitis. Third Internat. Congress Microbiology, New York 1939. Abstracts of Communications. Baltimore: Waverly Press, Inc. 1939.

SMADEL, J. E., and M. J. WALL: A soluble antigen of lymphocytic choriomeningitis. III. Independence of anti-soluble substance antibodies and neutralizing antibodies, and the rôle of soluble antigen and inactive virus in immunity to infection. J. exp. Med. **72**, 389—405 (1940).

SMADEL, J. E., and M. J. WALL: Identification of the virus of lymphocytic choriomeningitis. J. Bact. **41**, 421—430 (1941).

SMADEL, J. E., and M. J. WALL: Lymphocytic choriomeningitis in the Syrian hamster. J. exp. Med. **75**, 581—591 (1942).

SMADEL, J. E., M. J. WALL, and R. D. BAIRD: A soluble antigen of lymphocytic choriomeningitis. II. Characteristics of the antigen and its use in precipitin reactions. J. exp. Med. **71**, 43—53 (1940).

SMITH, R. C. F., and J. J. KINSELLA: Lymphocytic choriomeningitis in co. Durham. Lancet **II**, 882—883 (1951).

SMITH, S. B., K. ISAKOVIC, and B. H. WAKSMAN: Role of the thymus in tolerance. II. Transfer of specific unresponsiveness to BSA with thymus grafting. Proc. Soc. exp. Biol. (N. Y.) **121**, 1005—1008 (1966).

SMITHARD, E. H. R., and A. D. MACRAE: Lymphocytic choriomeningitis. Associated human and mouse infections. Brit. med. J. **I**, 1298—1300 (1951).

SMORODINTSEV, A. A.: Factors of natural resistance and specific immunity to viruses. Virology **3**, 299—321 (1957).

SOHIER, R., et J. BUISSIÈRE: Méningites et méningo-encéphalites à virus observées en France. Presse méd. **62**, 1248—1251 (1954).

SOHIER, R., J. BUISSIÈRE et I. ESSER: Recherches sur l'étiologie des méningites dites "lymphocytaires" à virus observées en France. Bull. Acad. nat. Méd. (Paris) **137**, 223—226 (1953).

SOUTHAM, C. M., and V. I. BABCOCK: Effect of cortisone, related hormones, and adrenalectomy on susceptibility of mice to virus infections. Proc. Soc. exp. Biol. (N. Y.) **78**, 105—109 (1951).

SPEEL, L. F., J. E. OSBORN, and D. L. WALKER: An immuno-cytopathogenic interaction between sensitized leukocytes and epithelial cells carrying a persistent noncytocidal myxovirus infection. J. Immunol. **101**, 409—417 (1968).

SREENIVASAN, B. R.: Lymphocytic choriomeningitis. Brit. med. J. **II**, 573—575 (1946).

STAPLES, P. J., I. GERY, and B. H. WAKSMAN: Role of the thymus in tolerance. III. Tolerance to bovine gamma globulin after direct injection of antigen into the shielded thymus of irradiated rats. J. exp. Med. **124**, 127—139 (1966).

STETSON, C. A.: Endotoxins and bacterial allergy. In: Cellular and Humoral Aspects of the Hypersensitive States. Ed.: H. S. LAWRENCE. New York: P. B. Hoeber, Inc. **1959**.

STEWART, S. E., B. E. EDDY, V. H. HAAS, and N. G. BORGESE: Lymphocytic choriomeningitis virus as related to chemotherapy studies and to tumor induction in mice. Ann. N.Y. Acad. Sci. **68**, 419—429 (1957).

STEWART, S. E., and V. H. HAAS: Lymphocytic choriomeningitis virus in mouse neoplasms. J. nat. Cancer Inst. **17**, 233—245 (1956).

STOCK, C. C., and T. FRANCIS: The inactivation of the virus of lymphocytic choriomeningitis by soaps. J. exp. Med. **77**, 323—336 (1943).

STRAUSS, E.: Discussion. Tex. St. J. Med. **44**, 367 (only) (1948).

STULBERG, C. S., L. BERMAN, and R. H. PAGE: Comparative viral susceptibilities of eight culture strains (Detroit) of human epithelial-like cells. Virology **2**, 844—845 (1956).

SUTER, E., and E. M. KIRSANOW: Hyperreactivity to endotoxin in mice infected with Mycobacteria. Induction and elicitation of the reactions. Immunology **4**, 354—365 (1961).

SYVERTON, J. T., O. R. McCOY, and J. KOOMEN: The transmission of the virus of lymphocytic choriomeningitis by *Trichinella spiralis*. J. exp. Med. **85**, 759—769 (1947).

SZERI, I., Z. BÁNOS, P. ANDERLIK, M. BALÁZS, and P. FÖLDES: Pathogenesis of the wasting syndrome following neonatal thymectomy. Acta microbiol. Acad. Sci. hung. **13**, 255—262 (1966/67).

TAYLOR, M. J., and E. C. MACDOWELL: Mouse leukemia. XIV. Freeing transplanted line I from a contaminating virus. Cancer Res. **9**, 144—149 (1949).

TAYLOR, R. B.: Immune paralysis of thymus cells by bovine serum albumin. Nature (Lond.) **220**, 611 (only) (1968).

THIEDE, W. H.: Cardiac involvement in lymphocytic choriomeningitis. Arch. intern. Med. **109**, 50—54 (1962).

TOBIN, J. O'H.: The growth of lymphocytic choriomeningitis virus in the developing chick embryo. Brit. J. exp. Path. **35**, 358—364 (1954).

TODOROVIĆ, K., M. MILOVANOVIĆ, A. KOSTIĆ, M. PETROVIĆ i R. MIRKOVIĆ: Prilog proučavanju etiologije i klinike limfocitnog meningoencefalita. Gl. srpske Akad. Nauka, Od. med. Nauka **248**, 27—41 (1961).

TOKUDA, S., and R. S. WEISER: Anaphylaxis in the mouse produced with soluble complexes of antigen and antibody. Proc. Soc. exp. Biol. (N. Y.) **98**, 557—561 (1958).

TOOMEY, J. A., and W. S. TAKACS: Chemotherapy of lymphocytic choriomeningitis in mice and guineapigs. J. Immunol. **48**, 49—55 (1944).

TRAUB, E.: A filterable virus recovered from white mice. Science **81**, 298—299 (1935 a).

TRAUB, E.: A filterable virus from white mice. J. Immunol. **29**, 69 (only) (1935 b).

TRAUB, E.: An epidemic in a mouse colony due to the virus of acute lymphocytic choriomeningitis. J. exp. Med. **63**, 533—546 (1936 a).

TRAUB, E.: Persistence of lymphocytic choriomeningitis virus in immune animals and its relation to immunity. J. exp. Med. **63**, 847—861 (1936 b).

TRAUB, E.: The epidemiology of lymphocytic choriomeningitis in white mice. J. exp. Med. **64**, 183—200 (1936 c).

TRAUB, E.: Immunization of guinea pigs with a modified strain of lymphocytic choriomeningitis virus. J. exp. Med. **66**, 317—324 (1937).

TRAUB, E.: Immunization of guinea pigs against lymphocytic choriomeningitis with formolized tissue vaccines. J. exp. Med. **68**, 95—110 (1938 a).

TRAUB, E.: Factors influencing the persistence of choriomeningitis virus in the blood of mice after clinical recovery. J. exp. Med. **68**, 229—250 (1938 b).

TRAUB, E.: Über die Immunität der Mäuse gegen die lymphozytische Choriomeningitis. Third Internat. Congress Microbiology, New York 1939. Abstracts of Communications. Baltimore: Waverly Press, Inc. 1939 a.

TRAUB, E.: Epidemiology of lymphocytic choriomeningitis in a mouse stock observed for four years. J. exp. Med. **69**, 801—817 (1939 b).

TRAUB, E.: Choriomeningitis der Mäuse. In: E. GILDEMEISTER, E. HAAGEN und O. WALDMANN: Handbuch der Viruskrankheiten, 2. Band. Jena: Gustav Fischer 1939 c.

TRAUB, E.: Über den Einfluß der latenten Choriomeningitis-Infektion auf die Entstehung der Lymphomatose bei weißen Mäusen. Zbl. Bakt., I. Abt. Orig. **147**, 16—25 (1941).

TRAUB, E.: Über die aktive Immunität von Küken aus virusinfizierten Eiern. Zbl. Bakt., I. Abt. Orig. **164**, 412—423 (1955).

TRAUB, E.: Specific immunity as a factor in the ecology of animal viruses. In: Perspectives in Virology. Ed.: M. POLLARD. New York: John Wiley and Sons, Inc. 1959.

TRAUB, E.: Über die natürliche Übertragungsweise des Virus der lymphocytären Choriomeningitis (LCM) bei Mäusen und ihre Parallelen zum Übertragungsmodus gewisser muriner Krebsviren. Zbl. Bakt., I. Abt. Orig. **177**, 453—471 (1960 a).

TRAUB, E.: Über die immunologische Toleranz bei der lymphocytären Choriomeningitis der Mäuse. Zbl. Bakt., I. Abt. Orig. **177**, 472—487 (1960 b).

TRAUB, E.: Demonstration, properties and significance of neutralizing antibodies in mature mice immune to lymphocytic choriomeningitis (LCM). Arch. ges. Virusforsch. **10**, 289—302 (1961 a).

TRAUB, E.: Observations on immunological tolerance and "immunity" in mice infected congenitally with the virus of lymphocytic choriomeningitis (LCM). Arch. ges. Virusforsch. **10**, 303—314 (1961 b).

TRAUB, E.: Interference with eastern equine encephalomyelitis (EEE) virus in the brains of mice immune to lymphocytic choriomeningitis (LCM). Arch. ges. Virusforsch. **11**, 419—427 (1962 a).

TRAUB, E.: Multiplication of LCM virus in lymph node and embryo cells from non-tolerant and tolerant mice. Arch. ges. Virusforsch. **11**, 473—486 (1962 b).

TRAUB, E.: Can LCM virus cause lymphomatosis in mice? Arch. ges. Virusforsch. **11**, 667—682 (1962 c).

TRAUB, E.: Studies on the mechanism of immunity in murine LCM. Arch. ges. Virusforsch. **14**, 65—86 (1964).

TRAUB, E., and F. KESTING: Further observations on the behavior of the cells in murine LCM. Arch. ges. Virusforsch. **13**, 452—469 (1963).

TRAUB, E., and F. KESTING: Experiments on heterologous and homologous interference in LCM-infected cultures of murine lymph node cells. Arch. ges. Virusforsch. **14**, 55—64 (1964).

TRAUB, E., und W. SCHÄFER: Serologische Untersuchungen über die Immunität der Mäuse gegen die lymphozytische Choriomeningitis. Zbl. Bakt., I. Abt. Orig. **144**, 331—345 (1939).

TRAUMANN, K. J., A. SCHMID und U. WETZEL: Lymphozytäre Choriomeningitis mit weitgehend nachweisbarer Infektkette. Med. Klin. **57**, 300—301 (1962).

TREUSCH, J. V., A. MILZER, and S. O. LEVINSON: Recurrent lymphocytic choriomeningitis. Report of a case in which treatment was with pooled normal adult serum. Arch. intern. Med. **72**, 709—714 (1943).

TRIANDAPHILLI, I., J. L. BARLOW, and S. M. COHEN: Immunofluorescence in the serodiagnosis of lymphocytic choriomeningitis. A. R. for 1964, Div. Lab. Res., N. Y. St. Dep. Hlth (Albany) pp. 52—53, 1965.

TRUM, B. F., and J. K. ROUTLEDGE: Common disease problems in laboratory animals. J. Amer. vet. med. Ass. **151**, 1886—1896 (1967).

TUBAKI, S.: Studies concerning the cultivation of choriomeningitis virus in the developing chick embryo. Kitasato Arch. exp. Med. **17**, 242—249 (1940).

TURK, J. L., and J. H. HUMPHREY: Immunological unresponsiveness in guinea pigs. II. The effect of unresponsiveness on the development of delayed type hypersensitivity to protein antigens. Immunology **4**, 310—317 (1961).

TYUSHNYAKOVA, M. K.: K voprosu ob alimentarnom puti peredachi virusa limfotsitarnovo choriomeningita. Vop. Virus. **7**, 50—52 (1962).

TYUSHNYAKOVA, M. K., i M. S. ZAGROMOVA: Materialy issledovanij po limfotsitarnomu choriomeningitu v Tomskoj oblasti. Tr. Tomskovo Inst. Vaktsin i Syvorotok Min. Zdrav. SSSR **11**, 25—32 (1960).

UNANUE, E. R., and F. J. DIXON: Experimental glomerulonephritis: immunological events and pathogenetic mechanisms. Advanc. Immunol. **6**, 1—90 (1967).

UPHOFF, D. E., and V. H. HAAS: Immunologic response to lymphocytic choriomeningitis virus in lethally irradiated mice treated with bone marrow. J. nat. Cancer Inst. **25**, 779—786 (1960).

VEDDER, A.: Een geval van maligne lymphocytaire chorio-meningo-encephalitis. Ned. T. Geneesk. **92, IV**, 3532—3536 (1948).

VERLINDE, J. D.: Virusmeningitis. II. Virological part. Antonie v. Leeuwenhoek **11**, 180—185 (1946).

VERLINDE, J. D., en H. A. E. VAN TONGEREN: Ervaringen over de virologische en serologische diagnostiek van aseptische, lymphocytaire meningitis. Ned. T. Geneesk. **93, III**, 2512—2517 (1949).

VERLINDE, J. D., J. VAN DER WERFF, and W. BRIËT: An encephalitis epidemic caused by the virus of lymphocytic choriomeningitis. Antonie v. Leeuwenhoek **14**, 33—50 (1948 a).

Verlinde, J. D., J. van der Werff en W. Briët: Een encephalitisepidemie, veroorzaakt door een nauw met het chorio-meningitisvirus van Armstrong verwante smetstof. Ned. T. Geneesk. **92**, **III**, 2802—2809 (1948 b).

Vermeil, C., et J. Maurin: Toxoplasmose expérimentale et chorio-méningite lymphocytaire chez la souris. Ann. Parasit. hum. comp. **28**, 5—13 (1953).

Viets, H. R., and S. Warren: Acute lymphocytic meningitis. J. Amer. med. Ass. **108**, 357—361 (1937).

Volkert, M.: Studies on immunological tolerance to LCM virus. A preliminary report on adoptive immunization of virus carrier mice. Acta path. microbiol. scand. **56**, 305—310 (1962).

Volkert, M.: Studies on immunological tolerance to LCM virus. 2. Treatment of virus carrier mice by adoptive immunization. Acta path. microbiol. scand. **57**, 465—487 (1963).

Volkert, M.: Studies on immunologic tolerance to LCM virus. In: Perspectives in Virology. IV. Ed.: M. Pollard. New York: Hoeber Medical Division, Harper & Row, Inc. 1965.

Volkert, M., and J. Hannover Larsen: Studies on immunological tolerance to LCM virus. 3. Duration and maximal effect of adoptive immunization of virus carriers. Acta path. microbiol. scand. **60**, 577—587 (1964).

Volkert, M., and J. Hannover Larsen: Studies on immunological tolerance to LCM virus. 5. The induction of tolerance to the virus. Acta path. microbiol. scand. **63**, 161—171 (1965 a).

Volkert, M., and J. Hannover Larsen: Studies on immunological tolerance to LCM virus. 6. Immunity conferred on tolerant mice by immune serum and by grafts of homologous lymphoid cells. Acta path. microbiol. scand. **63**, 172—180 (1965 b).

Volkert, M., and J. Hannover Larsen: Immunological tolerance to viruses. Progr. med. Virol. **7**, 160—207 (1965 c).

Volkert, M., J. Hannover Larsen, and C. J. Pfau: Studies on immunological tolerance to LCM virus. 4. The question of immunity in adoptively immunized virus carriers. Acta path. microbiol. scand. **61**, 268—282 (1964).

Volkert, M., and C. Lundstedt: The provocation of latent lymphocytic choriomeningitis virus infections in mice by treatment with antilymphocytic serum. J. exp. Med. **127**, 327—339 (1968).

Wagner, R. R., and R. M. Snyder: Viral interference induced in mice by acute or persistent infection with the virus of lymphocytic choriomeningitis. Nature (Lond.) **196**, 393—394 (1962).

Wainwright, S., and C. A. Mims: Plaque assay for lymphocytic choriomeningitis virus based on hemadsorption interference. J. Virol. **1**, 1091—1092 (1967).

Walford, R. L.: Further considerations towards an immunologic theory of aging. Exp. Geront. **1**, 67—76 (1964).

Walford, R. L.: The general immunology of aging. Advanc. geront. Res. **2**, 159—204 (1967).

Walker, D. L.: The viral carrier state in animal cell cultures. Progr. med. Virol. **6**, 111—148 (1964).

Wallgren, A.: Une nouvelle maladie infectieuse du système nerveux central? (Méningite aseptique aiguë.). Acta paediat. (Uppsala) **4**, 158—182 (1925).

Wallis, C., and J. L. Melnick: Cationic stabilization — a new property of enteroviruses. Virology **16**, 504—506 (1962).

Warren, J.: Lymphocytic choriomeningitis virus. In: F. L. Horsfall and I. Tamm: Viral and Rickettsial Infections of Man. Fourth ed. Philadelphia: J. B. Lippincott Co. 1965.

Webb, P. A.: Properties of Machupo virus. Amer. J. trop. Med. Hyg. **14**, 799—802 (1965).

Weigand, H., and J. Hotchin: Studies of lymphocytic choriomeningitis in mice. II. A comparison of the immune status of newborn and adult mice surviving inoculation. J. Immunol. **86**, 401—406 (1961).

WEISER, R. S., O. J. GOLUB, and D. M. HAMRE: Studies on anaphylaxis in the mouse. J. infect. Dis. **68**, 97—112 (1941).

WENNER, H. A.: Isolation of LCM virus in an effort to adapt poliomyelitis virus to rodents. J. infect. Dis. **83**, 155—163 (1948).

WENNER, H. A., M. M. SWAN, and I. HEILBRUNN: Lymphocytic choriomeningitis — detection of virus in body fluids of a patient. J. Kans. med. Soc. **50**, 64—68 (1949).

WHITNEY, E.: Response of infant and adult mice to lymphocytic choriomeningitis virus infection. A. R. for 1951, Div. Lab. Res., N. Y. St. Dep. Hlth (Albany) p. 35, 1951 a.

WHITNEY, E.: Response of infant and adult mice to lymphocytic choriomeningitis virus infection. Proc. Soc. exp. Biol. (N. Y.) **78**, 247—250 (1951 b).

WHITNEY, E., G. M. GNESH, W. LAWSON, and I. GORDON: An ultraviolet inactivated complement-fixation antigen prepared from embryonated hens' eggs infected with lymphocytic choriomeningitis virus. A. R. for 1952, Div. Lab. Res., N. Y. St. Dep. Hlth (Albany) p. 35, 1952.

WHITNEY, E., L. M. KRAFT, W. B. LAWSON, and I. GORDON: Noninfectious complement-fixing antigen from embryonated hens' eggs infected with lymphocytic choriomeningitis virus. Bact. Proc. p. 50, 1953.

WIKTOR, T. J., M. V. FERNANDES, and H. KOPROWSKI: Detection of a lymphocytic choriomeningitis component in rabies virus preparations. J. Bact. **90**, 1494—1495 (1965).

WIKTOR, T. J., M. M. KAPLAN, and H. KOPROWSKI: Rabies and lymphocytic choriomeningitis virus (LCMV). Infection of tissue culture; enhancing effect of LCMV. Ann. Med. intern. Fenn. **44**, 290—296 (1966).

WIKTOR, T. J., E. KUWERT, and H. KOPROWSKI: Immune lysis of rabies virus-infected cells. J. Immunol. **101**, 1271—1282 (1968).

WILSNACK, R. E.: Lymphocytic choriomeningitis. In: Viruses of Laboratory Rodents. Nat. Cancer Inst. Monograph No. 20. Ed.: R. HOLDENRIED. Bethesda, Md.: U. S. Department of Health, Education, and Welfare 1966.

WILSNACK, R. E., and W. P. ROWE: Immunofluorescent studies of the histopathogenesis of lymphocytic choriomeningitis virus infection. J. exp. Med. **120**, 829—840 (1964).

WOOLEY, J. G.: The preservation of lymphocytic choriomeningitis and St. Louis encephalitis viruses by freezing and drying *in vacuo*. Publ. Hlth Rep. (Wash.) **54**, 1077—1079 (1939).

WOOLEY, J. G., C. ARMSTRONG, and R. H. ONSTOTT: The occurrence in the sera of man and monkeys of protective antibodies against the virus of lymphocytic choriomeningitis as determined by the serum-virus protection test in mice. Publ. Hlth Rep. (Wash.) **52**, 1105—1114 (1937).

WOOLEY, J. G., F. D. STIMPERT, J. F. KESSEL, and C. ARMSTRONG: A study of human sera antibodies capable of neutralizing the virus of lymphocytic choriomeningitis. Publ. Hlth Rep. (Wash.) **54**, 938—944 (1939).

YAMADA, R.: Honpō ni okeru myakurakunōmakuen-byōdoku no bunri to sono jikkenteki kenkyu. I. to II. Saikingakuzasshi number **530**, pp. 245—273 and number **531**, pp. 294—315 (1940 a).

YAMADA, R.: Experimental studies concerning isolation of choriomeningitis virus in Japan. Part 2. Kitasato Arch. exp. Med. **17**, Appendix p. 4, 1940b.

YOUN, J. K., and G. BARSKI: Interference between lymphocytic choriomeningitis and Rauscher leukemia in mice. J. nat. Cancer Inst. **37**, 381—388 (1966).

ŽÁČKOVÁ, Z., I. JASTROWOVÁ a K. ŽÁČEK: Komplement-fixační antigen u lymfocytární choriomeningitidy, připravený bentonitovou purifikaci. Čs. Epidem. **8**, 153—156 (1959).

ZGORNIAK-NOWOSIELSKA, I., W. D. SEDWICK, K. HUMMELER, and H. KOPROWSKI: New assay procedure for separation of mycoplasmas from virus pools and tissue culture systems. J. Virol. **1**, 1227—1237 (1967).

[illegible] M. D.: Studies on [illegible] in the mouse. [illegible] 96, 97—112 (1961).

[illegible]

[illegible]

[illegible]

W[illegible]: [illegible] and [illegible] from [illegible] lines, [illegible] with [illegible] (1962).

W[illegible], [illegible], and [illegible]: [illegible]

[illegible] (1966).

W[illegible]: [illegible] of tissue culture [illegible] (1966).

W[illegible], and [illegible] 101, 1231—1242 (1968).

W[illegible] Monograph No. 20. [illegible] U.S. [illegible] of Health, Education, and Welfare 1966.

W[illegible]

[illegible]

[illegible]

[illegible]

[illegible]

[illegible]

[illegible]

VIROLOGY MONOGRAPHS

ECHO Viruses

By H. A. Wenner and A. M. Behbehani

The Simian Viruses

By R. N. Hull

Herpes Simplex and Pseudorabies Viruses

By A. S. Kaplan

Polyoma Virus

By Dr. Bernice E. Eddy